Don't Crack the Screen: The Ultimate TV Guide

From Diagnostics to Delivery – Everything You Need to Know About Your TV

Nicholas Francis

Don't Crack the Screen: The Ultimate TV Guide
Author: Nicholas Francis
Published by: Nicholas Francis
ISBN: 978-1-969564-07-9
Paperback
First Published in 2025
First Printed in 2025
Cover design: Desfia Phillips

For permissions, inquiries, or to connect with the author:
Email: dontcrackthescreenebook@gmail.com
Website: www.dontcrackthescreen.com

Disclaimer

This book is for educational purposes only. Fixing TVs can be dangerous if not done correctly. Always unplug devices before attempting repairs and take proper safety precautions. The author and publisher are not responsible for any injuries, damage, or losses that may result from following the information in this book. If you are unsure, please seek help from a qualified professional.

Dedication

To my family, and my true friends who encouraged me to get this done.

To all well-wishers and supporters.

Table of Contents

Appendices

About the Author

Nicholas Francis
Entrepreneur - Innovator - Mentor
Managing Director - Modern Systems and Solutions Ltd

Nicholas Francis makes a living solving problems - and he's built a legacy doing just that.

A passionate tech enthusiast from Trinidad and Tobago, Nicholas is the founder of Modern Systems and Solutions Ltd, the parent company behind ventures like The TV Centre, AC Experts, The Juicy Express, and QikChk. His journey began with a fascination for dismantling electronics as a child, which evolved into an award-winning career in technology and innovation.

At age 21, Nicholas designed a national RFID tracking system and later developed a Motor Vehicle Insurance Verification platform, both of which were recognized under the Government's i2i Innovation Program. Despite setbacks, including having his work dismissed or uncredited, Nicholas persevered - driven by his deep faith, his children, and a vision to empower others through technology.

Today, Nicholas leads with humility and tenacity, creating businesses that offer real solutions to real people. His goal? To build one of the largest and most impactful repair centres in the Caribbean, and to show young people that purpose, not just academia, can lead to success.

This book is just one step in that mission - a practical guide, a legacy, and a voice for the people.

How to Use this Book

This guide has been carefully designed to be both practical and easy to follow, whether you are a professional technician, a student of electronics, or a hands-on do-it-yourself enthusiast. Modern televisions can be complex, but with the right approach, many problems can be diagnosed and repaired without unnecessary frustration. The layout of this book ensures that you always have the right information at your fingertips, presented in a compact, readable format.

Each chapter is structured to provide **step-by-step guidance**, starting from the most common issues and moving toward more advanced troubleshooting techniques. You will find clear explanations written in plain language, supported by **graphics, diagrams, tables, and photos** to help you quickly identify components, follow wiring paths, and visualize repair processes. These visuals are especially useful when working with different TV types, whether CRT, LCD, LED, or Smart TVs.

To make the book as practical as possible, we have included **Technician and Pro Tips** throughout the chapters. These tips share insider knowledge, shortcuts, and safety practices drawn from years of real-world experience. They highlight common mistakes to avoid and offer suggestions that can save both time and money during repairs.

You will also encounter **checklists** designed to simplify the repair process. These checklists allow you to move systematically through diagnostic steps, ensuring nothing is overlooked. Whether you are verifying power supply integrity, inspecting display panels, or testing remote sensor circuits, the checklists act as quick reminders to stay thorough and consistent.

A key feature of this guide is the **Problem–Solution format**. Here, common television symptoms such as "TV won't power on," "no sound," or "picture flickering" are paired with possible causes and recommended solutions. This format allows you to match the issue you are facing with practical steps to resolve it quickly, without having to search through multiple chapters.

We recommend starting with the introduction to familiarize yourself with essential safety practices before diving into repairs. After that, you can read sequentially or simply use the book as a **toolbox reference**, turning directly to the section that matches your immediate need.

By combining technician insights, structured checklists, and problem-solution strategies all supported by clear visuals, this guide is built to help you repair televisions with confidence and efficiency.

Part 1: Understanding Televisions

Chapter 1:

The Evolution of Television Technology

Television technology has come a long way from the bulky cathode ray tubes (CRT) of the 20th century to today's ultra-slim OLED and QLED displays. Understanding this evolution not only helps you appreciate improvements in image quality, size, and efficiency but also allows for smarter repair and maintenance decisions.

- Early Television Sets (Cathode Ray Tube (CRT) Era): CRT TVs dominated from the 1950s to the early 2000s. They used electron beams to activate phosphor dots on the inside of the screen. While reliable and long-lasting, they were heavy, deep, and offered limited resolution.

- Plasma Screens: Plasma TVs emerged in the 1990s and became popular in the early 2000s. They provided superior color and contrast compared to CRTs but were heavy, power hungry, and prone to image burn-in.

- LCD and LED Technology: LCD (Liquid Crystal Display) TVs replaced CRTs as the most common format. LED TVs are LCDs backlit by light-emitting diodes, offering better brightness and thinner form factors.

- OLED and QLED: OLED (Organic LED) screens use self-lighting pixels, allowing for perfect blacks and vibrant colors. QLED, developed by Samsung, uses quantum dot filters to enhance color and brightness but still relies on a backlight.

- Smart TVs and Beyond: Modern TVs are now full-fledged computers with built-in apps, Wi Fi, and voice control. Features like 4K/8K resolution, HDR (High Dynamic Range), and variable refresh rates have made TV viewing more immersive than ever.

Figure: 1.1 Evolution of Television Technology

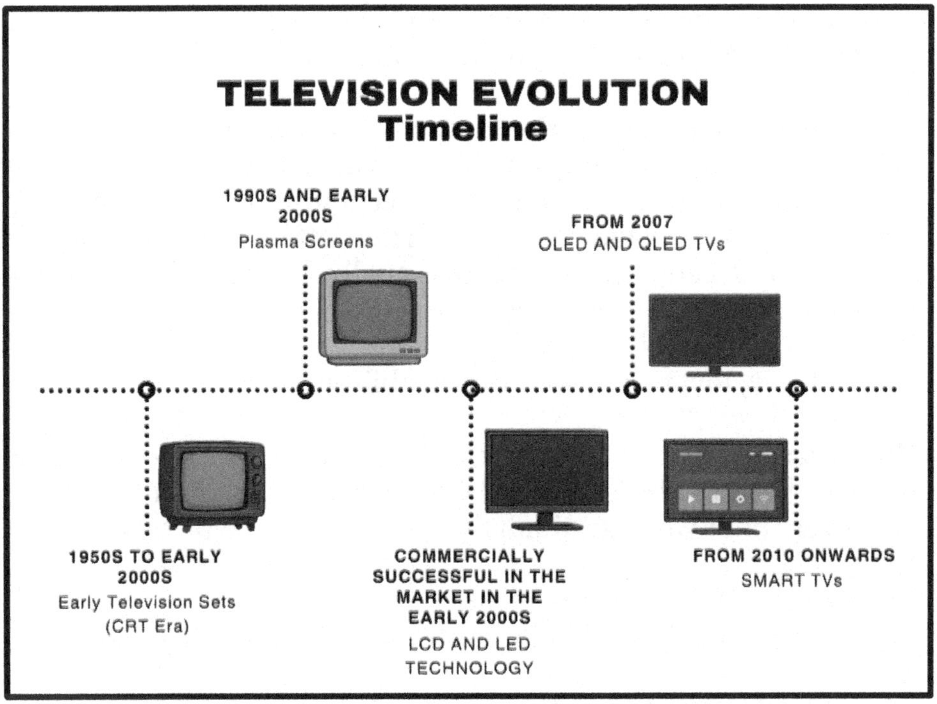

Chapter 2:

Types of TVs

Understanding the different types of televisions is essential for both diagnosing repairs and making informed purchasing decisions. Each display technology has its own strengths, weaknesses, and repair implications.

CRT (Cathode Ray Tube): Used in classic box-shaped TVs (1930s–2000s). Cathode Ray Tube (CRT) televisions were the first widely used TV technology, recognizable by their bulky design and curved glass screens. They offered reliable picture quality for decades but were eventually replaced by slimmer, more energy-efficient flat-screen technologies.
Pros: Durable, low burn-in.
Cons: Bulky, low resolution. Repairability: Medium.

Plasma: Popular in early 2000 and used gas-filled cells to produce bright, vibrant images with excellent color and contrast. However, they were gradually phased out in favor of LCD and LED TVs.
Pros: Deep blacks, great contrast.
Cons: Burn-in risk, heavy, discontinued. Repairability: Low.

LCD TVs (Liquid Crystal Display): LCDs became popular in the mid-2000s for their slim design, lighter weight, and lower power consumption compared to CRTs and plasma screens. They use CCFL backlighting. They offered sharp picture quality and quickly became the standard before being enhanced by LED backlighting technology.
Pros: Affordable, common.

Cons: Dimmer, backlight issues. Repairability: Moderate.

LED: LED TVs are an advanced form of LCD technology that use light-emitting diodes for backlighting, resulting in brighter displays and improved energy efficiency. They are thinner, longer lasting, and provide better contrast than traditional LCD TVs.
Pros: Slim, energy efficient.
Cons: LED strip failure. Repairability: High.

OLED: Premium display type TVs that use organic light-emitting diodes to deliver deeper blacks, vibrant colors, and superior picture quality in ultra-thin designs.
Pros: Perfect blacks, vibrant.
Cons: Expensive, burn-in risk. Repairability: Low.

Quantum Dot enhanced LED TVs (QLED): QLED use quantum dot technology with LED backlighting to produce brighter images, vivid colors, and excellent durability.
Pros: Bright, vivid color.
Cons: Similar issues to LED. Repairability: High.

SMART TVs: A smart TV is a television set with integrated Internet and interactive Web 3.0 features.
Pros: Streaming apps built-in (Netflix, YouTube, Disney+, etc.) – no need for extra devices.

Internet connectivity via Wi-Fi or Ethernet for browsing and updates.

Voice control and AI assistants (Google Assistant, Alexa, Siri in some models).

Screen mirroring and casting from smartphones, tablets, or laptops.

App store access for games and utilities.

High picture quality

Regular software updates to improve features and security.

Smart home integration (can connect with IoT devices like lights or thermostats).

Cons:

Privacy and security concerns – some models track viewing habits and internet usage and prone to hacking

TECHNICIAN TIP
For no-picture issues with sound present, check the backlight on LED TVs. Confirm display type before performing any high-cost diagnostics.

Software updates may stop after a few years, making apps obsolete.

Higher upfront cost compared to basic TVs.

Internet dependence – many features don't work offline.

Chapter 3:

Understanding Screen Sizes and Resolutions

When purchasing or repairing a television, understanding screen size and resolution is critical to both performance expectations and technical compatibility. Screen size affects the viewing experience, while resolution determines the clarity and sharpness of the image.

Screen Size: What Does It Really Mean?
The screen size of a TV is measured diagonally from one corner of the visible screen to the opposite corner, in inches (e.g., 32", 50", 65"). It includes the viewable screen only—not the frame or bezels.

Impact on Viewing:
A larger screen provides more immersive experience but requires more space. It must be noted that viewing distance should increase with size. For example:

- 32" TV: 3–5 ft away
- 50" TV: 6–8 ft away
- 65" TV: 8–10 ft away

Technician Insight: Sometimes customers believe "bigger is better," but larger screens with low resolution can appear pixelated up close.

Understanding Resolution:

Resolution refers to the number of pixels that make up the picture on a screen. More pixels equal a sharper image.

Resolution Types:
- 720p: 1280 x 720 (HD) – Basic cable, small TVs
- 1080p: 1920 x 1080 (Full HD) – Standard content
- 4K: 3840 x 2160 (Ultra HD) – Streaming, gaming, cinema
- 8K: 7680 x 4320 (Ultra HD 8K) – High-end, niche use

Resolution & Gaming:

In the world of gaming, resolution plays a pivotal role in shaping visual experience and overall immersion for players. Resolution refers to the number of pixels displayed on a screen, determining the clarity, sharpness, and detail of in-game graphics. Higher resolutions, such as 4K or 8K, offer more detailed environments, smoother textures, and a more lifelike gaming experience, while lower resolutions may result in blurrier or pixelated images but can improve performance on less powerful hardware. As games continue to push the boundaries of realism, understanding the impact of resolution is essential for both developers and players seeking the perfect balance between visual fidelity and gameplay performance.

Gamers often require the following features:
- 1080 pixels or higher
- Low input lag and high refresh rates
- A native resolution that matches the console output (e.g., PS5, Xbox Series X = 4K)

Tip: Some TVs upscale lower-resolution content to 4K. This helps with image clarity but may not look as sharp as native 4K.

TECHNICIAN TIP

When sourcing replacement screens or mainboards, always match the native resolution of the original panel. Installing a board from a different resolution variant can result in display distortion or partial functionality.

Misconceptions to Address:
- "4K always looks better than 1080p." Not necessarily true on small screens under 40" or if content is not native 4K.

- "Resolution is the only thing that matters." No—panel type, color processing, contrast ratio, and refresh rate are just as important.

Figure 3.1: Screen Size vs Room Size Chart

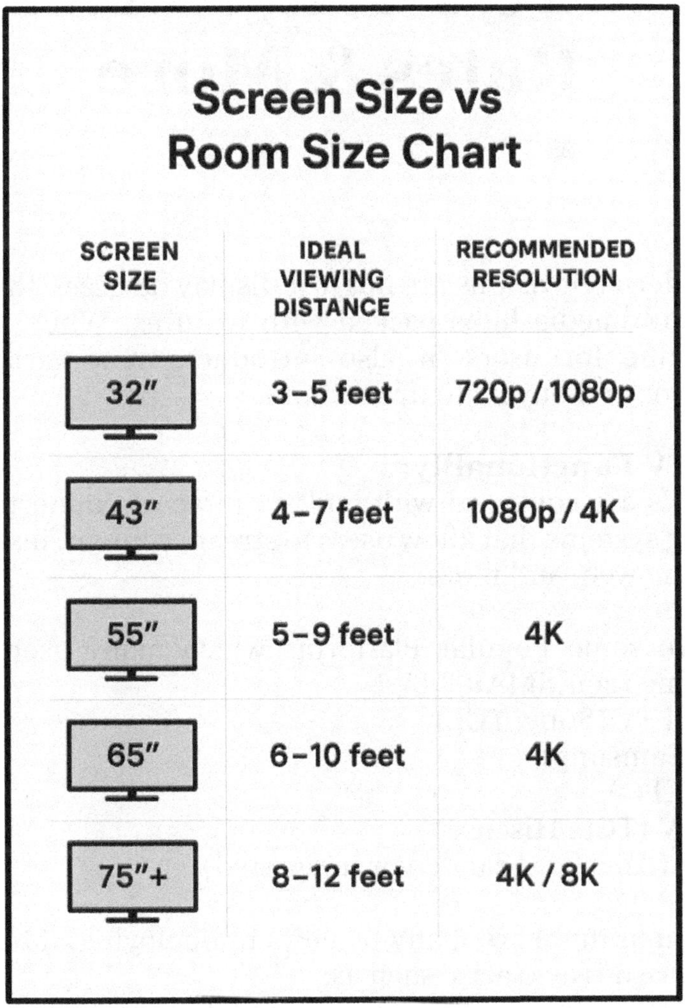

Screen Size vs Room Size Chart

SCREEN SIZE	IDEAL VIEWING DISTANCE	RECOMMENDED RESOLUTION
32"	3–5 feet	720p / 1080p
43"	4–7 feet	1080p / 4K
55"	5–9 feet	4K
65"	6–10 feet	4K
75"+	8–12 feet	4K / 8K

Chapter 4:

Common TV Features – Smart, HDR, Refresh Rates & More

Modern televisions are not just display devices—they are multimedia hubs packed with features. While this adds value for users, it also introduces new variables for technicians and buyers to understand.

Smart TV Functionality:
Smart TVs are equipped with built-in internet connectivity and operating systems that allow users to stream content, install apps, browse the web, and more.

There are some Popular Platforms which many users engage while using their SMART TVs:
- Android TV (Sony, TCL)
- Tizen (Samsung)
- webOS (LG)
- Roku TV (TCL, Hisense)
- Fire TV (Amazon-branded or integrated)

Even though there are many benefits to deploying SMART TVs, common issues also arise such as:
- Slow performance (usually due to outdated firmware or limited RAM)
- App crashes or failure to load

- Network disconnections

HDR (High Dynamic Range):

HDR enhances the contrast, brightness, and color range of content. It allows for darker blacks and brighter highlights, improving the overall picture quality.

There are various types of HDR:
- HDR10 (most common)
- Dolby Vision (premium TVs)
- HLG (broadcast HDR)
- HDR10+ (dynamic HDR format by Samsung)

There are benefits to HDR such as:
- Better detail in dark and bright scenes
- Enhanced color realism
- More immersive viewing, especially for movies and nature shows

Customer Misconception: Not all content is HDR even if the TV supports it. To truly experience HDR, you need HDR-compatible content and HDMI 2.0 or higher ports.

Refresh Rate:

The number of times per second (in Hertz or Hz) that a TV refreshes its image. Common rates are 60Hz, 120Hz, 240Hz. A higher refresh rate equals smoother motion, especially useful for:
- Fast-action sports
- Gaming (low latency)
- Reducing motion blur

Gaming Tip: Look for TVs with Variable Refresh Rate (VRR) and Auto Low Latency Mode (ALLM) for next-gen console compatibility (PS5, Xbox Series X).

HDMI and Connectivity:

Important HDMI Specs:
- HDMI 2.0: Supports 4K at 60Hz
- HDMI 2.1: Supports 4K at 120Hz and 8K content
- ARC/eARC: Enables audio pass-through to soundbars or receivers

Other Ports to Consider:
- USB (for media playback or updates)
- Optical audio
- Ethernet (for wired internet)
- Bluetooth (for wireless audio devices)

Voice Assistants and AI Features are now included in many Smart TVs such as:
- Google Assistant
- Amazon Alexa
- Samsung Bixby
- LG ThinQ

Smart TVs combine traditional television with internet-enabled features, offering capabilities such as streaming video and music, web browsing, accessing a variety of apps and games, controlling smart home devices via voice control, and mirroring content from phones and tablets to the big screen.

They run on operating systems like smartphones, allowing app installation and automatic updates for the latest features and content.

TECHNICIAN TIP
Always perform a factory reset and firmware update when troubleshooting Smart TV software problems. If the TV won't connect to Wi-Fi, check for MAC address blocking in the router or outdated network drivers.

Customer Tips When Shopping:
- Check refresh rate specs—avoid marketing tricks that inflate with "motion rate" numbers. - Look at the operating systems, some Smart TV platforms have poor app support.
- Ensure HDMI 2.1 for future-proofing gaming setups.

- Don’t overpay for features you won’t use—some users never touch Smart TV apps if they already use external streaming devices (like Roku or Firestick).

Part 2
Assessment and Diagnostics

Chapter 5:

How to Assess a Faulty TV

Proper assessment is the cornerstone of successful television repair. Whether you're a technician evaluating a unit or a customer trying to understand what's wrong, a structured diagnostic approach ensures accuracy, efficiency, and trust.

Visual Inspection First Clues:

> **TECHNICIAN TIP**
>
> If a Smart TV isn't booting or freezing on logo, the issue is likely with the mainboard or its embedded memory/storage. In some cases, reprogramming the eMMC chip with firmware can resolve it. Otherwise, a board replacement is required.

Before powering on the TV:
- Check the screen for cracks, discoloration, or lines.
- Inspect the frame and corners for signs of impact or bending.
- Examine the ports (HDMI, USB, power) for bent pins or looseness.
- Look for water damage or rust near ventilation grills or boards.
- Assess for pest infestation (ants, cockroaches) that often damage boards. Technician Tip: A cracked panel is not repairable

in most cases. The cost of replacement panels is often close to or more than the price of a new TV.

Power-On Behavior – What Happens When You Try?
Observe what the TV does when it is plugged in and turned on:
- No Power at All: May indicate a faulty power board, internal fuse, or dead mainboard.
- Standby Light Blinks: Check for error codes. Different brands (Sony, LG, Samsung) use blink patterns to signal faults.
- Backlight Comes on but there is no Picture: Could be T-con board, mainboard, or screen panel.
- Sound But No Picture: Typically LED backlight failure.
- Logo Then Freeze/Restart: Often a software or mainboard issue.
- Flashing Screen or Flicker: May indicate T-con or panel issue.

Basic Testing Tools:
You don't always need a lab to diagnose TVs. Start with the basics:
- Multimeter – for checking power supply voltages and continuity
- TV Tester Board/LED Tester for checking LED strips without disassembling the entire panel
- Remote Control Tester to verify IR signal
- HDMI Signal Generator to test input functionality
- Firmware USB for updating or reinstalling firmware (brand-specific)

Record the Findings:
Always log the following during an assessment:
- Serial number and model
- Reported symptoms
- Visible damage
- Power behavior
- Initial diagnosis
- Parts suspected (mainboard, power board, screen, etc.)
- Customer's input and complaint

Sample Assessment Workflow (Technician):
1. Visual inspection for physical or pest-related damage
2. Plug in and observe LED indicators or screen activity
3. Try power-on via remote and button
4. Listen for audio (e.g. startup chime, app sound, channel audio)

5. Shine a flashlight at the screen (for backlight check)
6. Test voltages at power board outputs
7. Swap known-good boards (if available)
8. Provide customers with diagnosis and estimate

For Customers: Quick Self-Check Tips:

- Ensure your TV is plugged directly into a working outlet (not a faulty power strip) - Try unplugging for 5 minutes and restart
- Use a flashlight to check for a faint image on the screen
- Test multiple inputs (HDMI 1, HDMI 2)
- Try another remote or power button

If none of this work, it's time to seek professional help.

When NOT to Proceed:

- TV physically cracked or smashed
- Burn marks or smoke smell from inside
- Water or chemical exposure (e.g. sprayed cleaner seeped in)
- No parts available for brand/model (very old or generic TVs)

Chapter 6:

Common Problems and Their Causes

Every TV failure tells a story. The key is to decode the symptoms and trace them back to the root cause. This chapter outlines the most common television issues across brands and technologies, along with likely culprits and repair considerations.

No Power / Dead TV:

Symptoms:
- No indicator light
- No sound or picture
- Unresponsive to remote or panel buttons

Likely Causes:
- Blown fuse or faulty internal power supply
- Mainboard failure
- Power surge damage
- Dead or shorted capacitors

Action:

Start with the power board. Use a multimeter to test voltage outputs. If voltages are present but the TV remains dead, suspect the mainboard.

Sound But No Picture:

Symptoms:
- You can hear Netflix, cable, or menu sounds
- Screen stays black or very dim

Likely Causes:
- Burned-out LED backlights
- Faulty T-con board
- Loose ribbon cables
- Panel malfunction

Action:
Shine a flashlight at the screen—if you see a faint image, the backlight is dead. Replace LED strips or test with an LED tester.

Picture But No Sound:

Symptoms:
- Clear image but no audio
- Volume level shows on screen but no output

Likely Causes:
- Blown audio IC on the mainboard
- Faulty speakers
- Muted source device
- Software glitch or settings misconfiguration

Action:
Check with headphones or external audio output (e.g., optical port). If headphones work, suspect the speaker circuit or audio IC.

TV Turns on Then off (Boot Loop):

Symptoms:
- TV powers up, shows logo, then shuts off
- Repeats endlessly

Likely Causes:
- Corrupt firmware
- Failing mainboard
- Shorted component (LEDs, T-con, or panel)

Action:
Try a firmware reflash via USB (if supported). Otherwise, test and isolate boards—start with the panel, then T-con, then main.

Colored Vertical or Horizontal Lines:
Symptoms:
- Red, green, or black lines across screen
- Stationary or flickering lines

Likely Causes:
- Damaged screen panel
- Loose ribbon cables
- Faulty T-con board

Action:
Reconnect all ribbon cables. If the problem persists, swap the T-con board. If lines remain, the panel may be defective.

White Screen / No Picture but Backlight On:
Symptoms:
- Screen glows white but shows no image
- Menus don't appear

Likely Causes:
- Dead T-con board
- Damaged LVDS cable
- Panel failure

Action:

Replace the T-con board or check if the mainboard is outputting proper signals to T-con. If confirmed, suspect panel.

TV Won't Respond to Remote or Buttons:

Symptoms:
- No reaction when pressing remote or TV buttons
- TV stuck on one screen/input

Likely Causes:
- Frozen software
- Defective IR sensor
- Mainboard issue

TECHNICIAN TIP
Many modern TVs use integrated systems, so failure in one area (e.g., a backlight short) can cause the entire TV to shut down or enter protection mode. Always disconnect the suspect circuit and retest to isolate the fault.

ACTION
Action:
Reset the TV. If there is no change, try replacing the IR sensor or reflowing the mainboard.

Signs of Pest or Moisture Damage:

Symptoms:
- Random shorts
- Burnt smell
-Inconsistent startup behavior

Likely Causes:
- Insect nests or dead pests bridging circuits
- Water damage corroding traces and ICs

ACTION
Action:
Open the unit and clean with isopropyl alcohol. Inspect for burnt tracks. Severe cases often require board replacement.

Chapter 7:

Understanding Error Codes, Lights, and Behavior

Modern televisions often include built-in diagnostics. These may appear as blinking lights, colored indicators, or error messages. Understanding these signals helps both technicians and informed customers quickly identify faults without full disassembly.

LED Blink Codes (Standby Lights):
Many brands use LED blink codes on the standby/power indicator light to communicate errors. These patterns vary depending on manufacturer.

Sony TVs:
- 2 Blinks: Power board issue (often overvoltage)
- 3 Blinks: Mainboard short
- 5 Blinks: T-con or panel failure
- 6/7 Blinks: Backlight or inverter failure
- 8 Blinks: Audio board or speaker issue

Samsung TVs:
Samsung often uses no blink codes, but a continuous flashing standby light can indicate a shorted LED or mainboard issue.

LG TVs:
Blinks usually occur during bootloop/failure; use flashlight test to check for backlight presence.

Interpreting Behavior Patterns:
Power On, Then Off (Auto Shutdown): Likely shorted LED, T-con, or panel — the TV enters protection mode.

Logo Appears, Then Freezes: Software corruption or mainboard memory failure.

Screen Flashes Then Stays Black: Often caused by LED backlight short or T-con error.

No Picture But Red Light Steady: Mainboard or screen fault; requires further probing.

Flashlight Test Technique:
Purpose: To determine whether the image is still being produced but not visible due to backlight failure.

TECHNICIAN TIP
Always document LED blink behavior and patterns before opening the TV. A simple code like 5 blinks can save hours of unnecessary board testing.

Steps:
1. Turn on the TV in a dark room.
2. Shine a flashlight at an angle across the screen.
3. If you can see faint images (logos, menus), your backlight is the issue.

Best Used When: TV has sound, powers on, but screen appears black.

Basic Testing Without Disassembly:
Signs You Can Check:
- Sound present = likely not the mainboard or power board.
- Remote responsiveness = mainboard booting.
- No lights or sound = test power supply first.

Brand-Specific Tools:

- Panasonic: Service mode via remote (hold Vol- and Input)
- LG: Use service remote or mobile app
- Samsung: Hold specific key combo on remote to enter service mode

NB. Caution: Service mode misuse can permanently damage or "brick" your TV.

Chapter 8:

Tools Every Technician (and Customer) Should Know

The right tools make all the difference between guesswork and precision. Whether you're a professional technician or a tech-savvy customer, having the proper tools ensures safer, faster, and more accurate diagnostics and repairs.

Core Tools for Every Technician:

1. Digital Multimeter (DMM)

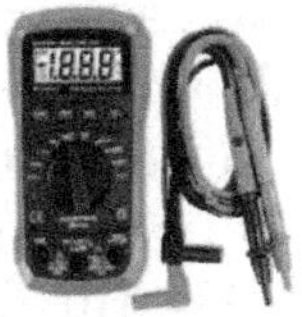

- Used to test voltage, resistance, and continuity
- Essential for verifying power board and LED voltages
- Must have sharp probes and auto-ranging

2. LED Tester

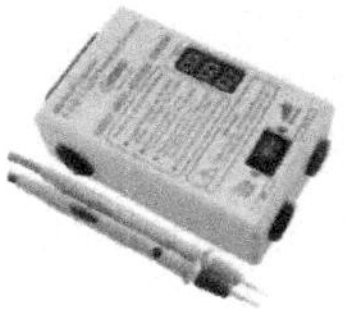

- Connects to backlight connector or strip
- Helps isolate failed LEDs without full disassembly
- Portable and low cost

3. TV Panel Light Tester

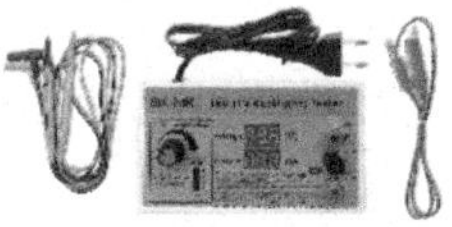

- Allows safe testing of individual LED strips or bars
- Shows real-time voltage and current draw

4. Screwdriver Set (Magnetic Tips)
- Multiple sizes for removing TV frames, boards, and screws
- Precision heads for handling delicate electronics

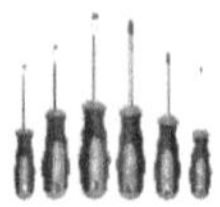

5. Soldering Iron & Soldering Station
- For component-level repairs like capacitor or IC replacement
- Use a temperature-controlled station for safety and accuracy

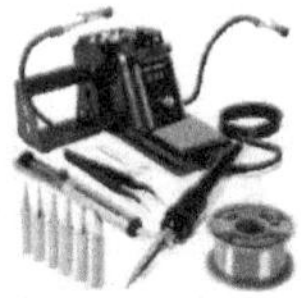

6. Hot Air Rework Station
- Essential for replacing surface-mounted components (SMDs)
- Often used with solder paste for chip replacement

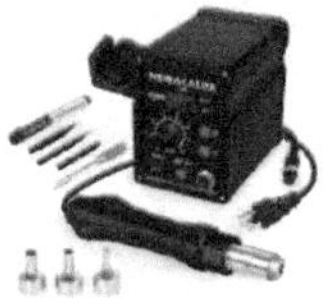

7. ESD Mat and Wrist Strap
- Prevents electrostatic discharge from damaging TV boards
- Mandatory when handling mainboards or T-con boards

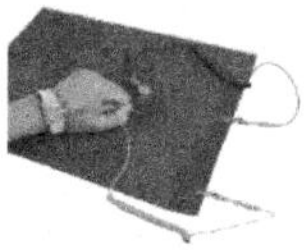

Advanced Tools for Diagnosis & Rework:

1. Oscilloscope
- For advanced signal tracing
- Useful for analyzing T-con and LVDS signals

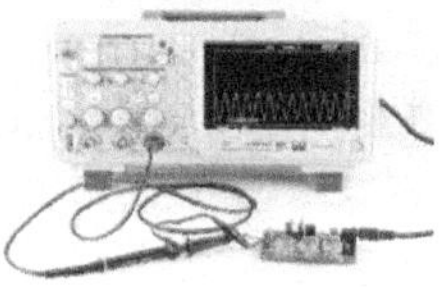

2. Infrared Thermometer / Thermal Camera
- Detects overheating components
- Great for locating short circuits or bad ICs

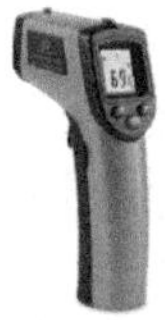

3. eMMC Programmer
- Used for reprogramming or flashing firmware onto mainboards
- Compatible with Samsung, LG, and Android-based TVs

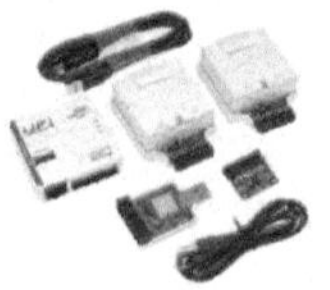

4. HDMI Signal Generator
- Verifies that HDMI ports are processing input
- Detects HDMI board or input switch issues

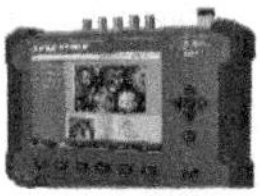

Diagnostic Aids for Field Technicians:

1. Flashlight or Headlamp – Helps spot cracked screens or faint images

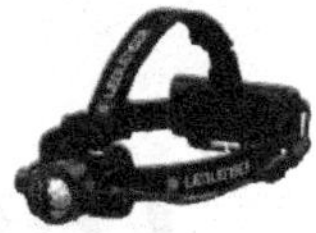

2. Smartphone Camera – Used to view IR signals from remotes

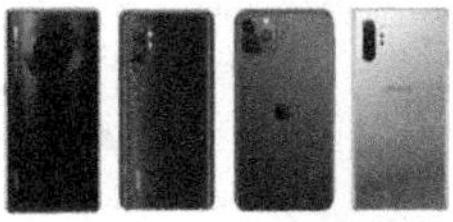

3. Portable Power Supply – For field diagnostics and safety isolation

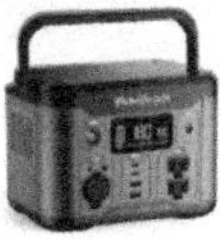

4. Universal Remote – For testing power-on and menu functions

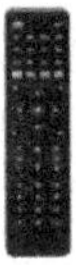

5. Labeling Tape or Pen – To tag and track removed connectors during disassembly

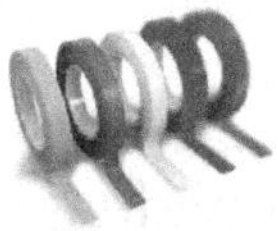

Essential Tools for Advanced Customers:

If you're a confident DIY user or enthusiast, the following tools can help you perform safe, basic checks:

- Digital Multimeter
- LED Tester
- Flashlight
- ESD Wrist Strap
- Basic Screwdriver Kit

TECHNICIAN TIP

Start with non-invasive tools first: flashlight test, multimeter, and LED tester. Only open the TV once you've gathered visual and power behavior clues. Always discharge capacitors before working inside!

Note: Avoid soldering unless you're trained. Improper soldering can destroy expensive components or pose a fire risk.

Chapter 9:

The Basics of Board-Level Repairs

Board-level repairs are one of the most valuable skills in television servicing. Instead of replacing an entire board, technicians can often fix individual faulty components – saving money and reducing e-waste.

What Are Board-Level Repairs:
Repairing individual components on a circuit board (power board, mainboard, T-con, etc.) rather than replacing the whole unit.

Common Boards in a TV:
- Power Board: Supplies voltage to other components
- Mainboard (Motherboard): Handles processing, video/audio signals, software - T-con Board: Controls screen timing and signal interpretation
- Inverter Board (older LCDs): Powers CCFL backlights
- Wi-Fi/Bluetooth Module: Handles wireless connectivity

Symptoms That Suggest Component-Level Failure:
- Blown capacitor bulging or leaking
- No power but fuse and voltage input are fine
- Vertical lines or distortion from T-con board
- TV reboots due to overheating ICs
- HDMI port not working on mainboard

Common Components Replaced:

Capacitors store and release energy
– Fail by bulging, leaking, or reduced capacity Diodes
– Direct current flow
– Fail by shorting or opening

Metal-Oxide-Semiconductor Field-Effect Transistors (MOSFETs) for power switching
– Fail from overheating or shorts

Integrated Circuits (IC) Chips handle logic and data
– Fail silently or from heat

Fuses provides Circuit protection
– Fail open (no continuity)

> **TECHNICIAN TIP**
>
> Sometimes the fault is not the obvious burned component but something upstream. Always check related components in the circuit path – especially when working with power rails or signal lines.

Connectors allow cable interface
– Fail from corrosion or damage

Required Skills and Tools:

Skills:
- Reading circuit diagrams
- Using a multimeter
- Soldering/desoldering
- Visual/electronic diagnosis of components

Tools:
- Soldering iron with fine tip
- Hot air rework station
- Flux and solder wick
- Tweezers, magnifier, and light
- Multimeter and ESR meter

Figure 9.1: Example Repair: Replacing a Blown Capacitor

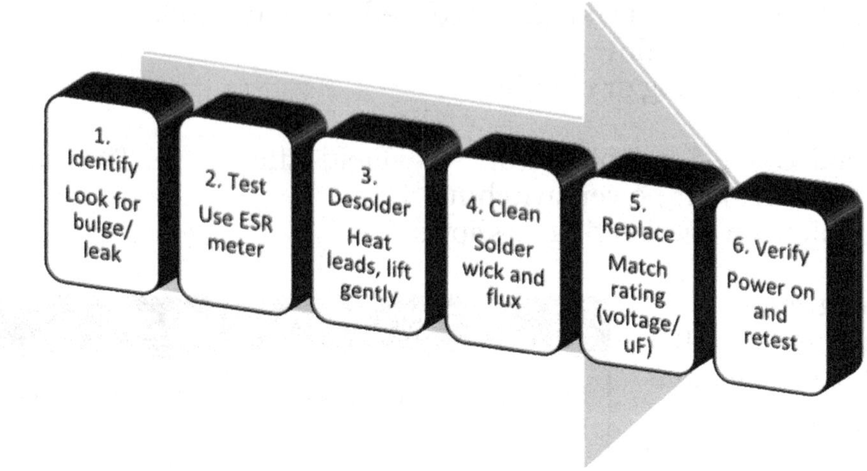

Safety Reminders:
- Always unplug the TV before opening
- Discharge capacitors properly
- Don't short capacitors directly
- Use ESD wrist strap on logic boards

Chapter 10:

When to Repair vs. Replace

Not all TV issues are worth repairing. Some problems cost more to fix than buying a new unit. This chapter provides a framework to help both technicians and customers decide whether a repair makes financial and practical sense.

Factors to Consider:
1. Cost of Repair vs. Replacement
- If the repair cost exceeds 50% of the current replacement cost, replacement is usually more economical.
- Example: If a new 55" Smart TV costs $3,500, and the repair estimate is $2,000+, it's often better to replace.

2. Age of the TV
- TVs over 5–7 years old are more likely to fail again due to aging components.
- Older TVs may lack modern features (HDR, 4K, Smart OS).

3. Availability of Parts
- If key components like screen panels or mainboards are discontinued or unavailable, replacement may be the only option.

4. Screen Damage
- Cracked or smashed screens are rarely worth fixing unless it's a high-end TV.

- LCD/OLED panels are the most expensive parts of the unit.

Common Scenarios: Repair or Replace?

- Cracked screen: Replace
- No power, repair < 40% of value: Repair
- Backlight failure: Repair (LED swap)
- Mainboard unavailable: Replace
- Burn-in on OLED: Replace
- Wi-Fi module failure: Repair
- Age over 8 years: Replace
- HDMI ports all dead: Repair (if affordable)

Repair Adds Value When...

- TV is under 5 years old
- Has high resolution (4K/8K) and premium features
- Customer prefers eco-friendly solutions
- Issue is a known and solvable fault (like backlight failure)
- Unit is wall-mounted and fits a specific decor or setup

Eco-Friendly Consideration:
Replacing a TV contributes to e-waste, which includes heavy metals, plastic, and non-biodegradable components. Responsible repair reduces your carbon footprint and promotes sustainability.

> TECHNICIAN TIP
>
> Always offer customers both options: repair quote and new TV recommendation. This builds trust and positions you as a transparent professional, not just a sales-driven service.

Part 3

Safe Handling and Transportation

Chapter 11:

How to Safely Move and Package a TV

Flat-screen TVs are delicate and expensive. Whether you're transporting one for repair, relocation, or delivery, improper handling can lead to screen cracks, internal component damage, or even voided warranties. This chapter outlines the safest way to move and package a TV to avoid costly accidents.

Why So Many TVs Get Damaged in Transit:

- Screens are extremely pressure-sensitive, especially edge-lit LED and OLED types.
- Many people lay TVs flat, which flexes the panel and can cause cracks.
- Wrapping with soft material only (like blankets) offers little protection against impact.
- Ports and boards can get jarred loose if the TV is not supported properly.

Pre-Transport Checklist:

A transportation checklist for television ensures safe packing, secure handling, and proper delivery without damage.

- Unplug and remove all cables
- Remove wall mount brackets if possible
- Take a photo of cable setup (for easy reconnection later)
- Check for visible damage or prior issues

- Clean the screen gently with a microfiber cloth

Packaging Materials:
Best Option: Original box with factory foam corners

If not available, use the following:
- Stiff cardboard box (as close to original size as possible)
- Foam padding or corner protectors
- Bubble wrap (especially for screen side)
- Plastic stretch wrap to hold padding in place
- Heavy-duty tape to secure flaps

TECHNICIAN TIP

If a TV arrives cracked and the customer claims it wasn't damaged when packed, inspect corner flex points and edge pressure marks often indicate poor transportation methods.

Proper Positioning:
Never lay a flat-screen TV face-down or flat on its back.
- Always transport upright, like a door
- Place screen side toward a padded surface (e.g., a car seat)
- If you use a vehicle, strap the TV in to prevent sliding
- Ensure the TV does not touch hard surfaces or metal parts

Temperature and Moisture Tips:
- Avoid transporting in extreme cold or hot environments
- Never store in a damp or wet space (e.g., trunk with leaks)
- Allow the TV to acclimate to room temperature before powering on

Chapter 12:

Common Damage from Improper Transport

Even if a TV appears fine after moving, hidden damage can surface later especially if transported incorrectly. Understanding the types of damage caused by poor handling helps both technicians and customers diagnose post-move issues more accurately.

Cracked or Pressurized Screens:
A cracked or pressurized TV screen can cause display damage, safety hazards, and may render the television unusable.

Most Common Issue:
- Cracks often begin at corners or along the bezel
- May not be visible until the screen is powered on
- Vertical or horizontal lines often indicate internal panel fractures caused by:
- Laying the TV flat
- Excessive pressure on one side
- Poor bracing in vehicle

Repair Status: Usually, non-repairable

Dislodged Boards and Loose Connections:
- Jarring or bumpy rides can loosen internal cable harnesses or flex connectors. This results in the following:
- No signal from HDMI

- T-con disconnection (no picture)
- Wi-Fi/Bluetooth modules disconnecting intermittently

How to Fix:
Open and reseat ribbon cables or board connectors

Puncture or Impact Damage:
- Occurs when TV contacts sharp or pointed objects
- May damage:
- LCD layer (causing bleeding or black spots)
- Frame/bracket
- Internal PCB

Tip: Always reinforce packaging around corners and screen face
Bent Frame or Warped Housing:
- If a TV frame is twisted or bent, the screen can flex and crack over time - Especially risky with ultra-slim LED and OLED TVs

Symptoms:
- Delayed line or crack appearance
- Uneven pressure causing display distortion

Moisture and Condensation Damage:
- Transporting in rain or humid conditions can introduce moisture

TECHNICIAN TIP
Corner cracks, loose ribbon cables, and signs of moisture are red flags for transport related damage.

Signs of moisture damage:
- Foggy screen corners
- Corroded connector pins
- Power failure due to short circuits

Prevention Tips: Use plastic wrap and silica gel packs in packaging.

Chapter 13:

Checklist for Customers: Do's and Don'ts

Many TV failures can be prevented or better managed if customers follow a few simple guidelines. This chapter offers a clear, practical checklist to help customers assess transport, and prepare their TVs for servicing or general use.

DO's – Best Practices:

Before Transporting a TV:
- Use original box and packaging if available
- Always transport upright — never flat
- Wrap corners and screen with bubble wrap and foam
- Secure TV in vehicle to prevent sliding
- Take photos of cable setup before unplugging
- Remove brackets and external devices (USB, HDMI)
- Cover with plastic wrap to protect from moisture

When Booking Repairs:
- Write down the model number and serial

- Note any visible symptoms (blinking light, sound, etc.)
- Explain what happened before the TV stopped working
- Take a picture or short video of the issue if possible
- Keep all accessories (remotes, power cords) handy

While Using the TV:
- Use a surge protector or voltage regulator
- Dust vents regularly to prevent overheating
- Keep drinks, sprays, and pets away from the screen
- Update firmware as recommended by the manufacturer
- Use screen cleaning cloths and avoid paper towels or alcohol

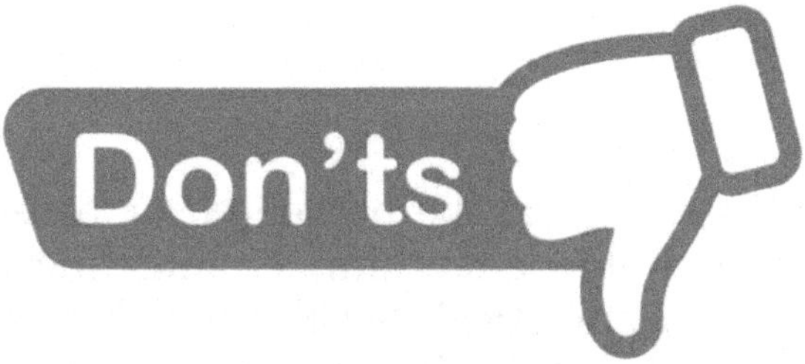

DON'Ts – Common Mistakes to Avoid:

During Transport:
- Don't lay the TV flat in a car
- Don't use only towels or sheets as padding
- Don't place items on top of the TV in storage
- Don't drag the TV by the corners or screen

Before Calling a Technician:
- Don't reset your TV multiple times unnecessarily
- Don't try to open the unit unless you're trained
- Don't spray cleaning liquid directly onto the screen
- Don't ignore blinking lights or unusual behavior, report them

TECHNICIAN TIP

Customers who follow these checklists often get quicker diagnoses, fewer repeat problems, and better pricing because the technician spends less time troubleshooting and more time repairing.

Daily Usage:
- Don't leave static images such as logos, paused games on-screen for hours to avoid burn-in
- Don't plug in during power surges or storms
- Don't run the TV in very dusty or humid environments
- Don't use unsupported apps or firmware hacks because they void warranties

Chapter 14:

How Technicians Should Log and Transport Units

Transporting a customer's television is not just a matter of loading it in a van. It's a critical phase where damage, confusion, or miscommunication can occur. A well-documented and standardized process protects both the technician and the customer.

Why Logging Matters:
Proper documentation:
- Ensures accountability
- Helps track repairs and parts usage
- Prevents disputes over pre-existing damage
- Improves service quality and professionalism

What to Log Before Transport:
Essential Information to Record:
- Customer name and contact details
- TV brand, model number, and size
- Serial number (photographed if possible)
- Reported issue(s)
- Physical condition upon pickup (note scratches, cracks, missing parts)
- Accessories collected (remote, power cable, base, wall brackets)
- Time/date of pickup and expected return

Optional: Take photos of the TV from all sides at pickup.

Packaging for Technician Transport:
- Use TV transport bags or custom foam sleeves if available
- Keep TVs upright, face-in toward padded wall or divider
- Secure using straps or tension bars to prevent tipping or movement
- Avoid loading TVs alongside heavy equipment or tools
- Never place TVs screen-to-screen and add cushioning in between

TECHNICIAN TIP

Use a triplicate service form (technician, office, customer) or digital app that captures all pickup and return details. It's your best protection against liability for damage not caused by your team.

Service Labels and Identification:
Place a temporary label or tag with:
- Job number or internal tracking code
- Technician name
- Repair center name/logo
- Clear "**HANDLE WITH CARE**" or "**SCREEN – DO NOT PRESS**" message This prevents confusion when handling multiple jobs.

Return Delivery Protocol:
Upon return:
- Re-inspect unit with customer
- Plug in and demonstrate fix if possible
- Have customers sign for received unit in good condition
- Provide repair summary/invoice detailing the fix
- Document any remaining issues (if applicable)

Part 4
TV
Maintenance and Longevity

Chapter 15:

How to Maintain Your TV for Long Life

Modern televisions are durable but still require basic maintenance to prevent overheating, image retention, and premature component failure. With proper care, your TV can perform like new for years.

Cleanliness and Environment:
Keep your TV in a clean, dust-free area. Dust buildup can block vents and overheat internal components.

Tips:
- Dust the screen and back vents weekly using a microfiber cloth
- Avoid using harsh cleaners; instead, use screen-safe sprays
- Never spray liquid directly onto the screen — spray onto cloth first
- Keep food, drinks, and pets away from the unit

Proper Ventilation:
All TVs generate heat, especially LED and OLED models. Poor airflow can lead to:
- Shortened LED lifespan
- Mainboard overheating
- Glitches or early shutdowns

As a result, ensure the following:
- At least 4–6 inches of space around vents
- Wall-mounted TVs are not flush against walls without airflow
- No blocked vents from dust, cabinets, or nearby objects

Use a Surge Protector:
Voltage fluctuations and lightning strikes can damage internal components. Always plug your TV into a surge protector or voltage regulator.

💡 Tip: Look for a protector with at least 1000 joules and indicator lights.

Safe Power Cycling and Usage:
Avoid frequent on/off switching in short intervals.

Instead:
- Use the standby/power button
- Turn off the unit when not in use for extended periods
- Don't unplug immediately after use; allow to cool naturally

Update Firmware Regularly:
Smart TVs run on internal operating systems. Manufacturers release updates to:
- Fix bugs
- Improve app support
- Add security patches

Check for firmware updates monthly via the settings menu.
- Avoid Static Images and Burn-In, especially on OLED panels.
- Static images can cause burn-in over time.

TECHNICIAN TIP

Many avoidable repairs stem from poor ventilation or power surges. Encourage customers to invest in proper installation, including brackets that support airflow and power protection equipment.

Tips:

- Avoid leaving pause screens on for hours
- Use screen savers or pixel shift features (if available)
- Turn down brightness for extended viewing

Chapter 16:

Voltage, Surge Protection, and Cooling Tips

Televisions are vulnerable to power-related damage and overheating, both of which are preventable. This chapter provides best practices to safeguard your investment from electrical spikes, brownouts, and thermal stress.

Voltage Risks to Your TV:

Common voltage problems:
- Surges from lightning or power grid switching
- Brownouts (low voltage) that stress power boards
- Power cuts leading to corrupt firmware or board failure
- Improper grounding that causes voltage to flow into AV ports

Symptoms of damage:
- No power after lightning storm
- HDMI or USB ports stop working
- TV randomly restarts or shuts down
- Burn marks on the power board

Choosing the Right Surge Protection:
Basic surge protectors are better than none but may not withstand major surges.

Look for:
- Energy Rating: 1000+ joules
- Indicator Lights: Show protection and grounding status
- Spaced Outlets: For oversized adapters
- USB Ports (optional): Charging smart remotes/devices
- Warranty: Some include equipment damage coverage

Better Option: Use a voltage regulator for consistent output.

Managing Heat and Airflow:
Heat is a silent killer of TV components. Over time, trapped heat causes:
- Backlight degradation
- Mainboard IC failures
- Power board burnouts
- Reduced panel brightness

> **TECHNICIAN TIP**
>
> When inspecting a dead or flickering TV, always check for cockroaches, corrosion on ribbon connectors and board discoloration, especially in the customer lives in a humid or pest prone area.

Cooling tips:
- Ensure wall-mounted TVs have space for airflow
- Avoid placing TVs in enclosed cabinets
- Don’t block rear vents with curtains, furniture, or décor
- Use a fan or AC in rooms that reach high temperatures

Seasonal Awareness:
- In rainy seasons, invest in surge protectors with lightning defense
- During dry seasons, dust builds up faster therefore clean vents weekly
- In hot climates, avoid leaving TVs on all day unattended

Chapter 17:

Environmental Risks: Dust, Moisture & Insects

Televisions are sensitive electronic devices. Exposure to poor environmental conditions like dust, moisture, and insects can significantly reduce their lifespan and reliability. This chapter explores how to protect TVs from these hidden dangers.

Dust – The Silent Clogger:

Risks:
- Blocks air vents and cooling fans
- Causes overheating and thermal shutdowns
- Builds static electricity on circuit boards
- Settles on T-con and mainboards, increasing short risk

Prevention Tips:
- Clean TV vents weekly using a soft brush or vacuum attachment
- Avoid placing TVs near open windows, fans, or vents
- Cover unused TVs with a breathable cloth (not plastic)

Moisture – Hidden Killer of Circuits:

Risks:
- Short circuits or corroded traces on boards
- Foggy screen corners and internal condensation
- Triggers rust in exposed metal parts and connectors
- Can result in full board failure or flickering

Prevention Tips:
- Keep TVs away from kitchens, bathrooms, or leaky roofs
- Avoid mounting above AC vents or humidifiers
- Use dehumidifiers in damp environments
- Don't clean with wet cloths or chemical sprays

Insects – Small but Destructive:
Cockroaches, ants, and other household insects are naturally drawn to the warmth, darkness, and electronic vibrations inside television sets, often nesting within the circuitry, which can lead to contamination, electrical shorts, unpleasant odors, and even permanent damage to sensitive components.

Risks:
- Short circuits from live roaches inside boards
- Burn marks and component failure
- Droppings causing corrosion or tracking issues
- Nesting inside power or mainboards

TECHNICIAN TIP

When inspecting a dead or flickering TV, always check for cockroaches, corrosion on ribbon connectors and board discoloration, especially in the customer lives in a humid or pest prone area.

Prevention Tips:
- Keep the TV area clean and crumb-free
- Use insect traps near entertainment units
- Seal wall penetrations and gaps in cabinetry
- Store TVs in clean, sealed environments during transport

Signs of Environmental Damage:
- Rust on HDMI or power ports
- Stains, droppings, or visible insect bodies
- Random shutdowns or power issues
- Flickering screen caused by board oxidation

Chapter 18:

Firmware Updates and Software Health

Modern TVs are essentially computers with screens. Their firmware (internal software) controls everything from power management to app performance. Keeping this software healthy is essential to long-term reliability.

What Is Firmware:
Firmware is the permanent software programmed into your TV's internal memory. It manages:
- Power sequencing
- Audio/video synchronization
- HDMI and USB port behavior
- Smart TV apps and system menus
- Network communication (Wi-Fi, Bluetooth, LAN)

Signs of Firmware Problems:
- TV freezes or reboots unexpectedly
- Smart apps crash or won't open
- HDMI ports stop detecting devices
- Settings won't save after restart
- Ghost inputs or lag in remote response
- Sound or picture issues not related to hardware

How to Check for Updates:

Most Smart TVs have an update option in the **Settings > About > Software Update** section.

Update Methods:

- Online (Wi-Fi): Quick and easy
- USB (manual): For models without internet access
- Technician-assisted: Using firmware recovery tools

Warning: Never turn off the TV during an update. This can corrupt the board.

> **TECHNICIAN TIP**
>
> Before replacing a mainboard for a "dead" TV, try to check if the firmware is corrupt. Many recoveries are possible with the correct USB tools especially for LG, Samsung, Sony and TCL.

What Happens If Firmware Is Corrupted:

- TV may get stuck in boot loop
- Screen may stay black with power light on
- May not respond to remote or buttons
- Can mimic dead mainboard symptoms

ACTION Solution: Reflash firmware using:

- USB recovery stick (manufacturer-provided)
- Factory jig tools
- Mainboard replacement if recovery fails

Preventative Tips for Software Health:

- Regularly restart your TV (don't leave it on for weeks)
- Clear app caches from settings (if available)
- Avoid installing unsupported third-party apps
- Ensure power is stable during updates
- Check manufacturer's website for the latest firmware file

Part 5 Buying the Right TV

Chapter 19:

Choosing the Best TV for Your Needs

Buying a new TV can feel overwhelming with so many models, terms, and price points. This chapter simplifies your decision-making by matching TV types to your needs, whether it's for gaming, cinema, or casual viewing.

Choosing the Right Size:
General rule of thumb for viewing distance (in feet): Multiply your seating distance by 7 for 1080p TVs or by 5 for 4K TVs.

Table 19.1: Seating Distance vs Best Screen Size

Seating Distance	Best Screen Size (4K)
4-5 ft	32-43"
6-8 ft	50-55"
9-10 ft	60-70"
11 + ft	75" and above

Tip: Bigger is better only if your space can accommodate it comfortably.

Here are some recommended used cases based on the purpose for the use of a television:

For Gaming:
- Look for 120Hz refresh rate or higher

- Input lag below 15ms
- HDMI 2.1 for PS5/Xbox Series X
- Game Mode and VRR (Variable Refresh Rate)
- Brands to consider: LG OLED, Samsung QLED, TCL 6-Series

For Movies:
- OLED for deep blacks and movie realism
- Dolby Vision and HDR10+ support
- Wide color gamut (WCG) panels
- Prefer a 55” or larger screen in a dark room
- Brands to consider: Sony Bravia, LG OLED, Hisense ULED

For Casual Watching:
- Affordable LED models work fine
- Smart TV apps (YouTube, Netflix) built-in
- Slim design with good power efficiency
- Brands to consider: Samsung, TCL, Skyworth, Vizio

Key Features to Consider:
When purchasing a television, it is important to evaluate several key features—including screen size, resolution, refresh rate, connectivity options, smart capabilities, and sound quality—to ensure the set matches both your viewing preferences and your room’s requirements

Table 19.2 Key Features of Different Types of TVs

Key Feature	Why it Matters
Resolution	4K is standard; 8K not yet widely supported
Panel Type **OLED** **QLED** **LED**	 Best blacks Bright and vibrant Basic
SMART Operating Systems (OS)	Roku, WebOS, Android TV affect speed & app support
Audio	Look for Dolby Audio or ARC support for soundbars
Connectivity	More HDMI ports equal better Bluetooth is a plus

Tips for Smart Buyers:
- Don't fall for just the brand — check panel specs and real reviews
- Avoid outdated ports (like Video Graphics Array (VGA) or Component)
- Look for local dimming zones for better contrast
- If wall mounting, make sure the TV supports Video Electronics Standards Association (VESA) standards
- Ask for manufacturer warranty and extended protection options

TECHNICIAN TIP

When customers ask for help choosing a TV, match their use case to features, not the hype. A gamer has different needs from a move lover or a senior who just watches cable.

Chapter 20:

Top TVs for Gaming, Movies, and Budget Buyers

With so many choices on the market, selecting the right TV can be daunting. This chapter provides a curated list of top-performing televisions categorized by Gaming, Cinema/Streaming, and Budget-Friendly Picks, all based on performance reviews, features, and price-to-value ratio.

Note: Prices and availability may vary by region and year. Always double-check with local vendors or updated tech review sources.

TECHNICIAN TIP

When customers ask, “Which TV should I get?” Always factor in:
- Usage scenario (gaming vs. streaming vs. news)
- Room lighting (OLEDs thrive in darker rooms)
- Warranty and repairability
-Power conditions in their area (recommend surge protection)

Best TVs for Gaming (2024–2025 Picks):
These models offer ultra-fast response times, HDMI 2.1 support, and high refresh rates — perfect for serious gamers using PS5, Xbox Series X, or gaming PCs.

Table 20.1 Best TVs for Gaming

Model and Features	Suggested cost (USD)
LG C3 OLED (42"–83"): 120Hz, VRR, G-SYNC, low input lag	$1,000–$2,500
Samsung QN90C Neo QLED (43"–85"): 144Hz, HDR10+, Game Bar, FreeSync	$1,100– $2,800
Sony A80L OLED (55"–77"): HDMI 2.1, Auto HDR Tone Mapping	$1,200–$2,200
TCL QM8 Series (55"–85"): 120Hz, Mini-LED, VRR support	$900–$1,700

Best TVs for Movies & Streaming:
These are ideal for cinematic viewing, home theaters, or streaming content with excellent color performance and black levels.

Table 20.2 Best TVs for Movies & Streaming

Model and Features	Suggested cost (USD)
LG G3 OLED Evo (55"–83"): OLED evo, Dolby Vision, perfect blacks	$1,600–$3,000
Sony X95L Mini-LED (65"–85"): XR Processor, X-Wide Angle, great HDR	$1,800–$3,500
Hisense U8K ULED (55"–75"): High brightness, Dolby Atmos, Google TV	$800–$1,500
- Samsung S90C OLED (55"–77"): QD-OLED, deep contrast	$1,300–$2,700

Best Budget-Friendly TVs (Smart + Reliable):
If you're looking for a solid smart TV without breaking the bank, these deliver good value and performance for everyday use.

Table 20.3 Budget Friendly TVs

Model and Features	Suggested cost (USD)
TCL 5-Series (50"–75") QLED screen, Roku/Google TV OS —	$400–$700
Vizio MQ6 Series (43"–75"): Quantum color, Apple AirPlay2/Chromecast	$350–$650
Samsung CU7000 (43"–85"): Good upscaling, decent HDR	$380–$800
Hisense A6 Series (43"–75"): Google TV, Dolby Vision	$300–$600

Chapter 21:

Frequently Asked Questions (FAQs) TV Owners Edition

This chapter compiles the most common questions asked by TV owners, both before and after purchase. These insights help consumers make smarter decisions and avoid unnecessary repairs or replacements.

Q1: "Is it safe to leave my TV on all day?"
A: It's not ideal. Prolonged use generates heat, which accelerates component wear and may lead to premature failure — especially for LED backlights and power boards. Turn off the TV when not in use or use timers/smart plugs.

Q2: "Do I really need a surge protector?"
A: Yes. Even minor voltage spikes can damage HDMI ports, mainboards, or power boards. Always plug your TV into a surge protector or voltage regulator especially in areas prone to lightning or grid instability.

Q3: "Can I lay my TV flat when transporting it?"
A: No. Always keep TVs upright in their original box with padding if possible. Laying flat can cause stress fractures in the panel, especially in large LED or OLED models.

Q4: "What's the best way to clean my screen?"

A: Use a microfiber cloth with a screen-safe spray. Never use alcohol, ammonia-based cleaners, or spray directly onto the screen. Always apply cleaner to the cloth first.

Q5: "Why does my smart TV freeze or restart randomly?"
A: Common causes:
- Outdated firmware
- Poor Wi-Fi connection
- Low internal storage (clear app cache)
- Software bugs or overheating

Try updating the firmware and restarting the TV. If problems persist, a factory reset may help.

Q6: "What size TV should I get for my room?"
A: Measure your seating distance and apply the rule:
- For 4K TVs: multiply distance in feet by 5
- For 1080p TVs: multiply by 7

This gives an ideal screen size range.

Q7: "How often should I update my TV firmware?"
A: Check once a month. Updates fix bugs, add new app compatibility, and patch security flaws. It's quick and worth it just to ensure the power doesn't go off during the process.

Q8: "Is it better to wall mount or use a stand?"
A: Both are fine but wall mounting saves space, reduces tipping hazards, and looks cleaner. Use quality mounts and install them properly (see Chapter 21). Stands work well for flexibility or rental homes.

Q9: "Can insects damage my TV?"
A: Yes. Roaches and ants often crawl into vents seeking warmth, causing shorts and corrosion. Keep the area clean and use traps or deterrents.

Q10: "Why does my TV keep saying 'No Signal'?"
A: Some causes include:
- Loose HDMI cable
- Wrong input selected
- Dead set-top box or gaming console

- Damaged HDMI port

You can also try another HDMI port or cable and verify if the source is powered on.

Chapter 22:

Technician Field Tips and Professional Advice

Experience in the field often teaches lessons no manual can. This chapter delivers a toolkit of real-world tips and best practices for TV repair professionals, installers, and service teams based on years of hands-on experience.

First Call Checklist (Before Visiting a Customer):
1. Confirm model and size of TV
2. Ask for photos of issue or error message
3. Verify wall mount vs. table-top setup
4. Ask if it was exposed to lightning, power cuts, or water
5. Confirm pick-up or on-site visit requirements

💡 Tip: A 2-minute pre-check call avoids unnecessary travel and prepares you with parts/tools in advance.

Initial Diagnosis Essentials:
- Check standby light behavior (solid, blinking, dead)
- Use flashlight test to rule out backlight vs. screen issue
- Check for signs of tampering or prior repair
- Bring a universal remote for menu/response testing
- Carry jumper wires to test power boards or T-con bypasses

Tools Every Technician Should Carry:
- Multimeter with diode and capacitance modes

- Mini screwdriver set (magnetic recommended)
- Power supply tester and universal AC cord
- LED backlight tester
- Flashlight and small mirror for angle checks
- Heat gun and flux for minor board work
- USB with test firmware (LG, TCL, Samsung, etc.)

Transport & Handling Best Practices:

- Never lay flat — always transport upright
- Use foam corners, anti-slip mats, and straps
- Label each unit by job number and owner
- Remove stands and screws — store separately in labeled bags
- Avoid placing tools or cables directly on screen surfaces

Job Documentation Tips:

- Take "before" and "after" photos
- Document board swaps, voltages tested, and firmware versions
- Capture customer signature upon delivery or service completion
- Record model number, serial, and any sticker details for warranty

Customer Communication Advice:

- Be honest if a TV is uneconomical to repair
- Avoid jargon — explain clearly in everyday terms
- Offer written estimates and get approval before repairs
- Always recommend surge protectors and cooling practices
- Leave a "care guide" or checklist for post-service care

💡 Pro Tip:

A great technician doesn't just fix TVs — they build trust, prevent repeat issues, and educate customers. A well-informed customer is your best repeat client.

Chapter 23:

End-of-Life for TVs: Recycling, Disposal, and Reuse

Not all TVs can or should be repaired. Whether due to age, parts unavailability, or economic impracticality, some units reach the end of their usable life. This chapter explores smart, responsible, and even profitable ways to dispose of or repurpose them.

When Is a TV Considered End-of-Life?
- Severe screen damage (e.g. internal cracks or burn-in)
- Mainboard failure with no available replacements
- Power issues tied to panel shorting
- Excessive age (10+ years for LCDs, 7+ years for plasmas)
- Panel discolored or faded beyond calibration

💡 Technician Tip: If parts and labor exceed 60–70% of the cost of a new TV, recommend replacement.

Proper Disposal Methods:
- E-Waste Collection Points such as using certified recycling programs that safely extract valuable metals and components
- Manufacturer Take-Back Programs as some brands offer trade-in or disposal incentives

- Retailer Drop-offs as major electronics stores often accept old TVs for recycling (sometimes for a fee)
- Municipal Pickups are available so inquire with local waste management services for scheduled bulky item collections

NB. Never discard TVs in regular garbage bins as they contain lead, mercury, and flame retardants.

Parts Harvesting and Reuse:
Even if the screen is dead, other components may still be viable:
- Power boards
- Speakers
- Cables, remotes, stands
- T-con boards
- Casings (for custom enclosures or repairs)

You can:
- Sell them online (eBay, repair forums)
- Use for your own future repairs
- Donate to repair training schools or workshops

Creative Reuse Ideas:
Repurpose broken TVs into:
- Digital signage (if display works via HDMI)
- Custom mirror or picture frame (screen removed)
- DIY arcade cabinet (install Raspberry Pi or mini-PC)
- Decorative lighting panels (edge lighting repurposed)

Educate Customers About Lifecycle:
Encourage your customers to:
- Use surge protectors and cooling to prolong life
- Perform regular cleaning and updates
- Recycle responsibly if failure is terminal
- Replace before it becomes a hazard (e.g., smoke, swelling)

Final Thought:
A broken TV isn't just trash, it's an opportunity. With the right knowledge, even end-of-life units can be given a second life through recycling, parts harvesting, or creative projects all while reducing environmental harm

Chapter 24:

Final Checklist:

This final chapter is a one-stop reference to help TV owners manage their television effectively from installation to long-term care. It focuses on ownership, maintenance and safety summary. Use this checklist to prevent damage, extend lifespan, and ensure your TV continues to deliver top performance.

Ownership & Setup Checklist:

- Register warranty with manufacturer
- Record model and serial numbers
- Use surge protector or voltage regulator
- Mount securely or use a stable TV stand
- Confirm ventilation space (2"+ on all sides)

Maintenance Checklist:

- Clean screen monthly with microfiber cloth
- Avoid harsh chemicals or rough cloths
- Update firmware regularly (check settings)
- Disconnect during lightning storms
- Use dust covers if in storage or infrequent use

Safety Checklist:

- Keep cords away from walkways
- Anchor stands or use wall straps if not mounted

- Do not leave the TV on unattended for extended periods
- Keep children from climbing on furniture or stands
- Use child-safe outlet covers behind TV setup

Technical Service Reminder:

- Seek professional help for screen or board issues
- Document repairs and part changes
- Replace units over 8–10 years old if failing frequently
- Always transport TVs upright
- Recycle responsibly when replacing

Final Note:

A well-maintained TV not only lasts longer but saves you from costly repairs, unexpected hazards, and poor performance. Keep this checklist nearby and revisit it every few months to keep your system in peak condition.

Appendices

Appendix A – TV Terminology Glossary

Backlight – A lighting system inside LCD/LED TVs that provides brightness.

Inverter Board – Converts low-voltage DC into the high-voltage AC needed for backlights.

HDMI-CEC – Feature allowing devices connected via HDMI to control each other (e.g., TV remote controlling a soundbar).

Refresh Rate – Number of times per second a TV updates its image (60Hz, 120Hz, etc.).

Smart TV OS – Built-in software platforms (Android TV, webOS, Roku, Tizen, Fire TV).

Burn-in – Permanent ghost-like image retention on OLED screens.

Pixel Mapping – Proper alignment of pixels between source device and TV display

Appendix B – Common Error Codes

Brand	Error Code	Meaning	First Step
Samsung	Blinking red light (2x)	Power supply failure	Unplug TV, hold power button 30s, retry
LG	Error 201	Network connection failed	Reset WiFi/router, reconnect
Sony	4 red blinks	Mainboard issue	Disconnect all HDMI devices, restart
TCL	Error 014.30	Internet drop	Check WiFi password, restart router
Hisense	Blue screen with no signal	HDMI input issue	Swap cables/ports, try another device

Appendix C – Maintenance Checklist

☑ Weekly – Wipe screen gently with microfiber cloth.

☑ Monthly – Check ventilation (no dust blocking vents).

☑ Quarterly – Inspect cables for wear or fraying.

☑ Always – Use surge protectors.

☑ Transport – Always keep TV upright, never lay flat.

Appendix D – Safety Guidelines

- Never attempt repairs while TV is plugged in.
- Large TVs (55"+) require two people for lifting.
- Avoid placing TVs near windows, heat sources, or humid areas.
- Use certified wall mounts rated for your TV size and weight

Appendix E – Tools & Materials Reference

For Homeowners:

- – Microfiber cloth
- – Surge protector
- – Cable ties
- – Universal remote

For Technicians:

- – Multimeter
- – Backlight tester
- – Antistatic wrist strap
- – Suction cups (for large screens)
- – Screwdriver

Appendix F – Troubleshooting Flowcharts

Problem: Sound but No Picture

Option 1:

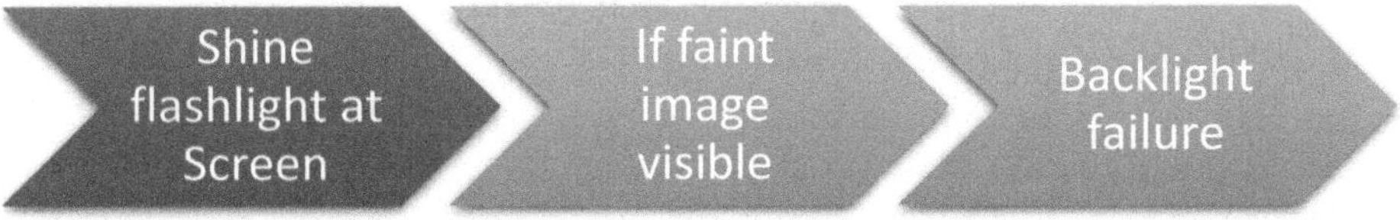

Option 2:

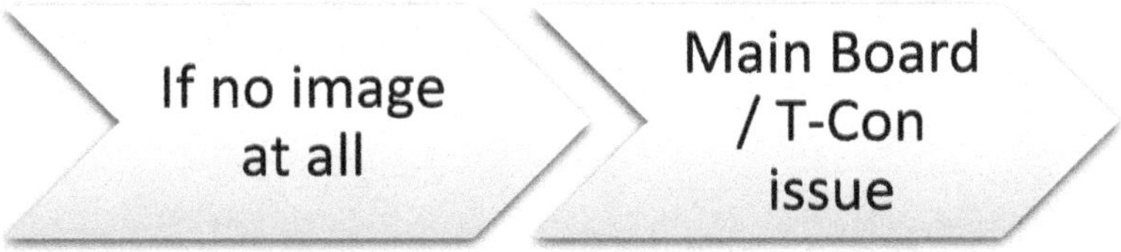

Problem: Lines on Screen

Option 1:

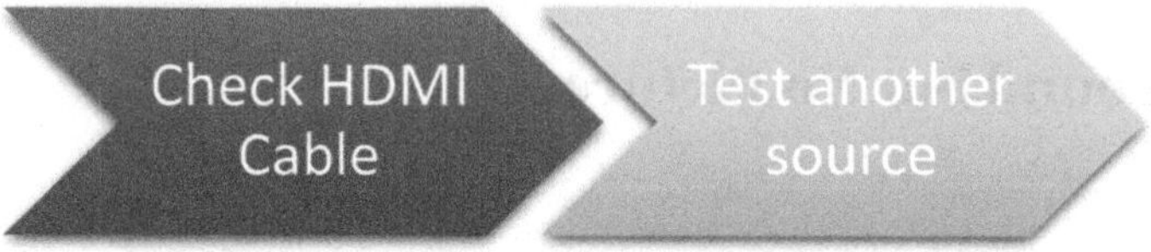

Option 2:

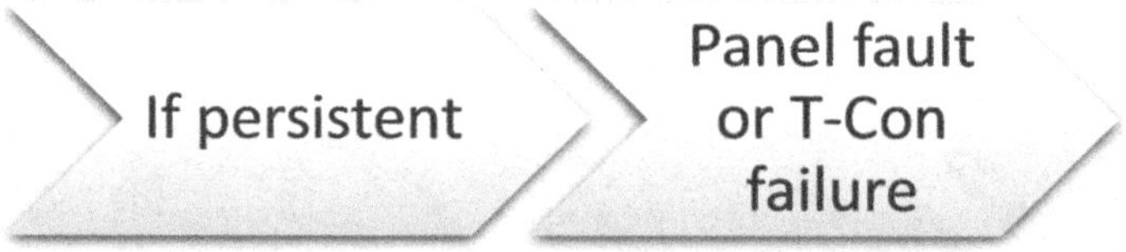

Problem: No Power

Option 1:

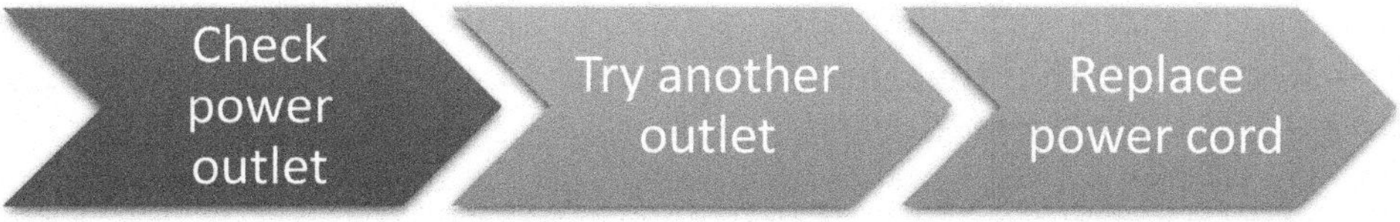

Option 2:

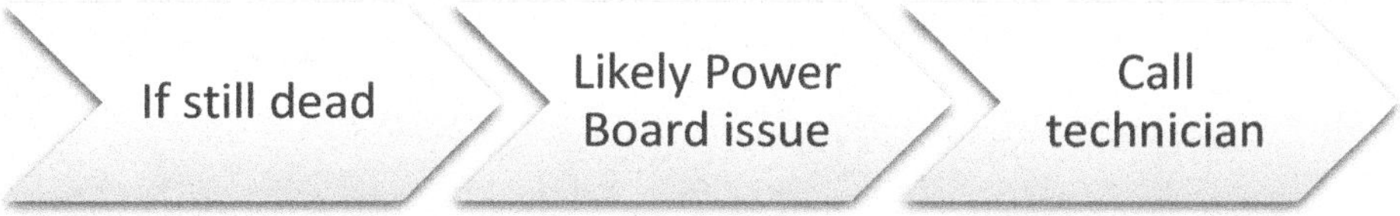

Appendix G – Transport & Setup Guide

- TVs must remain upright during transport.

- For vehicles: Secure with padding and straps.

- Allow TV to sit at room temperature for 1–2 hours before turning on (to avoid condensation damage).

- Recommended distance for viewing: Screen size ÷ 0.84 (e.g., 65" TV ≈ 6.5 feet)

Appendix H – Buyer's Guide & Recommendations

By Room Size:
– Small bedroom: 32–43"
– Living room: 55–65"
– Home theatre: 75–98"

By Use:
– Gaming: High refresh rate (120Hz+), low input lag.
– Movies: OLED or QLED with HDR support.
– Sports: Motion smoothing, wide viewing angles.

Future-Proof Features:
– HDMI 2.1
– 4K/8K resolution
– Dolby Vision + HDR10

Appendix I – Warranty & Service Records Template

Owner Name: ___________________________
TV Brand/Model: _______________________
Purchase Date: _________________________
Warranty Expiry: _______________________

Date	Service Done	Technician	Cost	Notes

Appendix J – Resources & Further Learning

• Official Manuals: Manufacturer websites (Samsung, LG, TCL, Sony).

• Communities: AV Forums, Reddit r/TV Repair, BadCaps.net.

• Professional Support: The TV Centre Ltd – www.tvcentrett.com

• AI Diagnostics: QikChk App – Coming Soon (TV Centre).

• Further Reading: Don’t Crack the Screen: Business Edition – for technicians and entrepreneurs.

Cancer and IgE

Manuel L. Penichet · Erika Jensen-Jarolim
Editors

Cancer and IgE

Introducing the Concept of AllergoOncology

Humana Press

Editors

Manuel L. Penichet
Associate Professor
Division of Surgical Oncology,
Department of Surgery,
and Department of Microbiology,
Immunology, and Molecular Genetics
David Geffen School of Medicine
University of California
at Los Angeles (UCLA)
10833 Le Conte Avenue
Los Angeles, CA 90095
USA
penichet@mednet.ucla.edu

Erika Jensen-Jarolim
Professor and Chair
Department of Pathophysiology
Center of Pathophysiology, Infectiology
and Immunology Medical University
of Vienna Waehringer G. 18-20,
1090 Vienna, Austria
erika.jensen-jarolim@meduniwien.ac.at

ISBN 978-1-60761-450-0 e-ISBN 978-1-60761-451-7
DOI 10.1007/978-1-60761-451-7
Springer New York Dordrecht Heidelberg London

Library of Congress Control Number: 2009939537

Cover illustration: The logo of AllergoOncology created by Dr. Erika Jensen-Jarolim and Mr. Walter Jarolim to promote the first "*1st International AllergoOncology Symposium*," which took place in Vienna, Austria, on April 16, 2007.

Printed on acid-free paper

Springer is part of Springer Science+Business Media (www.springer.com)

Contents

Contributors

Gernot Achatz Department of Molecular Biology, University of Salzburg, Salzburg, Austria

Gertrude Achatz-Straussberger Department of Molecular Biology, University of Salzburg, Salzburg, Austria

Wendy Cozen Departments of Preventive Medicine and Pathology, Keck School of Medicine, University of Southern California, Los Angeles, CA, USA

Maria A. Curotto de Lafaille Molecular Pathogenesis Program, The Kimmel Center for Biology and Medicine of the Skirball Institute and Department of Pathology, New York University School of Medicine, New York, NY, USA

Tracy R. Daniels Division of Surgical Oncology, Department of Surgery, University of California, Los Angeles (UCLA), Los Angeles, CA, USA

Victor C. de Vries Department of Microbiology and Immunology, Dartmouth Medical School, Lebanon, NH, USA

Julia I. Ellyard Division of Immunology and Genetics, John Curtin School of Medical Research, Australian National University, Canberra, ACT, Australia

Stefan Feichtner Department of Molecular Biology, University of Salzburg, Salzburg, Austria

Hannah J. Gould Randall Division of Cell and Molecular Biophysics, King's College London, Guy's Campus, London, UK

Gustavo Helguera Division of Surgical Oncology, Department of Surgery, University of California, Los Angeles (UCLA), Los Angeles, CA, USA

Erika Jensen-Jarolim IPP – Department of Pathophysiology, Center of Pathophysiology, Infectiology and Immunology, Medical University of Vienna, Vienna, Austria

Sophia N. Karagiannis NIHR Biomedical Research Centre at Guy's and St. Thomas's Hospitals and King's College London, Cutaneous Medicine and Immunotherapy, St. John's Institute of Dermatology, Division of Genetics and

Molecular Medicine, King's College London School of Medicine, Guy's Hospital, London, UK

Sebastian Koenigsberger Department of Molecular Biology, University of Salzburg, Salzburg, Austria

Juan J. Lafaille Molecular Pathogenesis Program, The Kimmel Center for Biology and Medicine of the Skirball Institute and Department of Pathology, New York University School of Medicine, New York, NY, USA

Marinus Lamers Max Planck Institute for Immunobiology, Freiburg, Germany

Stefan Lenz Department of Molecular Biology, University of Salzburg, Salzburg, Austria

Otoniel Martínez-Maza Departments of Obstetrics and Gynecology and Department of Microbiology, Immunology, and Molecular Genetics, Jonsson Comprehensive Cancer Center, AIDS Institute, David Geffen School of Medicine, University of California, Los Angeles (UCLA), Los Angeles, CA, USA

Diana Mechtcheriakova IPP – Department of Pathophysiology, Center of Pathophysiology, Infectiology and Immunology, Medical University of Vienna, Vienna, Austria

Alan Duane Moreno Department of Preventive Medicine, Keck School of Medicine, University of Southern California, Los Angeles, CA, USA

Frank O. Nestle NIHR Biomedical Research Centre at Guy's and St. Thomas's Hospitals and King's College London, Cutaneous Medicine and Immunotherapy, St. John's Institute of Dermatology, Division of Genetics and Molecular Medicine, King's College London School of Medicine, Guy's Hospital, London, UK

Elisa A. Nigro Department of Biology and Genetics, University of Milan and San Raffaele Scientific Institute, Milan, Italy

Randolph J. Noelle Department of Microbiology and Immunology, Dartmouth Medical School, Lebanon, NH, USA

Elizabeth C. Nowak Department of Microbiology and Immunology, Dartmouth Medical School, Lebanon, NH, USA

Elizabeth Ortiz-Sánchez Division of Surgical Oncology, Department of Surgery, University of California, Los Angeles (UCLA), Los Angeles, CA, USA

Isabella Pali-Schoell IPP – Department of Pathophysiology, Center of Pathophysiology, Infectiology and Immunology, Medical University of Vienna, Vienna, Austria

Christopher R. Parish Division of Immunology and Genetics, John Curtin School of Medical Research, Australian National University, Canberra, ACT, Australia

Doris Peckl-Schmid Department of Molecular Biology, University of Salzburg, Salzburg, Austria

Manuel L. Penichet Division of Surgical Oncology, Department of Surgery and Department of Microbiology, Immunology, and Molecular Genetics, Molecular Biology Institute, Jonsson Comprehensive Cancer Center, David Geffen School of Medicine, University of California, Los Angeles (UCLA), Los Angeles, CA, USA

José A. Rodríguez Division of Surgical Oncology, Department of Surgery and Molecular Biology Institute, University of California, Los Angeles (UCLA), Los Angeles, CA, USA

Antonio G. Siccardi Department of Biology and Genetics, University of Milan and San Raffaele Scientific Institute, Milan, Italy

Ljubov Simson Centre for Biomedical, Molecular and Chemical Research, University of Canberra, ACT, Australia

Michelle C. Turner McLaughlin Centre for Population Health Risk Assessment, Institute of Population Health, Faculty of Graduate and Post-Graduate Studies, University of Ottawa, Ottawa, ONT, Canada

Luca Vangelista Department of Biology and Genetics, University of Milan and San Raffaele Scientific Institute, Milan, Italy

Anna Wasiuk Department of Microbiology and Immunology, Dartmouth Medical School, Lebanon, NH, USA

Nadja Zaborsky Department of Molecular Biology, University of Salzburg, Salzburg, Austria

Chapter 1
Introduction

Erika Jensen-Jarolim and Manuel L. Penichet

1.1 Background

Infectious diseases, being the major burden in the history of mankind worldwide until the beginning of the 20th century, were important triggers in the understanding of immunological mechanisms. In contrast to infectious diseases, reports of allergies and cancers were less common, but increased tremendously within the last century. Based on the US mortality data of the National Center for Health Statistics, Centers for Disease Control and Prevention 2009, a recent report from the American Cancer Society indicated that the number of cancer deaths increased approximately from 100,000 to 550,000 per year between 1930 and 2006, paralleling the increase of the total population during this period. Leading causes of death from cancer are lung and bronchus cancer, in men prostate cancer, and in women breast cancer [1, 2]. Normalization to population size shows that the cancer death rate for most malignancies has been generally stable, although the mortality rate of certain malignancies, such as lung and bronchus cancer, has increased over the last 50 years [1-3].

In allergy, the situation is less clear, because for the time period around the turn of the 19th century, only imprecise information is available. However, within the last 30 years the incidences of allergies has doubled not only in industrial countries, but in developing countries as well [4]. From the diagnosed atopic state it is concluded that in some areas, such as in New Zealand, the incidence of skin and respiratory allergies increased as much as 40% in the population [5]. Thus, the cancer and allergy incidence parallel each other, whereas infectious diseases have decreased in industrialized countries. From an epidemiological point of view, the decreased parasite and bacterial burden may indirectly correlate with the increasing curves of allergy and cancer, being thus in accordance with the so-called hygiene hypothesis. This theory links the recent lower parasite and microbe burden to aberrant immune responses or failure of immune mechanisms [6, 7]. However, if allergies and malignancies both

---

E. Jensen-Jarolim (✉)
IPP-Department of Pathophysiology, Center of Pathophysiology, Infectiology and Immunology, Medical University of Vienna, Vienna, Austria
e-mail: erika.jensen-jarolim@meduniwien.ac.at

M.L. Penichet, E. Jensen-Jarolim (eds.), *Cancer and IgE*,
DOI 10.1007/978-1-60761-451-7_1,

increase, does that mean a linked positive association? This question is difficult to answer with epidemiology, as both diseases are correlated with a large number of genetic and environmental causative factors which again change continuously [8].

Based on clinical suspicion, multiple epidemiological studies have so far been undertaken to examine whether any, positive or negative association of allergies and cancer exist. Significant *p*-values demonstrating the inverse association between the incidence of allergies and/or levels of IgE and malignancies have been reported in several studies including a recent cohort study with a sample size above 1 million investigated persons [9, 10]. These results suggest a potential role of IgE in cancer immunosurveillance at least in certain tumors. Chapters 4 and 5 of this book give a comprehensive overview on these epidemiological approaches.

Although statistical methods are very helpful for capturing interrelationships, more experimental evidence is needed to find a cause and effect relationship. After evaluation of first tendencies by cohort studies, case–control studies and experimental in vitro and in vivo data must follow to achieve evidence-based medical statistics. Dependent on the development of modern laboratory technologies, knowledge about the immunological and molecular mechanisms of allergies and malignancies can be acquired. Interestingly, during the last decades a number of experimental approaches were developed to investigate whether factors and cells participating in the pathophysiology of allergy also are players in cancer. Let us move again one step back to history.

1.2 History of Allergy

Pioneers in medical history like John Bostock realized and were concerned about the increasing cases of hay fever from the beginning of the 19th century on, and Charles Bakely in 1869 invented skin testing as a diagnostic tool for specific sensitization [11]. However, much more focus was given to the major threats of this period, which were infectious diseases. Besides the continuous development of active immunization, passive applications of antisera raised in animals like horses were standard treatment options for infected patients. The so-called antitoxins were the first major success of therapeutic immunology, representing in fact specific immunoglobulins. Soon the risk of anaphylactic side reactions upon repetitive injection of antisera was recognized and feared: the death rates in 1890 were still 60%, in 1894 30%, and, after improvement of the industrial manufacturing of antitoxins, e.g., by ammonium precipitation, still in 1910 10% of the treated patients died as reported by the Metropolitan Asylums Board 1895–1910 [12]. During this time, Charles R. Richet and Paul Portier succeeded in imitating this immediate type hypersensitivity reaction by immunizing dogs with a protein extract of sea anemones (Actinaria). To describe this immediate type inflammatory reaction provoked by a specific antigen (which was considered to be a toxin), Richet and Portier coined the term anaphylaxis in 1902 [13]. The

word anaphylaxis is derived from the Greek words *ana* ("against") and *phylaxis* ("protection").

The pediatricians Clemens Freiherr von Pirquet from Vienna and Béla Schick, a Hungarian, were concerned about these sudden (anaphylactic) reactions and realized that by skin testing with the antiserum the (hyper) immune state of the patient could be predicted. This cognition led to the development of the Schick test for diphtheria and the Pirquet test for tuberculosis, routine tests which are still applied worldwide. Moreover, Pirquet eternized himself by coining the term "allergy" from the Greek words *allos* ("other") and *ergon* ("reaction") [14]. Thereby, he meant sensitization leading to hypersensitivity against toxins or infectious agents. Thus, the term "allergy" was in the beginning not associated with exogenous innocuous antigens like pollen or house dust mite. It took decades until it was understood that the key mechanism for "Pirquet's allergy" also accounts for allergy in its recent sense. And it took even longer until the key players were identified.

Focusing on a typical allergen, namely fish protein, Prausnitz and Küstner described in 1921 that a soluble, transferable "skin sensitizing factor" is responsible for hypersensitivities [15], which was shortly later nominated "atopic reagin" by Arthur F. Coca and Ella F. Grove [16]. These discoveries triggered research on "reagins" during the following five decades, analyzing their distribution [17], demonstrating their specificity for allergens [18, 19] and helminth antigens [20–22], attempting to purify them [23], and identifying them as a prototype of cytophilic antibodies, i.e., antibodies preferentially fixed to cells in contrast to free antibodies [24]. Coincidently, eosinophilic and basophilic granulocytes were detected in atopic skin [25].

The simultaneous discovery of IgE myelomas in two independent laboratories [26–29], closely followed by a third [30] identified reagins as being the fifth class of immunoglobulins with a key role in the pathophysiology of immediate type hypersensitivity. Finally, the detection of high- and low-affinity IgE receptors, being the last missing link between the effector cells and IgE antibodies became the explanatory mechanism of the anaphylactic reaction [31–34]. The molecular events restraining potentially dangerous high serum levels of IgE is reviewed in Chapter 2, the high specification of the IgE maturation program in Chapter 3, and the interplay of secreted IgE with its receptors determining its functional properties in Chapters 7 and 8.

The mechanism of the anaphylactic reaction is thus a consequence of allergens crosslinking IgE bound to its high-affinity receptor. Thereby, molecular patterns displayed by the allergens seem to be important and could be a common feature of allergenic molecules (Chapter 10). The released mediators as a consequence of the anaphylactic reaction have strong proinflammatory effects and are possibly effective in worm expulsion, but clearly detrimental in allergy when harmless allergens can produce mild to severe anaphylactic reactions in sensitized patients. Thus, it is accepted today that elevated specific and/or total IgE and Th2-type responses in general are hallmarks of allergies and parasitic diseases. However, as opposed to allergies, in helminth infection typically no anaphylactic shock is observed [35].

1.3 History of AllergoOncology

It is more or less neglected today that the association of tumor occurrence and allergic inflammation has been discussed since the first half of the twentieth century [36, 37] and continuously ever since (Table 1.1). Possibly the first publication on "Allergy against cancer" stems from E.G. Martin and was published in 1935 [36]. He investigated why "one person will develop carcinoma, while another does not," and his unanswered question was whether "the conception of allergy or idiosyncrasy could be broadened to include this mysterious fact?" Well, one has to admit that his usage of the term "allergy" was related to a rather imprecise scientific and clinical definition at that time. Still, in 1952 the view had not changed much when Bienengraber investigated "Tumor metastasis in the light of allergology" [37]. He analyzed the stages of metastasis and found that individually different dynamics of vascularization and transudation could be observed during the nesting phase of the tumor cells. Dependent on the sensitization state of the patient he categorized normergic, hypergic, anergic, and eu-ergic reactions. He found that these observations in tumor tissues paralleled the inflammatory reaction seen toward parasites, microbes, and self-antigens. Even though he likely meant "specific inflammation" he termed the phenomenon "tumor allergy".

Table 1.1 AllergoOncology is tightly connected with the history of allergy. This table gives an overview of selected key publications

Authors	Title	Reference
Definition of allergy and era of reagins		*1906*
Von Pirquet	Allergy	[14]
Martin	Predisposing factors and diagnosis of rectal cancer: a discussion of allergy	[36]
Bienengraber	Tumor metastasis in the light of allergology	[37]
Molomut et al.	The effect of an allergic inflammatory response in the tumor bed on the fate of transplanted tumors in mice	[38]
Berdel et al.	Mechanism of tumor allergy and its importance in tumor pathogenesis	[39]
Schlitter	Is there an allergy against malignant tumor tissue and what can it signify in regard to the defense of the body against cancer?	[41]
Identification of IgE		*1967*
Ishizaka and Ishizaka	Identification of gamma-E-antibodies as a carrier of reaginic activity	[27]
Johansson	Raised levels of a new immunoglobulin class (IgND) in asthma	[28]
Ure	Negative association between allergy and cancer	[44]
McCormick et al.	A study of allergy in patients with malignant lymphoma and chronic lymphocytic leukemia	[45]
Augustin and Chandradasa	IgE levels and allergic skin reactions in cancer and non-cancer patients	[46]

Table 1.1 (continued)

Authors	Title	Reference
Nagy et al.	Growth inhibition of murine mammary carcinoma by monoclonal IgE antibodies specific for the mammary tumor virus	[57]
Kershaw et al.	Tumor-specific IgE-mediated inhibition of human colorectal carcinoma xenograft growth	[56]
Gould et al.	Comparison of IgE and IgG antibody-dependent cytotoxicity in vitro and in a SCID mouse xenograft model of ovarian carcinoma	[55]
Reali et al.	IgEs targeted on tumor cells: therapeutic activity and potential in the design of tumor vaccines	[63]
Karagiannis et al.	Activity of human monocytes in IgE antibody-dependent surveillance and killing of ovarian tumor cells	[64]
Turner et al.	Cancer mortality among US men and women with asthma and hay fever	[9]
Riemer et al.	Active induction of tumor-specific IgE antibodies by oral mimotope vaccination	[58]
Definition of AllergoOncology		*2006*
Jensen-Jarolim et al.	AllergoOncology: the role of IgE in tumor defense	[62]
Karagiannis et al.	IgE-antibody-dependent immunotherapy of solid tumors: cytotoxic and phagocytic mechanisms of eradication of ovarian cancer cells	[54]
Bracher et al.	Three-colour flow cytometric method to measure antibody-dependent tumour cell killing by cytotoxicity and phagocytosis	[65]
Fu et al.	Immunoglobulin E antibodies from pancreatic cancer patients mediate antibody-dependent cell-mediated cytotoxicity against pancreatic cancer cells	[51]
Jensen-Jarolim et al.	AllergoOncology: the role of IgE-mediated allergy in cancer	[10]
Karagiannis et al.	Characterisation of an engineered trastuzumab IgE antibody and effector cell mechanisms targeting HER2/*neu*-positive tumour cells	[66]

The concept was, however, taken up again in the 1950s, when Molomut in a pioneer study constructed an in vivo model for examining the "allergic response" toward tumors [38]. He applied tumor transplants in two different strains of ovalbumin-sensitized inbred mice, fibrosarcoma S621 in C/Scott mice, and sarcoma I in DBA1/Jax mice. In this large experimental setup allergen challenges at the tumor sites could not prevent the growth of the transplants and he concluded "...that the localized allergic inflammatory response at the site of a tumor implantation per se has no effect upon the development of the graft." However, there might have been several sources of error in his experiment: (1) the transplanted tumor cells were driven by a dominant oncogene signal, (2) too many

cells within the "tiny tumor graft" and/or most importantly, and (3) the complete neglect of antigen-specificity. Taken together, we can conclude from this study that antigenic crossreactivity between ovalbumin and fibrosarcoma S621 and the used sarcoma cells does not exist. On the other hand, it should be noted that Molomut in his work used the current definition of the "allergy" term.

In the study entitled "Mechanism of tumor allergy and its importance in tumor pathogenesis" [39], Berdel and coworkers investigated the responses to tumor transplants and reported that upon repetitive injections of tumor cells in mice anaphylaxis in the sense of hyperacute transplant rejection can occur. Simultaneously the authors reported the phenomenon of tolerance when mice with spontaneous tumors are not able to reject tumor transplants. Based on previous observations for tuberculosis and pollen allergy, they concluded that a tumor-specific cytotoxic antibody must be formed in the first phase, followed by a second antibody with a neutralizing effect, later termed a blocking antibody [40]. The authors suggested that antigenic changes of the tumor cells are responsible for the specificity of the events.

Eosinophils were at that time recognized as a hallmark of allergic and parasitic diseases, and their appearance in tumor tissues had also been noticed. In the publication "Is there an allergy against malignant tumor tissue and what can it signify in regard to the defense of the body against cancer?", H.E. Schlitter compared tumors with parasitic microorganisms and analyzed the association of eosinophilia in the blood and tissues with the formation of metastases [41]. In his review he cites work of K. Ebhardt [42] and W. Fischer 1952 [43] who interpreted the eosinophilia in malignancies as a sign of a "special allergic condition." According to Schlitter's pathological experience tumor patients with hypereosinophilia were typically characterized with a high burden of metastases. On the other hand, he referred to studies in the elderly where too low numbers of eosinophils were disadvantageous and associated with rapid growth of the tumor. Thus, in his view the eosinophil could either be promoting tumor progression or be a regulatory counter-reaction to metastasis.

Shortly after the discovery of IgE in 1967 [27, 28], namely in 1969 D.M. Ure announced a negative association between atopy and gynecologic malignancies [44]. Thereafter, IgE determinations were already included in the following "allergooncological" examinations. For example, the group around Terry and Kimi Ishizaka was performing "A study of allergy in patients with malignant lymphoma and chronic lymphocytic leukemia" [45]. Interestingly, among Hodgkin's disease, reticulum cell sarcoma, lymphosarcoma, and chronic lymphatic leukemia (CLL), only in CLL decreased incidences of allergic symptoms throughout the lives associated with lowered IgE levels were found. Generally, in the lymphoma patients a large number of patients had noted that they lost allergic symptoms with the onset of the malignancy. The authors concluded that CLL patients might have a hereditary immunologic defect becoming apparent only later in life.

The discovery of IgE immunoglobulins made it possible to design more precise studies investigating the relationship of allergy or atopy and cancer [46, 47]. When Jacobs et al. studied circulating IgE levels they found that in 200 untreated cancer patients approximately half had very low levels (20–680 units per ml) and, on the contrary, others had exceptionally high levels (above 100,000 units per ml)

determined by radioimmunoassay but not by radial immunodiffusion. The authors suggested that cancer patients might form certain inhibitor substances from the tumors which interfere with the precipitation of IgE in the radial immunodiffusion assay, the results thus might, "...be considered as indicating the absence of IgE." They observed this phenomenon in sera as well as in blood samples from vessels draining tumors. The identity of this putative factor remains elusive to this day.

Coming back to epidemiology, for example, Joseph Allegra et al. described that there was a 15-fold decrease in prevalence of atopy in the cancer population in a Lancet paper in 1976 [48]. Atopic dermatitis patients also have a lower risk of developing melanoma and this may be due to the enhanced surveillance function of IgE being increasingly bound to the IgE receptors of the skin being overexpresssed in this disease [49].

Finally, Neuchrist et al. were the first who histologically detected natural IgE within tumor tissues of head and neck cancer patients; however, the function of these IgE antibodies was not determined [50]. Surprisingly, IgE was the most abundant and pronounced immunoglobulin isotype and appeared clustered on dendritic-like cells within the epithelial tumor tissues. Only a very recent study re-examined this subject again by isolating natural IgE from the serum of pancreatic carcinoma patients [51]. Indeed, high tumoricidic properties could be demonstrated pointing toward a defence function of these natural antitumor IgE antibodies. Similarly, as in atopic dermatitis where autoreactive IgE against keratinocyte antigens is found [52], anaphylaxis was not reported in any of the pancreatic cancer patients [51]. With respect to the mechanisms of antitumor IgE, antibody-dependent cell-mediated cytotoxicity (ADCC) and antibody-dependent cell-mediated phagocytosis (ADCP) seem to be especially important [53, 54], as described in Chapters 7 and 8. These chapters also discuss a variety of effector cells involved in ADCC and/or ADCP such as basophils, dendritic cells, Langerhans cells, and monocytes/macrophages. In this context, the role of mast cells and eosinophils in cancer, as well as of Th2 immunity in general, is discussed in Chapters 6 and 11, respectively.

Advancements in molecular biology and genetic engineering enabled several groups in the 1990s to design antitumor antibodies also of the IgE class [55–57]. Importantly, IgE antibodies can be used as direct therapeutics in passive immunotherapy of cancer (Chapters 7 and 8) and also as adjuvant of cancer vaccines (Chapter 9). Chapter 7 also describes an alternative strategy based on the induction of endogenous IgE antitumor response based on an oral mimotope vaccination [58]. The recombinant antibodies are not only useful for experimentally studying the effects of IgE-targeting of cancer cells, but they could be useful biologicals in cancer therapy of patients in the future. Undoubtedly, targeted therapy using chimeric, humanized, or fully human IgG antibodies has been a world success [59–61].

However, as discussed in Chapter 7, antibodies of the IgE class have several properties that may be advantageous for cancer therapy such as the fact that IgE binds to its Fc epsilon receptors (FcϵRs) with much higher affinity compared to that of IgG for the Fc gamma receptors (FcγRs), and the very low serum levels of IgE that provide minimal competition for Fc receptor occupancy further facilitating ADCC/ADCP. Therefore, in contrast to IgG, IgE could be applied in lower dosages

reducing the economic costs and increasing the efficacy. In fact, the large total doses of the therapeutics antibodies that are often required have been described as a limitation in their use as drugs [59]. However, it is important to stress that the use of antibodies of the IgG and IgE classes in cancer therapy is not necessarily mutually exclusive, as both classes of antibodies could be used in combination (simultaneously or sequentially) potentially maximizing their efficacy in certain cases through the engagement of different Fc receptors and effector cells.

1.4 Synopsis

So far numerous studies have evaluated the question of whether the same immunological mechanisms could be shared in malignancies and allergic disorders, either promoting or inhibiting disease. Nevertheless, until now a relationship between the two fields has not been officially acknowledged. This may be due to the fact that experts in IgE biology are today home to allergological societies. Vice versa, the oncology scene is dominated today by search for small molecules interfering with signaling, or attempts to activate antitumor cytotoxic T-lymphocytes, or by passive immunotherapy with IgG antibodies. Therefore, we strongly believe that there is a rationale for a platform where allergological and oncological know-how can be exchanged for the benefit of the patient. AllergoOncology can be defined as a field that aims to reveal the function of IgE-mediated immune responses against tumor cells in order to enhance the understanding of its biology and develop novel IgE-based treatment options against malignant diseases.

The term AllergoOncology was first proposed at the 2006 Malta-Meeting of the Collegium Internationale Allergologicum (CIA) [62]. The oral presentation was entitled "AllergoOncology, the role of IgE in tumor defense" and the audience was not ready for this provocation. Professor Johannes Ring, then president of the CIA, subsumed the event in the minutes of the meeting as follows: "*. . .a novel subject was presented at this meeting – AllergoOncology, a topic so hot that the discussion was immediately interrupted after the first question. . ..*"

Encouraged by equally many positive comments during this meeting the story went on [10]. To date, two International AllergoOncology Symposia have taken place in Vienna, and an AllergoOncology task force was officially approved by the World Allergy Organization in 2008, succeeding in implementing the subject into the World Allergy Congress 2009 for the first time. Therefore, we felt it is the right time to venture the first AllergoOncology book.

References

1. Jemal A, Siegel R, Ward E, Hao Y, Xu J, and Thun MJ (2009) Cancer Statistics, 2009. CA Cancer J Clin 59:225–49
2. American Cancer Society (2009) American Cancer Statistics 2009. http://www.cancer.org/docroot/STT/STT_0.asp

3. Wingo PA, Cardinez CJ, Landis SH, Greenlee RT, Ries LA, Anderson RN, and Thun MJ (2003) Long-term trends in cancer mortality in the United States, 1930–1998. Cancer 97:3133–275
4. Pearce N and Douwes J (2006) The global epidemiology of asthma in children. Int J Tuberc Lung Dis 10:125–32
5. Sly RM (1999) Changing prevalence of allergic rhinitis and asthma. Ann Allergy Asthma Immunol 82:233–48
6. Strachan D (2000) Family size, infection and atopy: the first decade of the "hygiene hypothesis". Thorax 55:2–10
7. Namazi MR (2007) Extension of the "Hygiene Hypothesis" to the negative association between acne and atopy, hematological malignancies, and malignant melanoma. Medical Hypotheses 69:960–961
8. Karhausen LR (2000) Causation: the elusive grail of epidemiology. Med Health Care Philos 3:59–67
9. Turner MC, Chen Y, Krewski D, Ghadirian P, Thun MJ, and Calle EE (2005) Cancer mortality among US men and women with asthma and hay fever. Am J Epidemiol 162:212–21
10. Jensen-Jarolim E, Achatz G, Turner MC, Karagiannis S, Legrand F, Capron M, Penichet ML, Rodriguez JA, Siccardi AG, Vangelista L, Riemer AB, and Gould H (2008) AllergoOncology: the role of IgE-mediated allergy in cancer. Allergy 63:1255–66
11. Emanuel MB (1988) Hay fever, a post industrial revolution epidemic: a history of its growth during the 19th century. Clinical Allergy 18:295–304
12. Biggs JP (1912) London Evidence Against Anti-Toxin (Chapter 107). In: Sanitation Versus vaccination. Leicester
13. Richet CR and Portier P (1902) De l'action anaphylactique de certain venins. Comptes rendus de la Société de biologie, Paris 54:170–2
14. Pirquet C (1906) Allergy. Münchener Medizinische Wochenschrift 53:1457–8
15. Prausnitz C and Kustner H (1921) Studien über die Ueberempfindlichkeit. Zentralbl Bakteriol 86:160–9.
16. Coca AF and Grove EF (1925) A study of the atopic reagins. J Immunol 10:445–64
17. Scherrer E (1930) The distribution of reagins in the blood plasma. J Allergy 2:467
18. Layton LL and Yamanaka E (1962) Demonstration of human reagins to foods, cat dander, an insect, and ragweed and grass pollens. J Allergy 33:271–5
19. Augustin R (1967) Demonstration of reagins in the serum of allergic subjects. From WEIR, Handbook of experimental immunology Oxford-Edinburgh: Blackwell, p. 1076
20. Kailin EW, Rossbach EA, and Walzer M (1950) Factors influencing reagin formation in experimental human sensitization to ascaris lumbricoides antigen; the influence of a previous sensitization on rate of sensitization. J Allergy 21:225–31
21. Ogilvie BM (1964) Reagin-like antibodies in animals immune to helminth parasites. Nature 204:91–2
22. Zvaifler NJ, Sadun E, and Becker EL (1966) Anaphylactic (reaginic) antibodies in helminthic infections. Clin Res 14:336
23. Vaerman JP, Epstein W, Fudenberg H, and Ishizaka K (1964) Direct demonstration of reagin activity in purified gamma 1a globulin. Nature 203:1046–8
24. Augustin R, Connolly R, and Lloyd G (1964) Atopic reagin as a prototype of cytophilic antibodies. Aus: Protides Biol. Fluids, Proc. 11th Coll. Bruges 1963, p. 56, H. Peeters (ed.). Amsterdam: Elseviers
25. Felarca AB and Lowell FC (1971) The accumulation of eosinophils and basophils at skin sites as related to intensity of skin reactivity and symptoms in atopic disease. J Allergy Clin Immunol 48:125–33
26. Ishizaka K and Ishizaka T (1966) Physicochemical properties of reaginic antibody. 1. Association of reaginic activity with an immunoglobulin other than gammaA- or gammaG-globulin. J Allergy 37:169–85
27. Ishizaka K and Ishizaka T (1967) Identification of gamma-E-antibodies as a carrier of reaginic activity. J Immunol 99:1187–98

28. Johansson SG (1967) Raised levels of a new immunoglobulin class (IgND) in asthma. Lancet 2:951–3
29. Johansson SG and Bennich H (1967) Immunological studies of an atypical (myeloma) immunoglobulin. Immunology 13:381–94
30. Fishkin BG, Orloff N, Scaduto LE, Borucki DT, and Spiegelberg HL (1972) IgE multiple myeloma: a report of the third case. Blood 39:361–7
31. Carson DA and Metzger H (1974) Interaction of IgE with rat basophilic leukemia cells. IV. Antibody-induced redistribution of IgE receptors. J Immunol 113:1271–7
32. Metzger H, Rivnay B, Henkart M, Kanner B, Kinet JP, and Perez-Montfort R (1984) Analysis of the structure and function of the receptor for immunoglobulin E. Mol Immunol 21:1167–73
33. Nakajima T and Delespesse G (1986) IgE receptors on human lymphocytes. I. Identification of the molecules binding to monoclonal anti-Fc epsilon receptor antibodies. Eur J Immunol 16:809–14
34. Ludin C, Hofstetter H, Sarfati M, Levy CA, Suter U, Alaimo D, Kilchherr E, Frost H, and Delespesse G (1987) Cloning and expression of the cDNA coding for a human lymphocyte IgE receptor. Embo J 6:109–14
35. Mangan NE, Fallon RE, Smith P, van Rooijen N, McKenzie AN, and Fallon PG (2004) Helminth infection protects mice from anaphylaxis via IL-10-producing B cells. J Immunol 173:6346–56
36. Martin EG (1935) Predisposing factors and diagnosis of rectal cancer: a discussion of allergy. Ann Surg 102:56–61
37. Bienengraber A (1952) Tumor metastasis in the light of allergology. Zentralbl Chir 77: 1873–81
38. Molomut N, Spain DM, Kreisler L, and Warshaw LJ (1955) The effect of an allergic inflammatory response in the tumor bed on the fate of transplanted tumors in mice. Cancer Res 15:181–3
39. Berdel W, Nass G, and Wiedemann G (1956) Mechanism of tumor allergy and its importance in tumor pathogenesis. Int Arch Allergy Appl Immunol 9:200–21
40. Loveless M and Cann JR (1955) Distribution of blocking antibody in human serum proteins fractionated by electrophoresis-convection. J Immunol 74:329–39
41. Schlitter HE (1961) Is there an allergy against malignant tumor tissue and what can it signify in regard to the defense of the body against cancer? Strahlentherapie 114:203–24
42. Ebhardt K (1937) Mschr. Krebsbekämpfung: 33
43. Fischer W (1952) Zbl. Path. 89:129
44. Ure DM (1969) Negative association between allergy and cancer. Scott Med J 14:51–4
45. McCormick DP, Ammann AJ, Ishizaka K, Miller DG, and Hong R (1971) A study of allergy in patients with malignant lymphoma and chronic lymphocytic leukemia. Cancer 27:93–9
46. Augustin R and Chandradasa KD (1971) IgE levels and allergic skin reactions in cancer and non-cancer patients. Int Arch Allergy Appl Immunol 41:141–3
47. Jacobs D, Landon J, Houri M, and Merrett TG (1972) Circulating levels of immunoglobulin E in patients with cancer. Lancet 2:1059–61
48. Allegra J, Lipton A, Harvey H, Luderer J, Brenner D, Mortel R, Demers L, Gillin M, White D, and Trautlein J (1976) Decreased prevalence of immediate hypersensitivity (atopy) in a cancer population. Cancer Res 36:3225–6
49. Synnerstad I, Fredrikson M, Ternesten-Bratel A, and Rosdahl I (2008) Low risk of melanoma in patients with atopic dermatitis. J Eur Acad Dermatol Venereol 22:1423–8
50. Neuchrist C, Kornfehl J, Grasl M, Lassmann H, Kraft D, Ehrenberger K, and Scheiner O (1994) Distribution of immunoglobulins in squamous cell carcinoma of the head and neck. Int Arch Allergy Immunol 104:97–100
51. Fu SL, Pierre J, Smith-Norowitz TA, Hagler M, Bowne W, Pincus MR, Mueller CM, Zenilman ME, and Bluth MH (2008) Immunoglobulin E antibodies from pancreatic cancer patients mediate antibody-dependent cell-mediated cytotoxicity against pancreatic cancer cells. Clin Exp Immunol 153:401–9

52. Altrichter S, Kriehuber E, Moser J, Valenta R, Kopp T, and Stingl G (2008) Serum IgE autoantibodies target keratinocytes in patients with atopic dermatitis. J Invest Dermatol 128:2232–9
53. Karagiannis SN, Bracher MG, Beavil RL, Beavil AJ, Hunt J, McCloskey N, Thompson RG, East N, Burke F, Sutton BJ, Dombrowicz D, Balkwill FR, and Gould HJ (2008) Role of IgE receptors in IgE antibody-dependent cytotoxicity and phagocytosis of ovarian tumor cells by human monocytic cells. Cancer Immunol Immunother 57:247–63
54. Karagiannis SN, Bracher MG, Hunt J, McCloskey N, Beavil RL, Beavil AJ, Fear DJ, Thompson RG, East N, Burke F, Moore RJ, Dombrowicz DD, Balkwill FR, and Gould HJ (2007) IgE-antibody-dependent immunotherapy of solid tumors: cytotoxic and phagocytic mechanisms of eradication of ovarian cancer cells. J Immunol 179:2832–43
55. Gould HJ, Mackay GA, Karagiannis SN, O'Toole CM, Marsh PJ, Daniel BE, Coney LR, Zurawski VR, Jr, Joseph M, Capron M, Gilbert M, Murphy GF, and Korngold R (1999) Comparison of IgE and IgG antibody-dependent cytotoxicity in vitro and in a SCID mouse xenograft model of ovarian carcinoma. Eur J Immunol 29:3527–37
56. Kershaw MH, Darcy PK, Trapani JA, MacGregor D, and Smyth MJ (1998) Tumor-specific IgE-mediated inhibition of human colorectal carcinoma xenograft growth. Oncol Res 10: 133–42
57. Nagy E, Berczi I, and Sehon AH (1991) Growth inhibition of murine mammary carcinoma by monoclonal IgE antibodies specific for the mammary tumor virus. Cancer Immunol Immunother 34:63–9
58. Riemer AB, Untersmayr E, Knittelfelder R, Duschl A, Pehamberger H, Zielinski CC, Scheiner O, and Jensen–Jarolim E (2007) Active induction of tumor-specific IgE antibodies by oral mimotope vaccination. Cancer Res 67:3406–11
59. Carter PJ (2006) Potent antibody therapeutics by design. Nat Rev Immunol 6:343–57
60. Maggon K (2007) Monoclonal antibody "gold rush". Curr Med Chem 14:1978–87
61. Reichert JM and Valge-Archer VE (2007) Development trends for monoclonal antibody cancer therapeutics. Nat Rev Drug Discov 6:349–56
62. Jensen-Jarolim E, Untersmayr E, Knittelfelder R, Zielinski CC, Scheiner O, Duschl A, and Riemer AB (2006) Allergo-Oncology: the role of IgE in tumor defense. 26th Symposium of the Collegium Internationale Allergologicum. May 5–10, Malta.
63. Reali E, Greiner JW, Corti A, Gould HJ, Bottazzoli F, Paganelli G, Schlom J, and Siccardi AG (2001) IgEs targeted on tumor cells: therapeutic activity and potential in the design of tumor vaccines. Cancer Res 61:5517–22
64. Karagiannis SN, Wang Q, East N, Burke F, Riffard S, Bracher MG, Thompson RG, Durham SR, Schwartz LB, Balkwill FR, and Gould HJ (2003) Activity of human monocytes in IgE antibody-dependent surveillance and killing of ovarian tumor cells. Eur J Immunol 33: 1030–40
65. Bracher M, Gould HJ, Sutton BJ, Dombrowicz D, and Karagiannis SN (2007) Three-colour flow cytometric method to measure antibody-dependent tumour cell killing by cytotoxicity and phagocytosis. J Immunol Methods 323:160–71
66. Karagiannis P, Singer J, Hunt J, Gan SK, Rudman SM, Mechtcheriakova D, Knittelfelder R, Daniels TR, Hobson PS, Beavil AJ, Spicer J, Nestle FO, Penichet ML, Gould HJ, Jensen-Jarolim E, and Karagiannis SN (2009) Characterisation of an engineered trastuzumab IgE antibody and effector cell mechanisms targeting HER2/*neu*-positive tumour cells. Cancer Immunol Immunother 58:915–30

Chapter 2
The Biology of IgE: Molecular Mechanism Restraining Potentially Dangerous High Serum IgE Titres In Vivo

Gernot Achatz, Gertrude Achatz-Straussberger, Stefan Feichtner, Sebastian Koenigsberger, Stefan Lenz, Doris Peckl-Schmid, Nadja Zaborsky, and Marinus Lamers

Abstract Our knowledge about the regulation of the expression of IgE and its biological function is at best limited. We do, however, know that the production of IgE is tightly regulated which is reflected by the fact that the steady-state serum levels of IgE in mice and humans are 3–4 orders of magnitude lower if compared to IgG1, which is an immunoglobulin isotype expressed in response to the same cytokine milieu. What are the rate-limiting steps responsible for this discrepancy? In the following chapter six molecular mechanisms restraining IgE levels will be discussed in detail. The understanding of these mechanisms, combined with the analysis of the biological function of the IgE molecule during an immune response, is the prerequisite for the establishment of new systemic IgE-targeted therapeutic strategies in the future.

2.1 Introduction

IgE is an evolutionary conserved member of the immunoglobulin (Ig) family. Compared to all other Ig classes, which are present in concentrations of micrograms to milligrams per ml serum, the titre of IgE is very low (nano- to micrograms per ml range) in plasma of normal healthy individuals and of normal laboratory mouse strains. IgE is most prominent in epitheliae and mucosae where it is bound to specific receptors on highly potent effector cells like eosinophilic granulocytes and mast cells. Bound to these cells IgE has a long half-life (weeks to months), while free in plasma the half-life is very short (~6 hours). This suggests that IgE plays a role in local immune defence mechanisms. However, the core function for IgE is still unknown. From an evolutionary point of view, IgE is conserved and can be found in all mammalia, including monotremata [1]. It therefore originated at least 160 million years ago, possibly even more than 300 million years ago [2], from a gene duplication of IgY, in which the anaphylactic and opsonic activities of IgY were separated,

---

G. Achatz (✉)
Department of Molecular Biology, University of Salzburg, Salzburg, Austria
e-mail: gernot.achatz@sbg.ac.at

M.L. Penichet, E. Jensen-Jarolim (eds.), *Cancer and IgE*,
DOI 10.1007/978-1-60761-451-7_2,

giving rise to IgE and IgG, respectively [3]. Apparently, in an evolutionary sense, anaphylactic defence mechanisms are needed but at a potentially high price to the organism. The division of anaphylactic and opsonic activities in separate genes allowed principally a tighter and more specific control of both immune mechanisms. In these days IgE is best known for its strong, unwanted effector functions, in the form of allergic reactions [4]. These can range from annoying, local symptoms, like hay fever, to life-threatening, systemic reactions like anaphylactic shock. This underlines the potential hazard of high systemic IgE titres. Remarkably, over the last four decades the incidence of allergic disease has risen. This represents an intriguing problem from a medical, epidemiological, immunological, genetic and evolutionary view. Unfortunately, it is also a major socio-economic problem. One interpretation of these data is that control mechanisms, which were adequate in the past and honed in evolution, are failing.

In the recent past others and we have described several B-cell-specific control mechanisms that indicate a tight control of the IgE response, in agreement with the arguments mentioned above, and that are different from the opsonic type of response (Fig. 2.1):

1. Reduced IL-4-dependent class switch recombination (CSR) to the ε heavy chain (ε-HC) locus in comparison to the γ-1 (γ1)-HC locus [5].
2. Short half-life of free IgE in serum, limiting the risk of a systemic anaphylactic reaction [6].
3. Negative feedback function of CD23, the "low" affinity receptor for IgE, resulting in an in-time and quantity-restricted response [7].
4. Direct impact of the membrane (m)IgE receptor on the quality and quantity of the IgE response in vivo [8, 9].
5. Poor expression of mRNA for the membrane form of both the murine and the human ε-HC, but not for the murine γ1- and the corresponding human γ4-HC [8, 10], resulting in limited expression of IgE as a membrane-bound, antigen-receptor-type molecule [8, 9, 11].
6. Lower chance to contribute to the long-lived plasma cell pool and thus to humoral immunologic memory [12].

In the present review we want to describe these molecular mechanisms and discuss their biological impact on the IgE level in detail.

2.2 Reduced Class Switch Frequency to the IgE Locus

During an immune response, B lymphocytes can switch the Ig isotype from IgM to IgG, IgE, or IgA. This Ig-CSR is based on a DNA recombination event that results in an exchange of the gene segments coding for the constant region of the Ig heavy chain, while retaining the Ig heavy chain variable region. This process changes the effector functions of the corresponding antibody. Much of our current

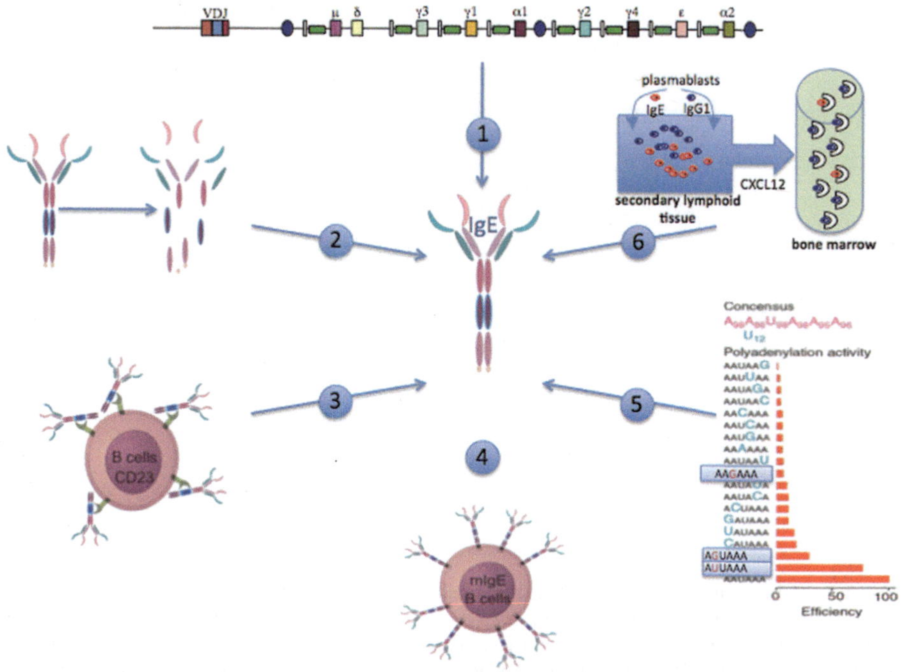

Fig. 2.1 Schematic overview of B-cell-specific control mechanisms, tightly regulating IgE expression in vivo (1) class switch recombination: Although class switching to IgE and IgG1 is induced by the same cytokine milieu followed by similar signal transduction pathways, a 6-fold reduced switching frequency to IgE is observed. (2) Serum half-life: IgE was reported to degrade between 5 and 12 hours, thus displaying the shortest half-life of all immunoglobulin isotypes. (3) Negative feedback regulation by CD23: CD23-knockout mice show a 6-fold increase in serum IgE level. (4) The IgE antigen receptor: Regulation of quantity and quality of the IgE response directly correlates with the surface expression of mIgE. (5) Alternative polyadenylation: In contrast to all other isotypes, the mIgE-RNA gets polyadenylated by three cryptic poly(A) sites. (6) Plasmablast migration: IgE plasmablasts have an intrinsic lower chance to contribute to humoral memory than IgG1 plasmablasts

understanding of the molecular mechanisms of CSR is based on the analysis of in vitro switched B cells where murine and human naïve B cells can be activated by bacterial lipopolysaccharides (LPS), anti-CD40, or CD40L to undergo CSR. Cytokine signals can direct CSR to distinct classes, e.g. interleukin-4 (IL-4) will target murine IgG1 and IgE, and human IgG4 and IgE, respectively. Class switch to IgE is a very rare process [5], which is tightly regulated and can thus be considered as a further means to keep serum IgE low.

CSR (Fig. 2.2) requires transcription of the S regions, which are located upstream of each isotype constant exon and which subsequently become a substrate for the activation-induced deaminase (AID). AID was first discovered by Muramatsu et al. [13] and soon turned out to be the central enzyme in CSR and hypermutation [14]. AID belongs to the RNA editing deaminase family. It could be shown that AID actually acts on DNA of Ig VDJ and S regions rather than on RNA, thereby deaminating

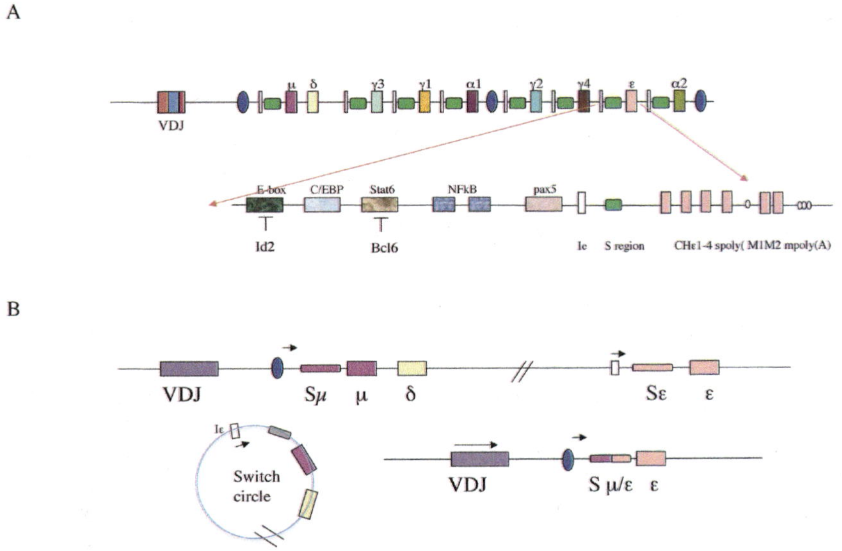

Fig. 2.2 The human immunoglobulin locus exhibits an upstream VDJ arrangement followed by several constant regions of different isotypes (**A**). Each isotype (except IgD) consists of a switch region, which has an upstream promoter/I exon region and downstream constant exons for the secreted Ig molecule followed by a poly(A) site for secreted antibody followed by exons M1 and M2 coding for transmembrane and cytoplasmic domains of the respective isotype and a poly(A) site for the membrane version. Also indicated are the promoters of the V, D and I exons and the internal enhancer elements as well as the 3′ enhancer. Identified transcription factor sites for the Iε promoter are indicated. (**B**) Upon transcription of the S region, RNA and DNA form a stable R-loop and AID gets access to the S regions and deaminates them causing U/G lesions. These lesions are causing DNA breaks, which ultimately lead to DNA recombination and excision of the intervening DNA as a switch circle

C to U [15]. The generated uracils are subjected to general repair mechanisms, which cause single- and double-stranded DNA breaks [16]. Joining of these ends, presumably by non-homologous end joining mechanisms, ultimately leads to CSR and the excision of the intervening DNA in a switch circle [17]. The central role for AID in CSR and hypermutation was not only shown in AID knockout mice [14] but also in patients who harbour defective AID gene expression or non-functional AID mutants [18]. Further elements are thought to contribute to the Ig isotype-specific targeting of CSR, such as the exact composition of the S region—including stem loop structures, chromatin and DNA modifications, promoter regions and germline transcription (GLT) levels (*cis*-acting elements) – as well as *trans*-acting factors that target the CSR machinery to distinct S regions.

Evidence for the necessity of GLT preceding CSR has come from studies in which deletion of promoter elements that abolished GLT also impaired CSR [19]. Vice versa, enforced transcription of S regions by constitutive or inducible promoter elements leads to induced CSR. This could be shown in knock-in experiments [20] as well as in artificial switch substrates introduced into B-cell lines and even in non-B cells that ectopically express transgenic AID [21]. In any S region, GLT initiates

from a promoter upstream of the germline CSR region (S region). The GLTs comprise a small 5′ exon—termed I exon, which is located upstream of the respective S region—spliced to the normal constant heavy chain exons with the intervening S region spliced out from the primary transcript [22]. To exploit GLT as a regulatory mechanism in isotype specificity of CSR, each germline promoter consists of a unique set of transcription factor (TF)-binding sites. In case of the ε germline promoter, it could be shown that treatment of primary B cells with the mitogen LPS and IL-4 is sufficient to trigger GLT from IgE [23].

Mitogenic signals like LPS or stimulation of CD40 [24] or signals transmitted by BAFF/April interacting with BAFFR/TACI/BCMA on B cells [25] lead to activation of NF-κB, which binds to the ε promoter together with the TF Stat6 that becomes activated upon IL-4/IL-13 signalling [26]. As shown in Fig. 2.2, several other TFs were identified, which can bind to the ε GL promoter like B-cell-specific activation protein (BSAP or Pax5) [27], c-Rel [28], C/EBP and AP1. AP1 only transactivates ε GLT from the mouse, but not from the human promoters [29]. TFs that repress transcription from the ε promoter are B-cell lymphoma 6 (Bcl-6) and Id2. Bcl-6 was shown to repress IL-4-induced CSR by competing for Stat6-binding sites within the ε and γ1 promoters [30] and Id2 binds to E2A TFs, thereby inhibiting their binding to ε promoter elements [31]. Possibly, TFs of the E2A group (E12 and E47) might also play a role in targeting AID to distinct promoter elements of the Ig locus [32] where AID might interact with the transcriptional complex to deaminate S regions [33]. In mouse cell lines, also the TF Ikaros was shown to dampen IgE and IgG GLT by binding to the germline promoter [34]. Schaffer et al. [35] showed that the homeodomain proteins HoxC4 and Oct-1 could bind to Iγ and Iε promoters to decrease levels of GLT and thus diminish CSR to IgG and IgE [35, 36]. There is also evidence for the 3′ enhancer of the Ig locus to selectively interact with promoter regions of the GLTs, in particular with the GL ε and γ2b promoters, which might help to target the recombination machinery to the distinct switch regions [37–39]. However, GLT without splicing of the primary transcript is not sufficient to target switch recombination as deletion of the splice donor site of the Iγ1 exon impaired CSR to IgG1.This shows that CSR also requires processing of the GLTs [40]. Stimulation of B cells with mitogenic signals and IL-4 not only induces GLT from the IgE—but also from IgG1–promoter, which exhibits similar TF-binding sites in its promoter region [41].

The observation that in single B cells more than one isotype-S regions are transcribed [42], together with the fact that AID-mediated DNA deamination is primarily restricted to the Ig locus and is not coupled to all genes that are transcribed in the B cell [22], implies that there have to be further levels of isotype-specific CSR regulation. Initially, it was proposed that due to the high GC contents, S regions are forming stable RNA–DNA hybrids (R-loops) upon transcription, in which the non-template strand remains single stranded and thus serves as a substrate for AID-mediated deamination [43]. However, AT-rich S regions, which are not prone to stable R-loop formation, are also effectively targeted by the CSR machinery, which implies the existence of R-loop-independent AID-recruiting mechanisms [44]. Larson et al. [45] propose that the tertiary G4 DNA structure of transcribed S regions allows specific attraction of repair proteins to S regions, thereby promoting

DNA synapsis and recombination. In addition, histone modifications such as phosphorylation, acetylation and methylation were found to occur in S regions accessible for CSR [33, 46, 47], which were not necessarily coupled to changes in the level of GLT [48]. Additionally, S region length was shown to affect the efficiency of CSR [49]. From these data, it is tempting to speculate that slight differences in S region length, composition and tertiary structures might generate isotype-specific protein-binding sites responsible for isotype-specific targeting of AID to individual S regions. In addition, the C-terminal domain of AID was found to be important for CSR but not for hypermutation, which leads to the assumption that CSR-specific factors might interact with the C-terminal domain of AID to either target AID to specific S regions or to mediate specific DNA synapsis and recombination [50]. Currently, the only published interaction partner for AID is the DNA-binding protein RPA (replication protein A) [51], which binds to AID upon phosphorylation by protein kinase A [52]. Binding of RPA to AID in vitro enhances the ability of AID to deaminate cytidines within transcribed double-stranded DNA and probably targets AID to the S region DNA. Further factors that are important in regulating CSR by yet obscure mechanisms, which do not exclude physical interaction with AID/CSR machinery, are the TF bach2 [53], E47 [32] and swap70, the latter could be shown to have a positive effect specifically on the IgE response in mice [54].

The puzzling phenotype of patients with Job′s or hyper IgE syndrome [55–57] (chronic eczematous dermatitis, recurrent skin and sinopulmonary tract infections, mucocutaneous candidiasis, coarse facies and a remarkably elevated serum IgE level) now seems to be solved and sheds additional light on the complexity of IgE immune response. Job′s syndrome is caused by mutations in the DNA-binding domain or the SH2 domain of the TF Stat3 [58, 59]. Whereas the infectious traits of Job′s syndrome can be explained by a deficiency in Th17-cell development [60, 61], which severely impairs immune responses to certain bacteria and fungi, the extremely high IgE levels are more diversely discussed. Stat3 is involved in many signalling pathways [62] and the most important TF in IL-21 signalling. In the mouse IL-21 or IL-21R deficiency has been correlated with low levels of serum IgG1 and high levels of IgE [63]. This may be due to an inhibition of CSR to IgE, because IL-21 induces ID2 expression [64]. Stat3, however, also transduces signals for the IL-6 family and the IL-10 family of cytokines and can induce several effector cells, like T and NK cells to produce IFN-γ [62]. All these factors can by themselves influence CSR to the IgE locus and influence the amount of IgE produced [62]. The influence of many ILs and cytokines on the level of expression of IgE clearly incorporates IgE in ongoing immune responses, yet without a clear hint to its core function.

2.3 Serum IgE Has the Shortest Half-Life of All Serum Immunoglobulins

The half-lives of several sets of murine monoclonal antibodies (mAbs) expressing the same V region in combination with all isotypes of serum Igs were determined by Vieira et al. [6] (Table 2.1). IgE was reported to degrade between 5 and 12 hours

Table 2.1 Serum half-lives of immunoglobulins in rodents and humans

	Serum half-life ($t\frac{1}{2}$)		
Immunoglobulin isotype	Mouse[a]	Rat	Human[c]
IgM	2 days	1 days[e]	5–10 days
IgG1	6–8 days	2 days[e], 9–10 days[f]	21–24 days
IgG2	–	–	21–24 days
IgG2a	6–9 days	4–5 days[e], 9–10 days[f]	–
IgG2b	4–6 days	2–3 days[f]	–
IgG2c	–	4 days[f]	–
IgG3	6–8 days	–	7–8 days
IgG4	–	–	21–24 days
IgA	17–22 hours	27 hours[e]	–
IgA1	–	–	5.9 days
IgA2	–	–	4.5 days
IgE	12 hours[a], 5–8 hours[b]	13.1 ± 5.7 hours[d]	1–5 days

[a]Vieira et al. [6], [b]Haba et al. [65], [c]Leffell et al. [168], [d]Hanashiro et al. [67], [e]Peppard and Orlans [169] and [f]Medesan et al. [170].

[6, 65], thus displaying the shortest half-life of all Ig isotypes. Additionally, alterations in the half-life of IgE were reported in dependency of the site of application. Hirano et al. [66] published that intravenously injected murine anti-DNP-IgE persisted for 12 hours whereas intradermally injected IgE was stable for at least 6 days. Similar half-lives for rat IgE (13.1 ± 5.7 hours) were published by Hanashiro et al. [67].

Waldmann et al. [68] hypothesized that an increased catabolic rate of IgE is dependent on the existence of intravascular and/or extravascular compartments. Human IgE is metabolized mainly in the extravascular compartment and the catabolism of IgE is related to the interaction of IgE with Fcε-receptor (FcεR)-bearing cells. In contrast, it has also been speculated that the vascular endothelium represents a site of catabolism of IgE. Interestingly, an FcRn (Brambell receptor [69]) knockout reduced the serum half-life of IgG1 in mice from 9 to 1.4 days. Thereby, IgG1 in FcRn-knockout mice has roughly the same half-life as all other Ig isotypes in mice [70]. Moreover, Lu et al. [71] generated transgenic mice that overexpressed the bovine FcRn (bFcRn) in their lactating mammary glands. Significantly increased IgG levels were observed in the sera and milk from transgenic animals, suggesting that the overexpressed bFcRn binds and protects endogenous mouse IgG and thus extends its life span. These results indicate that the main reason for the difference in the half-life time between IgG and IgE is explained by the stabilizing interaction between IgG and FcRn. Additionally, the MHC class I-related protein FcRn, originally identified by Simister and colleagues [72, 73] plays a critical role in IgG homeostasis by protecting IgG from normal protein catabolism, which results in a substantial increase in the half-life of IgG.

Similarly, the interaction between IgE and FcεRI stabilizes both partners, increasing the half-life of cell-bound IgE to months. The decreased sensitivity to decay

is accompanied by a conformational change in the three-dimensional structure of IgE: binding to the FcεRI causes the protein to open up from a bent shape into a more stretched shape, leaving the antigen-binding sites intact [4]. The majority of IgE in the body is probably bound to FcεRI on basophils and mast cells, whereas IgG is primarily found in the free, circulating form. Nevertheless, the short half-life of unbound (free) IgE in the blood limits the danger of a systemic anaphylactic reactions.

2.4 CD23 Influences IgE Expression by a Negative Feedback Inhibition

In humans two isoforms, CD23a and CD23b, differing in the first six cytoplasmic amino acids [74, 75] were described. While CD23a is constitutively expressed on B cells and follicular dendritic cells, CD23b, after IL-4 stimulation, is expressed on a variety of hematopoietic cell types like B cells, monocytes, eosinophils and Langerhans cells [75–77]. For a long time only one CD23 isoform was known in mouse, corresponding to human CD23a, but recent studies also described the existence of the CD23b isoform. However, CD23 expression in mouse is restricted to B cells (CD23a) and follicular dendritic cells (CD23a and CD23b) [78–80].

Unlike other Fc receptors, CD23 does not belong to the Ig superfamily of proteins, but is a 45 kDa type II transmembrane glycoprotein comprising a C-terminal lectin domain, followed by a stalk region, a transmembrane domain and a short cytoplasmic tail [81, 82]. The lectin domain binds IgE via the Cε3 domain in a calcium-dependent way [83, 84]. CD23 is expressed on the cell surface as trimers [82, 85]. Oligomerization mediates high-affinity binding to IgE, where two lectin heads bind to one IgE molecule [82]. CD23 binds IgE with both a medium affinity ($4–10 \times 10^7 M^{-1}$) and a low affinity ($4–10 \times 10^6 M^{-1}$) [86]. Besides this membrane-bound form (mCD23), CD23 also exists as soluble fragments of different sizes (sCD23) when cleaved by an autocatalytic mechanism mediated by the metalloprotease ADAM10 [87, 88]. With the exception of one soluble fragment, all of them contain the IgE-binding lectin domain and can bind IgE with low affinity in the range from 10^5 to $10^6 M^{-1}$ [89].

CD23 is a pluripotent molecule; its biological functions include cell activation and proliferation, cell adhesion, IgE-dependent antigen transport, processing and presentation as well as regulation of IgE synthesis and expression. However, the most striking phenomenon is CD23′s ambiguous function on IgE regulation, both in activation and/or inhibition of IgE production. Several studies with CD23-deficient and CD23-overexpressing mice clearly demonstrated CD23′s role as a negative feedback regulator of IgE production [90–95]. Yu et al. [7] showed that disruption of the CD23 gene led to increased specific IgE levels after immunization with TD antigens. While IgG1 levels were twice as high after immunization with 2,4-dinitrophenyl-ovalbumin (DNP-OVA), specific IgE levels were 6–12 times higher in these mice. In contrast, mice overexpressing CD23 produce much lower amounts of IgE, confirming CD23 as a potent regulator of IgE production. Experiments with

New Zealand black mice, which cannot form trimers of CD23 and therefore show impaired high-affinity binding of IgE, also have an exaggerated IgE response [96]. Furthermore, anti-CD23 antibody treatment inhibits specific IgE responses and anti-stalk antibodies enhance IgE production and promote cleavage of mCD23 [97–102]. This increase can be attributed to the prevention of cooperative association of the IgE-binding lectin domains, therefore interfering with oligomerization and high-affinity binding of CD23 [85, 98]. Kilmon et al. [98] demonstrated that RAS1, an anti-stalk antibody, not only prevents oligomerization of CD23 but also inhibits the release of mCD23 [98]. Mice treated with RAS1 and immunized with KLH-DNP/Alum with pertussis toxin also expressed higher levels of IgE, comparable to CD23$^{-/-}$ mice. mAB 19G5 also inhibited high-affinity IgE binding and led to increased IgE levels, but unlike RAS1, 19G5 favoured cleavage of mCD23, leading to elevated sCD23 levels (100–150-fold) [85, 103]. Kinetics of the IgE response were comparable with a primary immune response. Thus, here the elevated serum levels were simply the result of cytophilic release of CD23-bound IgE. Ford et al. [103] also showed that IgE levels are increased even in the absence of Ag-alum, indicating that CD23′s negative regulation of IgE can be abrogated by destabilizing CD23. These results clearly revealed CD23′s ambiguous function on IgE regulation: while stabilized mCD23 negatively regulates IgE production, destabilization of mCD23 leads to an increase of IgE.

Summarizing, in the early phase, IL-4 activates expression of both IgE and CD23, whereas later on, when IgE levels have reached a certain threshold, binding of IgE to CD23 stabilizes and prevents degradation of CD23. This inhibits ongoing IgE synthesis and dampens the immune reaction. However, CD23 seems to play only a role in regulating moderate amounts of IgE: first, helminth-infected wild-type and CD23$^{-/-}$ mice showed the same IgE response [7] and second, destabilization of mCD23 via 19G5 treatment did not lead to an increase of IgE in helminth-infected mice [103].

Many studies have been performed to address the mechanisms behind CD23′s regulatory function. Aubry et al. [104] showed that sCD23 enhances IgE synthesis by binding to CD21 on peripheral blood B cells. Christie et al. [105] prevented autocatalytic cleavage of mCD23 and measured reduced IgE levels. In contrast, Texido et al. [92] showed that transgenic mice for sCD23 exhibited no phenotype, indicating that it is the membrane-bound form of CD23 that regulates IgE production. Ford et al. [103] investigated the role of CD21, a natural ligand for CD23. By using CD21-deficient mice it could be demonstrated that the 19G5-induced IgE response is independent of CD21 signalling, suggesting that increased IgE levels can be attributed to the loss of mCD23 and the release of CD23-bound IgE and not to the accumulation of sCD23 [103]. Recent studies from McCloskey et al. [106] showed that sCD23 both inhibits and stimulates IgE production, depending on the structure of the fragments: while sCD23 monomers inhibit IgE synthesis in human B cells, oligomers stimulate synthesis by co-ligating IgE and CD21 on IgE^{+} B cells.

Summarizing, binding of IgE to mCD23 stabilizes the trimer and prevents its degradation, thus inhibiting the autocatalytic release of sCD23 fragments, which stimulate (in oligomeric form) IgE synthesis. Data from McCloskey et al. [106]

confirmed the competition model between CD23 and CD21 for membrane-bound IgE on the B-cell surface proposed by Hibbert et al. [107]. Co-cross-linkage of mCD23 and mIgE by an IgE/Ag complex results in a decrease of IgE; co-cross-linking of CD21 and mIgE by sCD23 leads to an increase of IgE [107]. Still, the mere absence of CD23, as we have seen, suffices to increase IgE responses.

2.5 The Biological Function of the mIgE Antigen Receptor on IgE Synthesis In Vivo

The B-cell receptor (BCR) is undoubtedly the most important component of a B cell′s interface regarding communication with the local environment. Main developmental steps taking place in the bone marrow like signalling through the pre-BCR as well as avoiding autoreactivity by clonal deletion or receptor editing utterly rely on the expression of a functional receptor. In the periphery, the BCR is one of the driving forces establishing antibody responses addressing invading pathogens and it has been shown to be essential for maintaining peripheral B-cell tolerance in the case of B-cell anergy [108]. Regarding mIgE, the relevance of the receptor seems restricted to responding secondary lymphoid organs like the spleen, lymph nodes and Peyer′s patches. Here, the decision to switch to $mIgE^+$ plasmablasts and finally to IgE-producing antibody-secreting cells (ASCs) is being made in an adequate cognate T-cell-help and cytokine context [109].

mIgE, in contrast to its soluble form, contains three additional structural features encoded by exon M1 and M2, namely the *EMPD* (extracellular membrane-proximal domain) domain, the *transmembrane domain*, which anchors the receptor in the cell membrane and serves as interaction domain for the CD79α/β sheath to form the BCR [110, 111] and the *cytoplasmic domain*. The EMPD regions of the five isotypes differ in length and amino acid composition. In human IgE two functional forms of ε_{EMPD}, namely ε_{short} and ε_{long}, exist composed of 14 and 66 amino acids, respectively [112–114]. According to a study of Poggianella et al. [115] carried out in the mature murine B cell line A20, the presence of the EMPD region is of critical importance for mobilizing intracellular Ca^{2+}, with the EMPD′s length apparently being the "sensor" of caspase-independent apoptosis sensitivity. A similar phenomenon of inhibition of proliferation has been reported in murine WEHI-231 cells transfected with the shorter human version of mIgE [116]. This study also showed that the rate of transport by which the two forms are brought to the cell surface as well as the association with CD79α and the kinetics of protein tyrosine phosphorylation in response to receptor cross-linking differs between the short and the long version. Thus, the form of the EMPD region might have an essential function in shaping the repertoire of $mIgE^+$ plasmablasts selected towards the long-lived plasma cell fate.

A step forward in the understanding of the role of mIgs other than mIgM or mIgD was achieved with two mouse lines with mutations in the ε-HC gene. In the first, the intracellular domain of IgE was removed except for three amino acids (Lys, Val and Lys) (KVKΔtail line). The cytoplasmic domain of IgE in these mice is the same as

that of mIgM and mIgD. In the second line both the intracellular and the transmembrane domains of IgE (ΔM1M2 line) are lacking [9]. In ΔM1M2 mice serum IgE is reduced to less than 10% of normal mice, while KVKΔ tail mice show a reduction of 50%, reflecting a serious impairment of the IgE-mediated immune response. Class switch to IgE was not impaired by the targeting event. Upon stimulation of isolated spleen cells of wild-type, ΔM1M2 and KVKΔtail mice with LPS and IL-4 in vitro, concentrations of IgE and IgG1 in the culture supernatants were comparable in wild-type and mutant mice. These results imply that the reduced IgE titres found in both mutant lines are solely a reflection of the loss of biological activities associated with the transmembrane and cytoplasmic domains of IgE. These data clearly show that the transmembrane domain of IgE is indispensable for a T-cell-dependent IgE-mediated immune response and that the cytoplasmic tail not only determines the absolute amount of IgE produced but also the quality of the antibodies. How does this work?

Two hypotheses can be brought forward. The first implies that signals generated via membrane-bound Ig are needed at all times, not only for the maturation process, but also for the expansion of antigen-specific cells. The second hypothesis postulates that antigen presentation to T-helper cells is necessary at all times during an antibody response and that the antigen receptor is the only device for an effective antigen presentation. The hypotheses are not necessarily mutually exclusive. All Ig classes can associate with the Ig-α/Ig-β heterodimer [117], the signal-transducing unit of the BCR. Recent experiments have shown that an intact antigen receptor on B cells is elementary for the survival of B cells [118]. It is not clear from these experiments which function the antigen receptor performs: interactions with external ligands, maintenance of a tonic signal generated by the mere presence of the receptor in the membrane, or capture of antigen. Both the Ig-α/Ig-β sheath and the cytoplasmic tail of mIg [119] have been implied in guiding antigen bound via the receptor to the antigen-processing compartments. Key residues for internalization are present in the tails in the form of an YxxI/M motif. This could be a prerequisite for processes that are highly dependent on T–B cell interactions like somatic mutation and affinity maturation and the generation of memory cells, but also processes like the rescue from apoptosis and the induction of plasma cells. These considerations predict that the results we obtained in the KVKΔtail and ΔM1M2 lines can be extended to the IgG isotypes and perhaps to IgA. Indeed, Kaisho et al. [120] reached matching conclusions, studying mice carrying similar mutations in the γ1 gene. The phenotype of the mIgG mutants is, however, more prominent.

Further studies showed that upon receptor ligation, the mere cytoplasmic tails of γ and ε but not μ, δ, or α are capable of inhibiting CD22 phosphorylation and SHP-1 recruitment [121, 122]. Due to the fact that none of the cytoplasmic tails of mIgs contain full ITAM/ITIM motifs [123], tail-interacting proteins may influence downstream B-cell signalling cascades. A study of Batista et al. [116] identified two proteins, namely εBAP37 and εBAP41, being exclusively associated with the cytoplasmic tail of mIgE. Those two molecules were shown to be glycosylated and form disulphide-bonded complexes, with each having an extracellular domain. Recently, we described another protein, involved in mIgE-mediated

signalling, HS1-associated protein X-1 (HAX-1). HAX-1 turned out to be associated with the mIgE tail, being indispensable for the internalization of the receptor by linking it to the cytoskeleton via its interaction with HS1 [124].

Additionally, Erazo et al. [125] suggested a model, in which IgE^+ cells exhibit a plasma cell programme from early onwards, with signs of somatic hypermutation despite their exclusion from GCs, with repression of Bcl6 and upregulation of Blimp-1, a central TF in plasma cell differentiation [126]. They further hypothesized that expression of mIgE requires an intermediate $IgG1^+$ cellular phase, leading to high-affinity IgE antibodies without requiring a prolonged IgE^+ GC phase. In contrast, Kelly et al. [127] claimed that in their system of administering phOx-BSA into the footpad of mice and monitoring the response in brachial lymph nodes, the majority of IgE^+ cells are localized in GCs. The notion that CSR to IgE is an actively inhibited process, as was revealed in IL-21- and IL-21R-knockout mice, which are characterized by low IgG and high IgE titres [63], does not support a consecutive switch model. In respect to additional partially controversial literature [128, 129] one can speculate that not only the type and the amount of administered antigen, but also the route of administration and the involved cytokines seem to be of critical importance concerning the nature of the response.

2.6 Impaired Splicing and Polyadenylation Restricts the Generation of a Mature mIgE Transcript

Both of the mRNAs for the secreted and the membrane form of IgHCs are generated from the same precursor mRNA by means of alternative splicing and polyadenylation. The third (IgD and IgGs) or fourth (IgM and IgE) constant exon, which is located 5′ of the transmembrane and the cytoplasmic exons, is a composite exon: it contains an internal splice donor site which is used when mRNA for membrane-bound Ig is made. It is also followed by an "internal" polyadenylation-addition site that is used when mRNA for secreted Ig is made. A 3′ "external" polyadenylation-addition site is found downstream of the membrane exons. With the exception of IgE, the consensus sequence AATAAA is used for the "internal" and the "external" polyadenylation signals. Looking at the mRNA levels of both forms in the course of B-cell development, a shift in the membrane-to-secreted ratio can be observed [130]. While resting B cells produce similar amounts of both mRNA′s, the ratio changes in favour of the secreted form in activated B lymphoblasts and in the terminally differentiated B cell, the plasma cell, mRNA for the secreted form is 20–100 times higher abundant than mRNA for the membrane form. This change in the membrane-to-secreted ratio does not seem to be caused by an increase in transcription rate, since the heavy chain enhancer is already completely active in the pre-B-cell stage [131]. This shift is far more likely generated by a selective increase in the processing rate and in the stability of secretory mRNA [132]. It is known for a long time that polyadenylation has a paramount effect on mRNA stability, nuclear export and translation. The process of polyadenylation requires numerous factors responsible for the

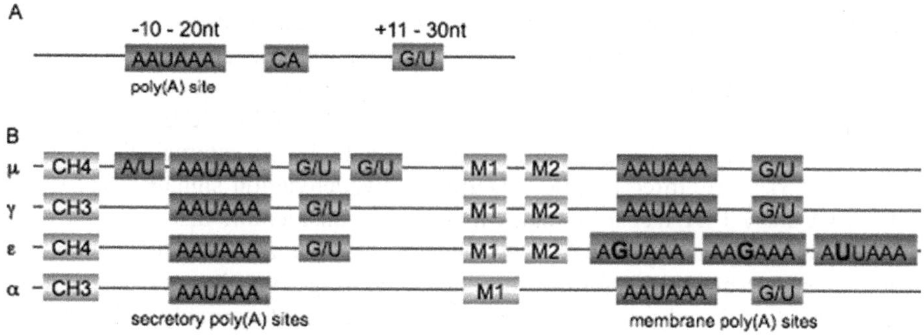

Fig. 2.3 Polyadenylation consensus sequences of mouse immunoglobulin isotypes. (**A**) An ideal polyadenylation consensus sequence (AAUAAA) and a perfectly positioned GU-rich region is shown. "CA" marks the site of actual cleavage and subsequent polyadenylation. (**B**) The secretory and membrane poly(A) sites of the immunoglobulin isotypes in mouse are shown. All sites except ε membrane poly(A) have a single AAUAAA consensus sequence. The ε membrane poly(A) site is made up of three "cryptic"-poly(A) sites. The μ secretory poly(A) site depicts a distinct dual structure, which is not found in the other isotypes. It has an upstream AU-rich region and two suboptimally placed GU-rich motifs, weakening the μ secretory poly(A) site

recognition, cleavage and addition of the poly(A) tail. Two multisubunit complexes, designated cleavage-polyadenylation specificity factor (CPSF) [133–135] and cleavage stimulation factor (CstF) [136], cooperate with each other to define the site of polyadenylation [137, 138]. They recognize the highly conserved AAUAAA hexanucleotide (Fig. 2.3) [137, 139] and a more divergent GU-rich sequence located downstream of the actual cleavage site [140–142]. Two additional factors, cleavage factor I and II (CFI and CFII), are further necessary for the cleavage reaction [135]. For the poly(A) synthesis itself, CPSF and poly(A) polymerase [143–145], together with poly(A)-binding protein II (PAB II), are sufficient, although CstF was recently shown to enhance this reaction [146]. A subunit of the CstF, CstF-64, was shown to be expressed in a stage-specific manner in B cells expressing IgM [141, 147]. It was speculated that in resting B cells, where CstF-64 is less abundant, the poly(A) site for the membrane form of μ (μm poly(A) site) is preferred over that of the secreted form (internal or μs poly(A) site). The higher amount of CstF in activated plasma cells leads to the better recognition of the "weaker" internal μs poly(A) site [147]. A supposed mechanism for this phenomenon is that polyadenylation of the μs poly(A) site takes place before transcription over the μm poly(A) site can proceed. However, this phenomenon was found to be valid for IgM [148–150] but not for IgG and IgA [151–153]. For IgG2b, not the increasing amount of CstF-64 during B-cell development is important but rather the improved binding and polyadenylation efficiency [154]. Further, Yan et al. [44] postulated a specific activity in B-cell extracts that selectively impairs the formation of a μs poly(A) site processing complex, suggesting that the function of this poly(A) site may be regulated by both positively and negatively acting factors. Additionally, the sequence of the intron 5′ of the M1 exon can influence the polyadenylation/splicing balance. For IgA a specific sequence in

the Cα3-Mα1 intron is recognized by a 58 kDa protein and leads to a predominant usage of the αs poly(A) site [153, 155]. In this special case, the ratio of αs-to-αm IgA in resting B cells is about 2. Therefore it is possible that *cis*-acting elements unique to each HC gene act upon a common mechanism regulation Ig mRNA processing.

The ε-HC gene differs from the Ig genes as to its 3′ external εm poly(A) site (Fig. 2.3). Here, three kryptic "external" polyadenylation signals (AGTAAA, AAGAAA and ATTAAA) are found, which are in considerable disagreement with the consensus sequence (AATAAA). As we have seen, the ratio of transcripts for the secreted and the membrane form of Ig reflects the usage of either polyadenylation signal. The poor 3′ polyadenylation sites in the ε gene unfavourably influence the production of mRNA for the membrane form of ε [10]. One of the consequences of the restricted polyadenylation of the εm transcript is a limited stable pool of εm mRNA which further influences the poor expression of the membrane-associated IgE-BCR on switched B cells. Surface expression of the membrane form of IgE is paramount to the survival of IgE switched B cells [9]. Therefore, weak 3 ṕrocessing of mε-mRNA seems to be a way to keep numbers of IgE-positive B cells and thus the titre of secreted IgE in the serum low.

Another interesting feature is that the human ε gene in vitro generates more than two mRNAs for the secretory and the membrane-associated forms, generated via alternative splicing and polyadenylation. Burrone et al. have found and characterized two functional membranes and two functional secretory isoforms out of six possible isoforms. All four heavy chains seem to assemble into proper Igs, although with different kinetics, and are functionally active as a receptor or as a mediator of a humoral immune response [116, 156, 157].

2.7 IgE Plasmablasts Have an Intrinsic, Lower Chance to Contribute to the Long-Lived Plasma Cell Pool

It is generally accepted that the switch of B cells expressing membrane-bound Igs, which serve as antigen receptors, to antibody-secreting plasmablasts and finally non-dividing, long-lived plasma cells, marks the terminal differentiation of a B cell. Thus, besides memory B cells, antibody-secreting plasma "memory" cells represent the key cell type for the maintenance of humoral immunological memory. Although some populations of long-lived plasma cells persist in the spleen, most of them return to their "place of birth" and invade the bone marrow or inflamed tissues where they survive as resident, immobile cells in survival niches up to several months [158–160]. However, the life span of plasma cells is limited by the immigration of newly formed migratory plasmablasts that compete with old plasma cells for their survival niches. In these niches, resident long-lived plasma cells are resistant to therapies targeting activated and/or proliferating lymphocytes, for example, by radiation [161] or cyclophosphamide [162]. The permanent and antigen-independent secretion of antibodies specific for allergens or autoantigens makes these cells key players in allergic and autoimmune diseases and obviously key targets for possible therapeutic interference.

The migration of plasmablasts to the bone marrow is a critical differentiation step for long-lived plasma cells. Little is known about the migration of ASCs in general and ASCs of IgE in particular. Chemokines and their receptors are crucially involved in the control of lymphocyte trafficking. Hauser et al. [163, 164] showed that migratory cells lose responsiveness to many chemokines, with the exception of chemokine ligand (CXCL) 12 and CXCL9. The corresponding receptors, sensitive for CXCL12 and CXCL9, were identified as chemokine receptor (CXCR) 4 and CXCR3, respectively. It has recently been suggested that the chemokine receptor CXCR4 is required for normal accumulation of plasma cells in the bone marrow [165], as demonstrated by the increased sensitivity of the CXCR4 receptor for its ligand CXCL12, which is mainly expressed in the splenic red pulp, the lymph node medullary cords and the bone marrow.

Muehlinghaus [166] first pointed out the importance of the antigen receptor for migration behaviour of memory B cells. It was shown that CXCR3 is preferentially expressed on a fraction of human memory B cells, in particular on those expressing IgG1. Further, $CXCR3^-$ memory B cells upregulate CXCR3 and migrate towards concentration gradients of its ligand only when co-stimulated with interferon γ but not with IL-4.

In order to analyse the migratory behaviour of memory B cells in the dependence of the isotype of the antigen receptor, we constructed "knock-in" mouse strain KN1, where we completely exchanged the membrane ε-genomic region downstream of the secretory poly(A) site for the membrane γ1-region [167]. Thus, in KN1 the IgE immune response develops under the regulation of γ1-specific cytoplasmic signalling. KN1 not only showed a significant increase in mRNA for the membrane and secreted ε-transcripts, but also a 6-fold increase in serum IgE. The continually accumulating serum IgE titre is the result of a selection advantage of chimeric mIgE-expressing B cells in KN1 mice for their immigration to the bone marrow. The γ1-based signalling in chimeric mIgE-B cells indicates the existence of an isotype-specific, antigen-receptor-dependent developmental programme for B cells to become long-lived plasma cells.

Summarizing, our data strongly support the concept that BCR-mediated signalling continues in the plasmablast stage and has an isotype-specific component: γ1-like signalling, in contrast to ε-like signalling, facilitates migration of plasmablasts towards the chemokine CXCL12, allowing them to settle in plasma cell niches, like in the bone marrow, and (thus) more efficiently induces progression towards the fully matured plasma cell stage. Our observations also lead to the conclusion that during a Th2-mediated immune response, in normal wild-type mice, IgE plasmablasts have an intrinsic lower chance to contribute to the long-lived plasma cell pool and thus to humoral immunologic memory than IgG1 plasmablasts.

2.8 Conclusions

Our knowledge about the regulation of the expression of IgE is at best limited. Unfortunately, a similar statement can be made regarding the function of membrane-bound IgE. We do, however, know that the production of IgE is tightly regulated.

This regulation is evident on the level of DNA (switch) recombination, transcription and RNA processing. It is not inconceivable that also post-translational processes may influence the expression of membrane-bound IgE. The consequences of a possible disregulation, i.e. uncontrolled IgE secretion, warrant an in-depth study of these processes.

Summarizing, IgE antibodies may have strong effector functions, but this contrasted with the slow IgE response and the limited development of memory responses. Together these observations represent mechanisms to restrain potentially dangerous, but apparently necessary, because present, high serum IgE titres at many different levels in a biological process.

Acknowledgements Experimental work and publication charges were supported by the Austrian Science Foundation (P19017-B13), the Austrian National Bank (OENB grant: 11710) and the Christian Doppler Laboratory for Allergy Diagnosis and Therapy.

References

1. Vernersson M, Aveskogh M, Hellman L (2004) Cloning of IgE from the echidna (Tachyglossus aculeatus) and a comparative analysis of epsilon chains from all three extant mammalian lineages. Dev Comp Immunol 28:61–75
2. Kumar S, Hedges SB (1998) A molecular timescale for vertebrate evolution. Nature 392:917–920
3. Warr GW, Magor KE, Higgins DA (1995) IgY: Clues to the origins of modern antibodies. Immunol Today 16:392–398
4. Gould HJ, Sutton BJ, Beavil AJ, Beavil RL, McCloskey N, Coker HA, Fear D, Smurthwaite L (2003) The biology of IGE and the basis of allergic disease. Annu Rev Immunol 21: 579–628
5. Siebenkotten G, Esser C, Wabl M, Radbruch A (1992) The murine IgG1/IgE class switch program. Eur J Immunol 22:1827–1834
6. Vieira P, Rajewsky K (1988) The half-lives of serum immunoglobulins in adult mice. Eur J Immunol 18:313–316
7. Yu P, Kosco-Vilbois M, Richards M, Kohler G, Lamers MC (1994) Negative feedback regulation of IgE synthesis by murine CD23. Nature 369:753–756
8. Achatz G, Luger E, Geisberger R, Achatz-Straussberger G, Breitenbach M, Lamers M (2001) The IgE antigen receptor: a key regulator for the production of IgE antibodies. Int Arch Allergy Immunol 124:31–34
9. Achatz G, Nitschke L, Lamers MC (1997) Effect of transmembrane and cytoplasmic domains of IgE on the IgE response. Science 276:409–411
10. Karnowski A, Achatz-Straussberger G, Klockenbusch C, Achatz G, Lamers MC (2006) Inefficient processing of mRNA for the membrane form of IgE is a genetic mechanism to limit recruitment of IgE-secreting cells. Eur J Immunol 36:1917–1925
11. Luger E, Lamers M, Achatz-Straussberger G, Geisberger R, Infuhr D, Breitenbach M, Crameri R, Achatz G (2001) Somatic diversity of the immunoglobulin repertoire is controlled in an isotype-specific manner. Eur J Immunol 31:2319–2330
12. Achatz-Straußberger G, Königsberger S, Karnowsky A, Lamers M, Achatz G (2007). Elevated histamine release in chimeric IgE/IgG1 antigen receptor knock-in mice. Allergy Clin Immunol Int Hogrefe & Huber Supp 2:121–123
13. Muramatsu M, Sankaranand VS, Anant S, Sugai M, Kinoshita K, Davidson NO, Honjo T (1999) Specific expression of activation-induced cytidine deaminase (AID), a novel member of the RNA-editing deaminase family in germinal center B cells. J Biol Chem 274: 18470–18476

14. Muramatsu M, Kinoshita K, Fagarasan S, Yamada S, Shinkai Y, Honjo T (2000) Class switch recombination and hypermutation require activation-induced cytidine deaminase (AID), a potential RNA editing enzyme. Cell 102:553–563
15. Petersen-Mahrt SK, Harris RS, Neuberger MS (2002) AID mutates E. coli suggesting a DNA deamination mechanism for antibody diversification. Nature 418:99–103
16. Di Noia J, Neuberger MS (2002) Altering the pathway of immunoglobulin hypermutation by inhibiting uracil-DNA glycosylase. Nature 419:43–48
17. Kenter AL (2005) Class switch recombination: an emerging mechanism. Curr Top Microbiol Immunol 290:171–199
18. Durandy A, Taubenheim N, Peron S, Fischer A (2007) Pathophysiology of B-cell intrinsic immunoglobulin class switch recombination deficiencies. Adv Immunol 94:275–306
19. Linehan LA, Warren WD, Thompson PA, Grusby MJ, Berton MT (1998) STAT6 is required for IL-4-induced germline Ig gene transcription and switch recombination. J Immunol 161:302–310
20. Xu L, Gorham B, Li SC, Bottaro A, Alt FW, Rothman P (1993) Replacement of germ-line epsilon promoter by gene targeting alters control of immunoglobulin heavy chain class switching. Proc Natl Acad Sci USA 90:3705–3709
21. Yoshikawa K, Okazaki IM, Eto T, Kinoshita K, Muramatsu M, Nagaoka H, Honjo T (2002) AID enzyme-induced hypermutation in an actively transcribed gene in fibroblasts. Science 296:2033–2036
22. Di Noia JM, Neuberger MS (2007) Molecular mechanisms of antibody somatic hypermutation. Annu Rev Biochem 76:1–22
23. Rothman P, Li SC, Gorham B, Glimcher L, Alt F, Boothby M (1991) Identification of a conserved lipopolysaccharide-plus-interleukin-4-responsive element located at the promoter of germ line epsilon transcripts. Mol Cell Biol 11:5551–5561
24. Grewal IS, Foellmer HG, Grewal KD, Xu J, Hardardottir F, Baron JL, Janeway CA, Jr., Flavell RA (1996) Requirement for CD40 ligand in costimulation induction, T cell activation, and experimental allergic encephalomyelitis. Science 273:1864–1867
25. Claudio E, Brown K, Park S, Wang H, Siebenlist U (2002) BAFF-induced NEMO-independent processing of NF-kappa B2 in maturing B cells. Nat Immunol 3:958–965
26. de Vries JE, Punnonen J, Cocks BG, de Waal Malefyt R, Aversa G (1993) Regulation of the human IgE response by IL4 and IL13. Res Immunol 144:597–601
27. Thienes CP, De Monte L, Monticelli S, Busslinger M, Gould HJ, Vercelli D (1997) The transcription factor B cell-specific activator protein (BSAP) enhances both IL-4- and CD40-mediated activation of the human epsilon germline promoter. J Immunol 158:5874–5882
28. Agresti A, Vercelli D (2002) c-Rel is a selective activator of a novel IL-4/CD40 responsive element in the human Ig gamma4 germline promoter. Mol Immunol 38:849–859
29. Shen CH, Stavnezer J (2001) Activation of the mouse Ig germline epsilon promoter by IL-4 is dependent on AP-1 transcription factors. J Immunol 166:411–423
30. Harris MB, Chang CC, Berton MT, Danial NN, Zhang J, Kuehner D, Ye BH, Kvatyuk M, Pandolfi PP, Cattoretti G, Dalla-Favera R, Rothman PB (1999) Transcriptional repression of Stat6-dependent interleukin-4-induced genes by BCL-6: specific regulation of iepsilon transcription and immunoglobulin E switching. Mol Cell Biol 19:7264–7275
31. Sugai M, Gonda H, Kusunoki T, Katakai T, Yokota Y, Shimizu A (2003) Essential role of Id2 in negative regulation of IgE class switching. Nat Immunol 4:25–30
32. Schoetz U, Cervelli M, Wang YD, Fiedler P, Buerstedde JM (2006) E2A expression stimulates Ig hypermutation. J Immunol 177:395–400
33. Nambu Y, Sugai M, Gonda H, Lee CG, Katakai T, Agata Y, Yokota Y, Shimizu A (2003) Transcription-coupled events associating with immunoglobulin switch region chromatin. Science 302:2137–2140
34. Strom L, Lundgren M, Severinson E (2003) Binding of Ikaros to germline Ig heavy chain gamma1 and epsilon promoters. Mol Immunol 39:771–782
35. Schaffer A, Kim EC, Wu X, Zan H, Testoni L, Salamon S, Cerutti A, Casali P (2003) Selective inhibition of class switching to IgG and IgE by recruitment of the HoxC4 and

Oct-1 homeodomain proteins and Ku70/Ku86 to newly identified ATTT cis-elements. J Biol Chem 278:23141–23150
36. Kim EC, Edmonston CR, Wu X, Schaffer A, Casali P (2004) The HoxC4 homeodomain protein mediates activation of the immunoglobulin heavy chain 3′ hs1,2 enhancer in human B cells. Relevance to class switch DNA recombination. J Biol Chem 279:42258–42269
37. Laurencikiene J, Deveikaite V, Severinson E (2001) HS1,2 enhancer regulation of germline epsilon and gamma2b promoters in murine B lymphocytes: evidence for specific promoter-enhancer interactions. J Immunol 167:3257–3265
38. Laurencikiene J, Tamosiunas V, Severinson E (2007) Regulation of epsilon germline transcription and switch region mutations by IgH locus 3′ enhancers in transgenic mice. Blood 109:159–167
39. Manis JP, van der Stoep N, Tian M, Ferrini R, Davidson L, Bottaro A, Alt FW (1998) Class switching in B cells lacking 3′ immunoglobulin heavy chain enhancers. J Exp Med 188:1421-1431
40. Hein K, Lorenz MG, Siebenkotten G, Petry K, Christine R, Radbruch A (1998) Processing of switch transcripts is required for targeting of antibody class switch recombination. J Exp Med 188:2369–2374
41. Mao CS, Stavnezer J (2001) Differential regulation of mouse germline Ig gamma 1 and epsilon promoters by IL-4 and CD40. J Immunol 167:1522–1534
42. Fear DJ, McCloskey N, O′Connor B, Felsenfeld G, Gould HJ (2004) Transcription of Ig germline genes in single human B cells and the role of cytokines in isotype determination. J Immunol 173:4529–4538
43. Selsing E (2006) Ig class switching: targeting the recombinational mechanism. Curr Opin Immunol 18:249–254
44. Zarrin AA, Alt FW, Chaudhuri J, Stokes N, Kaushal D, Du Pasquier L, Tian M (2004) An evolutionarily conserved target motif for immunoglobulin class-switch recombination. Nat Immunol 5:1275–1281
45. Larson ED, Duquette ML, Cummings WJ, Streiff RJ, Maizels N (2005) MutSalpha binds to and promotes synapsis of transcriptionally activated immunoglobulin switch regions. Curr Biol 15:470–474
46. Kaminski DA, Stavnezer J (2007) Stimuli that enhance IgA class switching increase histone 3 acetylation at S alpha, but poorly stimulate sequential switching from IgG2b. Eur J Immunol 37:240–251
47. Wang L, Whang N, Wuerffel R, Kenter AL (2006) AID-dependent histone acetylation is detected in immunoglobulin S regions. J Exp Med 203:215–226
48. Bradley SP, Kaminski DA, Peters AH, Jenuwein T, Stavnezer J (2006) The histone methyltransferase Suv39h1 increases class switch recombination specifically to IgA. J Immunol 177:1179–1188
49. Zarrin AA, Tian M, Wang J, Borjeson T, Alt FW (2005) Influence of switch region length on immunoglobulin class switch recombination. Proc Natl Acad Sci USA 102:2466–2470
50. Shinkura R, Ito S, Begum NA, Nagaoka H, Muramatsu M, Kinoshita K, Sakakibara Y, Hijikata H, Honjo T (2004) Separate domains of AID are required for somatic hypermutation and class-switch recombination. Nat Immunol 5:707–712
51. Chaudhuri J, Khuong C, Alt FW (2004) Replication protein A interacts with AID to promote deamination of somatic hypermutation targets. Nature 430:992–998
52. Basu U, Chaudhuri J, Alpert C, Dutt S, Ranganath S, Li G, Schrum JP, Manis JP, Alt FW (2005) The AID antibody diversification enzyme is regulated by protein kinase A phosphorylation. Nature 438:508–511
53. Muto A, Tashiro S, Nakajima O, Hoshino H, Takahashi S, Sakoda E, Ikebe D, Yamamoto M, Igarashi K (2004) The transcriptional programme of antibody class switching involves the repressor Bach2. Nature 429:566–571
54. Borggrefe T, Keshavarzi S, Gross B, Wabl M, Jessberger R (2001) Impaired IgE response in SWAP-70-deficient mice. Eur J Immunol 31:2467–2475

55. Buckley RH, Wray BB, Belmaker EZ (1972) Extreme hyperimmunoglobulinemia E and undue susceptibility to infection. Pediatrics 49:59–70
56. Davis SD, Schaller J, Wedgwood RJ (1966) Job's Syndrome. Recurrent, "cold", staphylococcal abscesses. Lancet 1:1013–1015
57. Grimbacher B, Holland SM, Gallin JI, Greenberg F, Hill SC, Malech HL, Miller JA, O'Connell AC, Puck JM (1999) Hyper-IgE syndrome with recurrent infections – an autosomal dominant multisystem disorder. N Engl J Med 340:692–702
58. Holland SM, DeLeo FR, Elloumi HZ, Hsu AP, Uzel G, Brodsky N, Freeman AF, Demidowich A, Davis J, Turner ML, Anderson VL, Darnell DN, Welch PA, Kuhns DB, Frucht DM, Malech HL, Gallin JI, Kobayashi SD, Whitney AR, Voyich JM, Musser JM, Woellner C, Schaffer AA, Puck JM, Grimbacher B (2007) STAT3 mutations in the hyper-IgE syndrome. N Engl J Med 357:1608–1619
59. Minegishi Y, Saito M, Tsuchiya S, Tsuge I, Takada H, Hara T, Kawamura N, Ariga T, Pasic S, Stojkovic O, Metin A, Karasuyama H (2007) Dominant-negative mutations in the DNA-binding domain of STAT3 cause hyper-IgE syndrome. Nature 448:1058–1062
60. de Beaucoudrey L, Puel A, Filipe-Santos O, Cobat A, Ghandil P, Chrabieh M, Feinberg J, von Bernuth H, Samarina A, Janniere L, Fieschi C, Stephan JL, Boileau C, Lyonnet S, Jondeau G, Cormier-Daire V, Le Merrer M, Hoarau C, Lebranchu Y, Lortholary O, Chandesris MO, Tron F, Gambineri E, Bianchi L, Rodriguez-Gallego C, Zitnik SE, Vasconcelos J, Guedes M, Vitor AB, Marodi L, Chapel H, Reid B, Roifman C, Nadal D, Reichenbach J, Caragol I, Garty BZ, Dogu F, Camcioglu Y, Gulle S, Sanal O, Fischer A, Abel L, Stockinger B, Picard C, Casanova JL (2008) Mutations in STAT3 and IL12RB1 impair the development of human IL-17-producing T cells. J Exp Med 205:1543–1550
61. Milner JD, Brenchley JM, Laurence A, Freeman AF, Hill BJ, Elias KM, Kanno Y, Spalding C, Elloumi HZ, Paulson ML, Davis J, Hsu A, Asher AI, O'Shea J, Holland SM, Paul WE, Douek DC (2008) Impaired T(H)17 cell differentiation in subjects with autosomal dominant hyper-IgE syndrome. Nature 452:773–776
62. Schindler C, Plumlee C (2008) Inteferons pen the JAK-STAT pathway. Semin Cell Dev Biol 122:401–408
63. Ozaki K, Spolski R, Feng CG, Qi CF, Cheng J, Sher A, Morse HC, 3rd, Liu C, Schwartzberg PL, Leonard WJ (2002) A critical role for IL-21 in regulating immunoglobulin production. Science 298:1630–1634
64. Kishida T, Hiromura Y, Shin-Ya M, Asada H, Kuriyama H, Sugai M, Shimizu A, Yokota Y, Hama T, Imanishi J, Hisa Y, Mazda O (2007) IL-21 induces inhibitor of differentiation 2 and leads to complete abrogation of anaphylaxis in mice. J Immunol 179:8554–8561
65. Haba S, Ovary Z, Nisonoff A (1985) Clearance of IgE from serum of normal and hybridoma-bearing mice. J Immunol 134:3291–3297
66. Hirano T, Hom C, Ovary Z (1983) Half-life of murine IgE antibodies in the mouse. Int Arch Allergy Appl Immunol 71:182–184
67. Hanashiro K, Tokeshi Y, Nakasone T, Sunagawa M, Nakamura M, Kosugi T (2001) Analysis of IgE turnover in non-sensitized and sensitized rats. Mediators Inflamm 10:217–221
68. Waldmann TA, Iio A, Ogawa M, McIntyre OR, Strober W (1976) The metabolism of IgE. Studies in normal individuals and in a patient with IgE myeloma. J Immunol 117: 1139–1144
69. Brambell FW (1966) The transmission of immunity from mother to young and the catabolism of immunoglobulins. Lancet 2:1087–1093
70. Roopenian DC, Christianson GJ, Sproule TJ, Brown AC, Akilesh S, Jung N, Petkova S, Avanessian L, Choi EY, Shaffer DJ, Eden PA, Anderson CL (2003) The MHC class I-like IgG receptor controls perinatal IgG transport, IgG homeostasis, and fate of IgG-Fc-coupled drugs. J Immunol 170:3528–3533
71. Lu W, Zhao Z, Zhao Y, Yu S, Zhao Y, Fan B, Kacskovics I, Hammarstrom L, Li N (2007) Over-expression of the bovine FcRn in the mammary gland results in increased IgG levels in both milk and serum of transgenic mice. Immunology 19:311–318

72. Simister NE, Mostov KE (1989) An Fc receptor structurally related to MHC class I antigens. Nature 337:184–187
73. Ahouse JJ, Hagerman CL, Mittal P, Gilbert DJ, Copeland NG, Jenkins NA, Simister NE (1993) Mouse MHC class I-like Fc receptor encoded outside the MHC. J Immunol 151:6076–6088
74. Sutton BJ, Gould HJ (1993) The human IgE network. Nature 366:421–428
75. Yokota A, Kikutani H, Tanaka T, Sato R, Barsumian EL, Suemura M, Kishimoto T (1988) Two species of human Fc epsilon receptor II (Fc epsilon RII/CD23): tissue-specific and IL-4-specific regulation of gene expression. Cell 55:611–618
76. Delespesse G, Sarfati M, Wu CY, Fournier S, Letellier M (1992) The low-affinity receptor for IgE. Immunol Rev 125:77–97
77. Delespesse G, Suter U, Mossalayi D, Bettler B, Sarfati M, Hofstetter H, Kilcherr E, Debre P, Dalloul A (1991) Expression, structure, and function of the CD23 antigen. Adv Immunol 49:149–191
78. Maeda K, Burton GF, Padgett DA, Conrad DH, Huff TF, Masuda A, Szakal AK, Tew JG (1992) Murine follicular dendritic cells and low affinity Fc receptors for IgE (Fc epsilon RII). J Immunol 148:2340–2347
79. Rao M, Lee WT, Conrad DH (1987) Characterization of a monoclonal antibody directed against the murine B lymphocyte receptor for IgE. J Immunol 138:1845–1851
80. Sukumar S, Conrad DH, Szakal AK, Tew JG (2006) Differential T cell-mediated regulation of CD23 (Fc epsilonRII) in B cells and follicular dendritic cells. J Immunol 176:4811–4817
81. Conrad DH (1990) Fc epsilon RII/CD23: the low affinity receptor for IgE. Annu Rev Immunol 8:623–645
82. Gould H, Sutton B, Edmeades R, Beavil A (1991) CD23/Fc epsilon RII: C-type lectin membrane protein with a split personality? Monogr Allergy 29:28–49
83. Chretien I, Helm BA, Marsh PJ, Padlan EA, Wijdenes J, Banchereau J (1988) A monoclonal anti-IgE antibody against an epitope (amino acids 367–376) in the CH3 domain inhibits IgE binding to the low affinity IgE receptor (CD23). J Immunol 141:3128–3134
84. Richards ML, Katz DH (1990) The binding of IgE to murine Fc epsilon RII is calcium-dependent but not inhibited by carbohydrate. J Immunol 144:2638–2646
85. Kilmon MA, Shelburne AE, Chan-Li Y, Holmes KL, Conrad DH (2004) CD23 trimers are preassociated on the cell surface even in the absence of its ligand, IgE. J Immunol 172:1065–1073
86. Dierks SE, Bartlett WC, Edmeades RL, Gould HJ, Rao M, Conrad DH (1993) The oligomeric nature of the murine Fc epsilon RII/CD23. Implications for function. J Immunol 150:2372–2382
87. Weskamp G, Ford JW, Sturgill J, Martin S, Docherty AJ, Swendeman S, Broadway N, Hartmann D, Saftig P, Umland S, Sehara-Fujisawa A, Black RA, Ludwig A, Becherer JD, Conrad DH, Blobel CP (2006) ADAM10 is a principal 'sheddase' of the low-affinity immunoglobulin E receptor CD23. Nat Immunol 7:1293–1298
88. Lemieux GA, Blumenkron F, Yeung N, Zhou P, Williams J, Grammer AC, Petrovich R, Lipsky PE, Moss ML, Werb Z (2007) The low affinity IgE receptor (CD23) is cleaved by the metalloproteinase ADAM10. J Biol Chem 282:14836–14844
89. Bartlett WC, Kelly AE, Johnson CM, Conrad DH (1995) Analysis of murine soluble Fc epsilon RII sites of cleavage and requirements for dual-affinity interaction with IgE. J Immunol 154:4240–4246
90. Stief A, Texido G, Sansig G, Eibel H, Le Gros G, van der Putten H (1994) Mice deficient in CD23 reveal its modulatory role in IgE production but no role in T and B cell development. J Immunol 152:3378–3390
91. Getahun A, Hjelm F, Heyman B (2005) IgE enhances antibody and T cell responses in vivo via CD23+ B cells. J Immunol 175:1473–1482
92. Texido G, Eibel H, Le Gros G, van der Putten H (1994) Transgene CD23 expression on lymphoid cells modulates IgE and IgG1 responses. J Immunol 153:3028–3042

93. Payet M, Conrad DH (1999) IgE regulation in CD23 knockout and transgenic mice. Allergy 54:1125–1129
94. Cho SW, Kilmon MA, Studer EJ, van der Putten H, Conrad DH (1997) B cell activation and Ig, especially IgE, production is inhibited by high CD23 levels in vivo and in vitro. Cell Immunol 180:36–46
95. Carlsson F, Hjelm F, Conrad DH, Heyman B (2007) IgE enhances specific antibody and T-cell responses in mice overexpressing CD23. Scand J Immunol 66:261–270
96. Lewis G, Rapsomaniki E, Bouriez T, Crockford T, Ferry H, Rigby R, Vyse T, Lambe T, Cornall R (2004) Hyper IgE in New Zealand black mice due to a dominant-negative CD23 mutation. Immunogenetics 56:564–571
97. Flores-Romo L, Shields J, Humbert Y, Graber P, Aubry JP, Gauchat JF, Ayala G, Allet B, Chavez M, Bazin H (1993) Inhibition of an in vivo antigen-specific IgE response by antibodies to CD23. Science 261:1038–1041
98. Kilmon MA, Ghirlando R, Strub MP, Beavil RL, Gould HJ, Conrad DH (2001) Regulation of IgE production requires oligomerization of CD23. J Immunol 167:3139–3145
99. Nakamura T, Kloetzer WS, Brams P, Hariharan K, Chamat S, Cao X, LaBarre MJ, Chinn PC, Morena RA, Shestowsky WS, Li YP, Chen A, Reff ME (2000) In vitro IgE inhibition in B cells by anti-CD23 monoclonal antibodies is functionally dependent on the immunoglobulin Fc domain. Int J Immunopharmacol 22:131–141
100. Sherr E, Macy E, Kimata H, Gilly M, Saxon A (1989) Binding the low affinity Fc epsilon R on B cells suppresses ongoing human IgE synthesis. J Immunol 142:481–489
101. Munoz O, Brignone C, Grenier-Brossette N, Bonnefoy JY, Cousin JL (1998) Binding of anti-CD23 monoclonal antibody to the leucine zipper motif of FcepsilonRII/CD23 on B cell membrane promotes its proteolytic cleavage. Evidence for an effect on the oligomer/monomer equilibrium. J Biol Chem 273:31795–31800
102. Wakai M, Pasley P, Sthoeger ZM, Posnett DN, Brooks R, Hashimoto S, Chiorazzi N (1993) Anti-CD23 monoclonal antibodies: comparisons of epitope specificities and modulating capacities for IgE binding and production. Hybridoma 12:25–43
103. Ford JW, Kilmon MA, Haas KM, Shelburne AE, Chan-Li Y, Conrad DH (2006) In vivo murine CD23 destabilization enhances CD23 shedding and IgE synthesis. Cell Immunol 243:107–117
104. Aubry JP, Pochon S, Graber P, Jansen KU, Bonnefoy JY (1992) CD21 is a ligand for CD23 and regulates IgE production. Nature 358:505–507
105. Christie G, Barton A, Bolognese B, Buckle DR, Cook RM, Hansbury MJ, Harper GP, Marshall LA, McCord ME, Moulder K, Murdock PR, Seal SM, Spackman VM, Weston BJ, Mayer RJ (1997) IgE secretion is attenuated by an inhibitor of proteolytic processing of CD23 (Fc epsilonRII). Eur J Immunol 27:3228–3235
106. McCloskey N, Hunt J, Beavil RL, Jutton MR, Grundy GJ, Girardi E, Fabiane SM, Fear DJ, Conrad DH, Sutton BJ, Gould HJ (2007) Soluble CD23 Monomers Inhibit and Oligomers Stimulate IGE Synthesis in Human B Cells. J Biol Chem 282:24083–24091
107. Hibbert RG, Teriete P, Grundy GJ, Beavil RL, Reljic R, Holers VM, Hannan JP, Sutton BJ, Gould HJ, McDonnell JM (2005) The structure of human CD23 and its interactions with IgE and CD21. J Exp Med 202:751–760
108. Gauld SB, Benschop RJ, Merrell KT, Cambier JC (2005) Maintenance of B cell anergy requires constant antigen receptor occupancy and signaling. Nat Immunol 6:1160–1167
109. McHeyzer-Williams LJ, Malherbe LP, McHeyzer-Williams MG (2006) Checkpoints in memory B-cell evolution. Immunol Rev 211:255–268
110. Grupp SA, Campbell K, Mitchell RN, Cambier JC, Abbas AK (1993) Signaling-defective mutants of the B lymphocyte antigen receptor fail to associate with Ig-alpha and Ig-beta/gamma. J Biol Chem 268:25776–25779
111. Shaw AC, Mitchell RN, Weaver YK, Campos-Torres J, Abbas AK, Leder P (1990) Mutations of immunoglobulin transmembrane and cytoplasmic domains: effects on intracellular signaling and antigen presentation. Cell 63:381–392

112. Batista FD, Efremov DG, Burrone OR (1995) Characterization and expression of alternatively spliced IgE heavy chain transcripts produced by peripheral blood lymphocytes. J Immunol 154:209–218
113. Peng C, Davis FM, Sun LK, Liou RS, Kim YW, Chang TW (1992) A new isoform of human membrane-bound IgE. J Immunol 148:129–136
114. Zhang K, Saxon A, Max EE (1992) Two unusual forms of human immunoglobulin E encoded by alternative RNA splicing of epsilon heavy chain membrane exons. J Exp Med 176:233–243
115. Poggianella M, Bestagno M, Burrone OR (2006) The extracellular membrane-proximal domain of human membrane IgE controls apoptotic signaling of the B cell receptor in the mature B cell line A20. J Immunol 177:3597–3605
116. Batista FD, Anand S, Presani G, Efremov DG, Burrone OR (1996) The two membrane isoforms of human IgE assemble into functionally distinct B cell antigen receptors. J Exp Med 184:2197–2205
117. Venkitaraman AR, Williams GT, Dariavach P, Neuberger MS (1991) The B-cell antigen receptor of the five immunoglobulin classes. Nature 352:777–781
118. Lam KP, Kuhn R, Rajewsky K (1997) In vivo ablation of surface immunoglobulin on mature B cells by inducible gene targeting results in rapid cell death. Cell 90:1073–1083
119. Patel KJ, Neuberger MS (1993) Antigen presentation by the B cell antigen receptor is driven by the alpha/beta sheath and occurs independently of its cytoplasmic tyrosines. Cell 74: 939–946
120. Kaisho T, Schwenk F, Rajewsky K (1997) The roles of gamma 1 heavy chain membrane expression and cytoplasmic tail in IgG1 responses. Science 276:412–415
121. Sato M, Adachi T, Tsubata T (2007) Augmentation of signaling through BCR containing IgE but not that containing IgA due to lack of CD22-mediated signal regulation. J Immunol 178:2901–2907
122. Wakabayashi C, Adachi T, Wienands J, Tsubata T (2002) A distinct signaling pathway used by the IgG-containing B cell antigen receptor. Science 298:2392–2395
123. Ravetch JV, Lanier LL (2000) Immune inhibitory receptors. Science 290:84–89
124. Oberndorfer I, Schmid D, Geisberger R, Achatz-Straussberger G, Crameri R, Lamers M, Achatz G (2006) HS1-associated protein X-1 interacts with membrane-bound IgE: impact on receptor-mediated internalization. J Immunol 177:1139–1145
125. Erazo A, Kutchukhidze N, Leung M, Christ AP, Urban JF, Jr., Curotto de Lafaille MA, Lafaille JJ (2007) Unique maturation program of the IgE response in vivo. Immunity 26:191–203
126. Shapiro-Shelef M, Lin KI, McHeyzer-Williams LJ, Liao J, McHeyzer-Williams MG, Calame K (2003) Blimp-1 is required for the formation of immunoglobulin secreting plasma cells and pre-plasma memory B cells. Immunity 19:607–620
127. Kelly KA, Butch AW (2007) Antigen-specific immunoglobulin E+ B cells are preferentially localized within germinal centres. Immunology 120:345–353
128. Auci DL, Chice SM, Heusser C, Athanassiades TJ, Durkin HG (1992) Origin and fate of IgE-bearing lymphocytes. II. Gut-associated lymphoid tissue as sites of first appearance of IgE-bearing B lymphocytes and hapten-specific IgE antibody-forming cells in mice immunized with benzylpenicilloyl-keyhole limpet hemocyanin by various routes: relation to asialo GM1 ganglioside+ cells and IgE/CD23 immune complexes. J Immunol 149:2241–2248
129. Wang CH, Richards EM, Block RD, Lezcano EM, Gutierrez R (1998) Early induction and augmentation of parasitic antigen-specific antibody-producing B lymphocytes in the non-Peyer's patch region of the small intestine. Front Biosci 3:A58–65
130. Galli G, Guise J, Tucker PW, Nevins JR (1988) Poly(A) site choice rather than splice site choice governs the regulated production of IgM heavy-chain RNAs. Proc Natl Acad Sci USA 85:2439–2443
131. Gerster T, Picard D, Schaffner W (1986) During B-cell differentiation enhancer activity and transcription rate of immunoglobulin heavy chain genes are high before mRNA accumulation. Cell 45:45–52

132. Phillips C, Jung S, Gunderson SI (2001) Regulation of nuclear poly(A) addition controls the expression of immunoglobulin M secretory mRNA. EMBO J 20:6443–6452
133. Christofori G, Keller W (1988) 3′ cleavage and polyadenylation of mRNA precursors in vitro requires a poly(A) polymerase, a cleavage factor, and a snRNP. Cell 54:875–889
134. Gilmartin GM, Nevins JR (1989) An ordered pathway of assembly of components required for polyadenylation site recognition and processing. Genes Dev 3:2180–2190
135. Takagaki Y, Ryner LC, Manley JL (1989) Four factors are required for 3′-end cleavage of pre-mRNAs. Genes Dev 3:1711–1724
136. Takagaki Y, Manley JL, MacDonald CC, Wilusz J, Shenk T (1990) A multisubunit factor, CstF, is required for polyadenylation of mammalian pre-mRNAs. Genes Dev 4:2112–2120
137. Murthy KG, Manley JL (1995) The 160-kD subunit of human cleavage-polyadenylation specificity factor coordinates pre-mRNA 3′-end formation. Genes Dev 9:2672–2683
138. Murthy KG, Manley JL (1992) Characterization of the multisubunit cleavage-polyadenylation specificity factor from calf thymus. J Biol Chem 267:14804–14811
139. Keller W, Bienroth S, Lang KM, Christofori G (1991) Cleavage and polyadenylation factor CPF specifically interacts with the pre-mRNA 3′ processing signal AAUAAA. Embo J 10: 4241–4249
140. Beyer K, Dandekar T, Keller W (1997) RNA ligands selected by cleavage stimulation factor contain distinct sequence motifs that function as downstream elements in 3′-end processing of pre-mRNA. J Biol Chem 272:26769–26779
141. Takagaki Y, Manley JL (1997) RNA recognition by the human polyadenylation factor CstF. Mol Cell Biol 17:3907–3914
142. MacDonald CC, Wilusz J, Shenk T (1994) The 64-kilodalton subunit of the CstF polyadenylation factor binds to pre-mRNAs downstream of the cleavage site and influences cleavage site location. Mol Cell Biol 14:6647–6654
143. Wahle E, Lustig A, Jeno P, Maurer P (1993) Mammalian poly(A)-binding protein II. Physical properties and binding to polynucleotides. J Biol Chem 268:2937–2945
144. Wahle E, Keller W (1996) The biochemistry of polyadenylation. Trends Biochem Sci 21:247–250
145. Raabe T, Bollum FJ, Manley JL (1991) Primary structure and expression of bovine poly(A) polymerase. Nature 353:229–234
146. Moreira A, Takagaki Y, Brackenridge S, Wollerton M, Manley JL, Proudfoot NJ (1998) The upstream sequence element of the C2 complement poly(A) signal activates mRNA 3′ end formation by two distinct mechanisms. Genes Dev 12:2522–2534
147. Takagaki Y, Seipelt RL, Peterson ML, Manley JL (1996) The polyadenylation factor CstF-64 regulates alternative processing of IgM heavy chain pre-mRNA during B cell differentiation. Cell 87:941–952
148. Galli G, Guise JW, McDevitt MA, Tucker PW, Nevins JR (1987) Relative position and strengths of poly(A) sites as well as transcription termination are critical to membrane versus secreted mu-chain expression during B-cell development. Genes Dev 1:471–481
149. Guise JW, Lim PL, Yuan D, Tucker PW (1988) Alternative expression of secreted and membrane forms of immunoglobulin mu-chain is regulated by transcriptional termination in stable plasmacytoma transfectants. J Immunol 140:3988–3994
150. Yan DH, Weiss EA, Nevins JR (1995) Identification of an activity in B-cell extracts that selectively impairs the formation of an immunoglobulin mu s poly(A) site processing complex. Mol Cell Biol 15:1901–1906
151. Flaspohler JA, Milcarek C (1990) Myelomas and lymphomas expressing the Ig gamma 2a H chain gene have similar transcription termination regions. J Immunol 144:2802–2810
152. Flaspohler JA, Boczkowski D, Hall BL, Milcarek C (1995) The 3′-untranslated region of membrane exon 2 from the gamma 2a immunoglobulin gene contributes to efficient transcription termination. J Biol Chem 270:11903–11911
153. Lebman DA, Park MJ, Fatica R, Zhang Z (1992) Regulation of usage of membrane and secreted 3′ termini of alpha mRNA differs from mu mRNA. J Immunol 148: 3282–3289

154. Edwalds-Gilbert G, Veraldi KL, Milcarek C (1997) Alternative poly(A) site selection in complex transcription units: means to an end? Nucleic Acids Res 25:2547–2561
155. Coyle JH, Lebman DA (2000) Correct immunoglobulin alpha mRNA processing depends on specific sequence in the C alpha 3-alpha M intron. J Immunol 164:3659–3665
156. Anand S, Batista FD, Tkach T, Efremov DG, Burrone OR (1997) Multiple transcripts of the murine immunoglobulin epsilon membrane locus are generated by alternative splicing and differential usage of two polyadenylation sites. Mol Immunol 34:175–183
157. Batista FD, Efremov DG, Burrone OR (1996) Characterization of a second secreted IgE isoform and identification of an asymmetric pathway of IgE assembly. Proc Natl Acad Sci USA 93:3399–3404
158. Manz RA, Hauser AE, Hiepe F, Radbruch A (2005) Maintenance of serum antibody levels. Annu Rev Immunol 23:367–386
159. Manz RA, Lohning M, Cassese G, Thiel A, Radbruch A (1998) Survival of long-lived plasma cells is independent of antigen. Int Immunol 10:1703–1711
160. Manz RA, Thiel A, Radbruch A (1997) Lifetime of plasma cells in the bone marrow. Nature 388:133–134
161. Holt PG, Sedgwick JD, O'Leary C, Krska K, Leivers S (1984) Long-lived IgE- and IgG-secreting cells in rodents manifesting persistent antibody responses. Cell Immunol 89: 281–289
162. Hoyer BF, Moser K, Hauser AE, Peddinghaus A, Voigt C, Eilat D, Radbruch A, Hiepe F, Manz RA (2004) Short-lived plasmablasts and long-lived plasma cells contribute to chronic humoral autoimmunity in NZB/W mice. J Exp Med 199:1577–1584
163. Hauser AE, Debes GF, Arce S, Cassese G, Hamann A, Radbruch A, Manz RA (2002) Chemotactic responsiveness toward ligands for CXCR3 and CXCR4 is regulated on plasma blasts during the time course of a memory immune response. J Immunol 169:1277–1282
164. Hauser AE, Muehlinghaus G, Manz RA, Cassese G, Arce S, Debes GF, Hamann A, Berek C, Lindenau S, Doerner T, Hiepe F, Odendahl M, Riemekasten G, Krenn V, Radbruch A (2003) Long-lived plasma cells in immunity and inflammation. Ann N Y Acad Sci 987:266–269
165. Hargreaves DC, Hyman PL, Lu TT, Ngo VN, Bidgol A, Suzuki G, Zou YR, Littman DR, Cyster JG (2001) A coordinated change in chemokine responsiveness guides plasma cell movements. J Exp Med 194:45–56
166. Muehlinghaus G, Cigliano L, Huehn S, Peddinghaus A, Leyendeckers H, Hauser AE, Hiepe F, Radbruch A, Arce S, Manz RA (2005) Regulation of CXCR3 and CXCR4 expression during terminal differentiation of memory B cells into plasma cells. Blood 105:3965–3971
167. Achatz-Straussberger G, Zaborsky N, Konigsberger S, Luger EO, Lamers M, Crameri R, Achatz G (2008) Migration of antibody secreting cells towards CXCL12 depends on the isotype that forms the BCR. Eur J Immunol 38:3167–3177
168. Leffell MS, Donnenberg AD, Rose NR. Handbook of Human Immunology. 1 ed. Boca Raton FL: CRC Press, 1997
169. Peppard JV, Orlans E (1980) The biological half-lives of four rat immunoglobulin isotypes. Immunology 40:683–686
170. Medesan C, Cianga P, Mummert M, Stanescu D, Ghetie V, Ward ES (1998) Comparative studies of rat IgG to further delineate the Fc:FcRn interaction site. Eur J Immunol 28: 2092–2100

Chapter 3
The Biology of IgE: The Generation of High-Affinity IgE Antibodies

Maria A. Curotto de Lafaille and Juan J. Lafaille

Abstract B cells can undergo affinity maturation through the process of somatic hypermutation (SHM) followed by selection for high-affinity variants. Affinity maturation occurs in germinal centers (GC) and requires T–B cell cooperation. Extra GC B-cell responses are associated with the production of low-affinity antibodies. B cells producing high-affinity IgE during T-dependent responses are not directly selected in GC but are produced by the sequential switching of GC-selected high-affinity IgG-producing B cells. In contrast, natural low-affinity IgE can be generated without cognate T–B cell interactions in lymphopenic conditions. Low- and high-affinity IgE may differentially affect mast cell survival and degranulation and thus determine whether mast cells contribute to a beneficial or pathogenic environment.

3.1 High-Affinity Versus Low-Affinity IgE Antibodies

B cells can undergo affinity maturation, a process that essentially entails two steps: (1) somatic hypermutation (SHM) of the immunoglobulin genes and (2) selection of the B cells displaying high-affinity variants. Years of evidence have established that affinity maturation occurs in GC. Affinity maturation results in antibodies displaying high-affinity binding for their ligands. However, not all antibody responses undergo affinity maturation, and low-affinity antibodies are also part of some immune responses.

"Natural" IgE antibodies recognize natural antigens such as phosphoryl choline and do not undergo affinity maturation; they are low-affinity IgE antibodies. Importantly, these low-affinity IgE antibodies can be generated without cognate T cell–B cell interactions and without GC, although their generation, like the generation of high-affinity IgE antibodies, is strictly IL-4 dependent [1]. Although the occurrence of natural IgE antibodies have been only demonstrated in conditions of lymphopenia in mice, it is likely that, in a normal individual exposed to antigens

---

M.A. Curotto de Lafaille (✉)
Molecular Pathogenesis Program, The Kimmel Center for Biology and Medicine of the Skirball Institute and Department of Pathology, New York University Scholl of Medicine, New York, NY, USA
e-mail: maria.lafaille@med.nyu.edu

M.L. Penichet, E. Jensen-Jarolim (eds.), *Cancer and IgE*,
DOI 10.1007/978-1-60761-451-7_3,

and allergens, the IgE compartment contains a mixture of natural low-affinity IgE antibodies and cognate T cell–B cell interaction-driven high-affinity IgE antibodies.

As we will discuss in detail later, high-affinity IgE antibodies are generated though a unique developmental pathway that entails the generation of high-affinity IgG1 cells in GC, followed by sequential switching of the IgG1$^+$ cells to IgE. Thus, the affinity maturation of the IgE response occurs during the IgG1 phase that precedes sequential switching. Cognate T cell–B cell interactions are essential for the generation of high-affinity IgE antibodies [2].

The functional differences between high- and low-affinity IgE antibodies are highly significant. High-affinity antibodies can be cross-linked by minute amounts of multivalent antigen, whereas low-affinity antibodies require a much higher antigen concentration of such antigens. Thus, antigens can easily cross-link B cells that display high-affinity membrane antibodies. High level of cross-linking of FcεRI receptors results in mast cell degranulation as well as cytokine/chemokine secretion by mast cells, whereas low level of cross-linking leads to cytokine and chemokine secretion by mast cells, but no degranulation [3, 4]. Furthermore, Yamasaki et al. expressed CD8/FcRγ chimeric molecules on mast cells from FcRγ-deficient mice (FcRγ is one of the components of FcεRI, also of CD16 and CD64). Strong cross-linking of the CD8/FcRγ chimeric receptor with anti-CD8 antibodies induced mast cell survival and degranulation, whereas weaker stimulation (in terms of anti-CD8 concentration and valency) resulted in survival but not degranulation [4]. As indicated above, cytokines such as IL-3 are produced by mast cells and are important for their own survival. Thus, both high- and low-affinity IgE antibodies are equally capable of carrying out the beneficial effect of IgE on mast cells. However, because of their differential affinity and specificity, the allergen-mediated cross-linking of IgE antibodies bound to FcεRI molecules can only be carried out by high-affinity IgE antibodies, which are driven by cognate T–B interactions. In targeting IgE response against cancer cells, it is important that this IgE response be of high affinity.

3.2 Switching to IgE and Its Control in B Lymphocytes

Of all secreted immunoglobulins, IgE is found at the lowest concentration in normal individuals, suggesting that the production of IgE is strongly regulated. Atopic diseases are characterized by the production of IgE antibodies to common non-infectious environmental or food proteins. The production of allergen-specific IgE antibodies is highly dependent on cognate T cell–B cell interactions involving the co-stimulatory molecules CD40/CD40L and on the cytokine IL-4 [5, 6]. Atopy is also associated with, and depends on, the presence of allergen-specific Th2 lymphocytes.

Naïve B cells express the constant region of IgM; switching to other constant regions (generating IgGs, IgE or IgA) is brought about by B-cell activation. B-cell stimulation with anti-CD40 + IL-4, soluble CD40L + IL-4, LPS + IL-4, or cognate

interaction with Th2 cells leads to IgG1 and IgE class switching in vitro. However, even under these favorable conditions, the percentage of cells switching to IgE is low compared to the percentage of cells switching to IgG1.

Class switching to IgE is preceded by the production of germline transcripts driven by the IL-4-responsive Iε promoter. Replacement of the Iε promoter and exon with an enhancer/promoter active in all B cells lead to constitutive expression of the Cε germline transcript and IL-4-independent switching to IgE [7], and downregulation of Iε transcription caused a reduction in IgE switching [8]. Activation of the Iε promoter requires binding of phosphorylated STAT6, NF-kB, Pax5, C/EBP, PU.1, and E2A transcription factors [5, 6, 9]. Switching ultimately occurs through recombination between S regions, repetitive sequences located 5′ of the first exon encoding the constant region (Fig. 3.1, S regions depicted in elliptical shape). Switching, thus, entails DNA recombination and is often abbreviated as CSR (class switch recombination, reviewed in [10–12]).

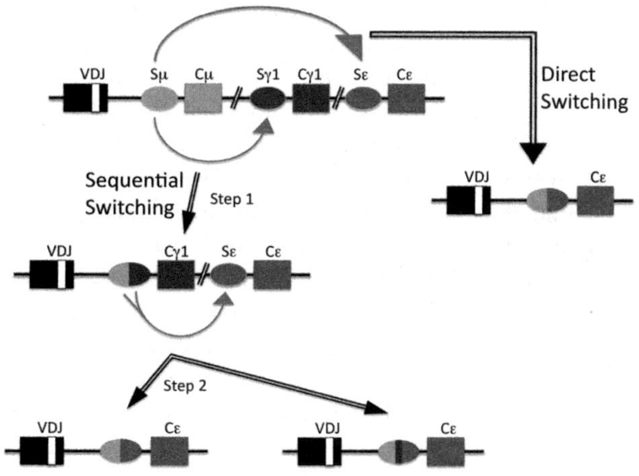

Fig. 3.1 Direct and sequential switching to IgE. Schematic representation of direct (IgM to IgE) and sequential (IgM to IgG1 to IgE) class switching to IgE. The figure depicts in simplified manner relevant elements of the heavy chain immunoglobulin locus: the rearranged VDJ gene, the switch regions (Sμ, Sγ1 and Sε) and the constant region genes (Cμ, Cγ1 and Cε)

Germline transcription of IgE and IgG1 in activated B cells can be inhibited by the combination of the cytokines IL-12 and IL-18 [13], IFN-γ [8, 14], TGF-β, bacterial CpG-rich sequences [15], or expression of the proto oncogene Bcl-6 [16]. IL-21 and Id2 also display inhibitory effects on IgE switching. IL-21 will be discussed later in the proposal. Id2 is a transcription factor of the Id family that is involved in the negative regulation of E proteins. Id2-deficient mice have increased IgE levels in serum, and Id2-deficient B cells preferentially switch to IgE in vitro. Id2 is induced by TGF-β in B lymphocytes and suppresses germline Iε transcription by interacting with E2A and Pax5 and inhibiting their DNA binding to the Iε promoter [9].

A recent study by the Mohrs laboratory showed beyond doubt that, under very strong Th2 stimulation such as the one triggered by helminth parasites, IgE could be induced in μMT KO mice, which lack mature B cells [17]. However, no IgE was generated in worm-infected J_H-deficient mice. μMT KO mice have a developmental defect that occasionally can be overcome by expression of other isotypes [18, 19], whereas rearrangement to J_H is physically obligatory for the generation of all immunoglobulins and cannot be overcome. Nevertheless, the result by Mohrs and colleagues indicates that, under strong stimulation, IgE antibodies can be generated without even a membrane IgM^+ cell phase (please see the section below for more discussion).

3.3 Sequential Switching to IgE in Mice and Humans

In mice and humans, the ε locus is downstream the γ loci (Fig. 3.1 is a schematic representation of the mouse locus). In humans there is a duplication of the heavy chain locus that is not found in the mouse. Analysis of the excision circles that occur upon CSR led to the surprising but now indisputable discovery that the switching to IgE in mouse B cells could occur sequentially, that is first a switch from IgM to IgG1, followed by a switch from IgG1 to IgE [20]. Soon after that, Mills et al. found that the switch to ε in a human lymphoid cell line was preceded by a Sμ-Sγ recombination [21]. There have been many subsequent reports in both human and mouse IgE cells [22]. Analysis of the murine chromosomal product Sμ-Sε showed that 30% of the recombined switch regions contained Sγ1 sequences, which represented remnants of a previous switch to γ1 [23]. As shown in Fig. 3.1, this frequency underestimates the real frequency of sequential switching, as many sequentially switched cells do not have an Sγ remnant (bottom left panel in Fig. 3.1 lacks IgG1 remnants, while bottom center panel in Fig. 3.1 retains a small segment of Sγ1 sequence, colored in blue, even though both are generated through sequential switching). In humans, the situation is more complex. Although IgG4 remnants (human IgG4 is considered the equivalent of mouse IgG1) have been found in IgE^+ cells [24], remnants of other IgGs have also been described [25, 26]. Incontrovertible evidence for direct IgM to IgE switching in humans, collected through the study of excised circles, has been presented [27], but the quantitative comparison of direct versus sequential switching is lacking. Despite the complexity of the situation in humans, the frequency of sequentially switched IgE is roughly the same, with 11 of 40 sequences (27.5%) obtained from patients with schistosomiasis showing IgG remnants [26]. As stated above, both mouse and human studies underestimate the proportion incidence of sequential switching. Importantly, all these molecular data did not address whether sequential switching from IgG1 to IgE occurred immediately or there was a true IgG1 phase on the life of these IgE^+ cells. Below we review the data indicating that a distinct IgG1 cellular phase can occur in cells that later will become IgE-producing cells.

3.4 Unique Pathway for the Generation of High-Affinity IgE Antibodies

3.4.1 Summary of Findings

Our data show that IgE^+ cells are exceptional because they are largely found outside germinal centers (GC) and express, from very early on, a genetic program of plasma cells (PCs). In contrast, $IgG1^+$ cells are found in GC and express genes characteristic of the GC stage. In spite of their extra-GC localization and PC phenotype, IgE^+ cells show signs of SHM and affinity maturation. Our data show that high-affinity IgE^+ cells are generated through a unique differentiation program that involves two phases: (1) a pre-IgE-switching phase in which a GC reaction involving SHM and affinity maturation takes place in $IgG1^+$ cells; (2) after sequential switching of high-affinity $IgG1^+$ cells to IgE, a post-IgE-switching phase in which IgE cells differentiate swiftly into PCs [28].

In contrast to high-affinity IgE antibodies, low-affinity IgE antibodies are generated outside GC, by direct switching from IgM to IgE. A model of high-affinity IgE versus low-affinity IgE generation is shown in Fig. 3.2. The data that were used to put together the model will be summarized in subsequent paragraphs. Further support for the model in Fig. 3.2 comes from the publication by Zinkernagel's lab in which the generation of natural IgE antibodies (which are low-affinity, poorly mutated antibodies) do not require the presence of organized secondary lymphoid tissue [1].

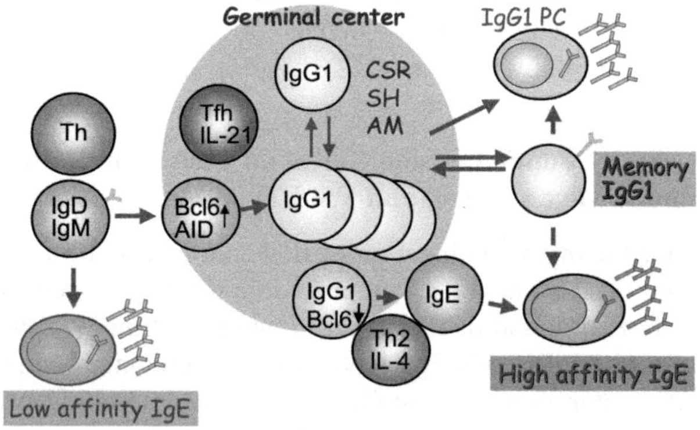

Fig. 3.2 A model of the differentiation of IgE^+ cells in vivo. B lymphocytes in the germinal centers (GC) upregulate Bcl-6, switch to IgG1 and undergo SHM and affinity maturation. Follicular helper T cells (Tfh) provide an IL-21-rich environment in the GC. Bcl-6 expression and signaling through the IL-21R inhibit class switching to IgE in most GC cells. Class switching to IgE can occur in GC cells that downregulate Bcl-6 function, and interact with Th cells in a high IL-4 and low IL-21 microenvironment. Switching to IgE is linked to a pathway of exit from the GC and differentiation to plasma cell. CSR, class switch recombination; SHM, somatic hypermutation; AM, affinity maturation; PB, plasmablast; PC, plasma cell; MC, memory cell

3.4.2 *Experimental Evidence*

The unique pathway involved in the generation of the high-affinity IgE response was uncovered using two mouse models of high IgE response. The first model consists of immunization of T-cell receptor transgenic B-cell knock-in mice, named T-Bmc mice [2]. The second model consists on the infection of wild-type BALB/c mice with the helminth parasite *Nippostrongylus brasiliensis* (Nb) [29, 30]. T-Bmc carry anti-chicken ovalbumin (OVA) T-cell receptor transgenes and anti-influenza hemagglutinin (HA) knocked in B-cell receptor genes on a RAG1-deficient background. The use of T-Bmc enables the tracking of antigen-specific B cells, while the helminth infection of wild-type mice allows the analysis of a broad repertoire response in a non-manipulated immune system.

Even with the availability of these two experimental systems, a technical difficulty remained that hampered the study of the IgE response in vivo. Every time there is a high IgE response, flow cytometry analysis using anti-IgE antibodies indicate the vast majority of B cells appear to be IgE$^+$ cells, even though molecular analysis show that the vast majority of these cells are not genuine IgE producers. This generalized false-positive result is due to the expression of CD23, the low-affinity ligand for IgE, by B cells. Circulating IgE antibodies, when present at high concentrations, bind via CD23 to genuine IgE$^+$ cells as well as IgE$^-$ cells, which are most B cells even in the midst of a hyper IgE response. The technical key to overcome the problems in studying IgE$^+$ cells was the use of a mild acid treatment that removes the cytophilic IgE antibodies that bind B cells via CD23 [28]. Now the experimental systems and the methodology were in place to reliably study the generation of the high-affinity IgE response in vivo.

These technical advantages enabled us to reach the following conclusions regarding the generation of the IgE response. What follows is a summary of the main findings in the manuscript by Erazo et al. [28].

3.4.2.1 IgE$^+$ Cells are Found Outside Germinal Centers in Both T/B Monoclonal Mice (T-Bmc) and Wild-Type Mice

This was concluded using a combination of flow cytometry and immunohistology techniques. At no time point after immunization were IgE$^+$ cells found in GC. Instead, IgE$^+$ cells were found in alternative locations within the spleen and lymph nodes. In contrast with IgE$^+$ cells, IgG1$^+$ cells were found mainly in GC. Although SHM and affinity maturation occur in GC, our findings do not imply that the IgE response is of low affinity, as we will discuss below.

3.4.2.2 IgE Antibodies Undergo Somatic Hypermutation and Affinity Maturation

The lack of GC localization of IgE$^+$ cells, together with their low or absent Bcl-6 and AID expression, raised the question of whether IgE antibodies did undergo SHM and affinity maturation. To study affinity maturation of IgE$^+$ cells, we used a variant

peptide that is recognized by the B cells in T-Bmc mice only after affinity maturation of the IgE response. Indeed, upon repeated immunizations we found IgE^+ cells that could bind to the variant peptide. Furthermore, the sequence of VDJ genes in the variant peptide-binding IgE^+ cells indicated the presence of three mutations whose presence confers high-affinity binding to the variant peptide.

It was interesting to note that variant peptide-specific antibody titers of both IgG1 and IgE increased over time, with the plateau in IgE titers lagging behind the plateau of IgG1 titers. In addition, IgG1 antibody genes displayed higher frequency of DNA mutations in the VDJ than IgE antibody genes from the same mice. Thus, the high-affinity IgE response lags behind the IgG1 response.

3.4.2.3 $IgG1^+$ B Cells can Generate IgE Antibodies by Sequential Switching

Up to this point our results had demonstrated that high-affinity IgE antibodies were produced during a Th2-mediated response in vivo, but a GC phase for IgE^+ cells could not be visualized, generating a potential paradox. Based on these results, and on previous findings of IgG1 switch region remnants on IgE^+ cells which demonstrated sequential switching from μ to $\gamma1$ to ε [20], we hypothesized that IgE^+ cells may not undergo SHM and affinity maturation, but rather they could inherit mutated and selected VDJ genes from precursor $IgG1^+$ cells. While molecular evidence supporting the existence of sequential switching was abundant, it was equally clear that sequential switching was not obligatory for all IgE responses [31]. Furthermore, it was possible that the second step of sequential switching ($\gamma1$ to ε) occurred immediately after the first step (μ to $\gamma1$) due to the simultaneous presence of both $\gamma1$ and ε sterile transcripts, without involving an $IgG1^+$ cellular phase. It was thus unknown whether cells with a memory $IgG1^+$ phenotype could give rise to IgE^+ cells. To test whether or not memory $IgG1^+$ cells could give rise to IgE^+ cells by sequential switching in vivo, we sorted $B220^+Fas^+IgG1^+IgD^-$ and $B220^+Fas^+IgG1^-IgD^-$ B cells from mice immunized with a variant peptide that does not bind to B cells in T-Bmc mice unless the B cells undergo affinity maturation. Sorted B cells were transferred together with naïve anti-OVA $CD4^+$ T cells into T-cell-deficient mice, and the recipient mice were immunized once with the variant peptide. Strikingly, a high-affinity IgE response could be detected only in sera from mice that received the $IgG1^+$ B-cell population. In the recipient mice, IgE molecules that, by the experimental design, must be derived from the transferred $IgG1^+$ cells carried affinity-enhancing somatic mutations, albeit at lower frequency than IgG1 molecules. These results confirmed that $IgG1^+$ cells can generate high-affinity IgE antibodies via sequential switching in vivo.

3.4.2.4 Interleukin-21 Inhibits the Sequential Switching of $IgG1^+$ Cells to IgE, Thus Inhibiting the High-Affinity IgE Response

While sequential switching to IgE was profoundly suppressed by IL-21, IgG1 production was not. The effect of IL-21 in the low-affinity IgE response was not determined. In GC, IL-21 is produced by follicular helper T cells (Tfh) [32–36].

Although there is disagreement as to some of the many functions of IL-21 (for instance it has been reported that IL-21 induces B-cell death and that it does not induce B-cell death), it has been reported that in vivo injection of IL-21 prevents antigen-specific IgE but not IgG2a production upon immunization [37]. Furthermore, IL-21R-deficient mice have higher production of IgE, but lower IgG1, than wild-type animals [38]. The inhibitory effect of IL-21 on IgE is interesting in that it affects ε but not $\gamma 1$ germline transcription. The mechanism by which IL-21 inhibits ε germline transcription remains unknown; however, it does not involve inhibition of STAT-6 or NF-κB activation [37] (Fig. 3.2). $IgG1^+$ cells from GC phase were able to produce much higher IgE in response to stimulation in short-time cultures (days 2–5) than purified IgD^+ cells from naïve or immunized mice. Production of IgE was dependent on stimulation with anti-CD40 antibodies and IL-4 since no IgE was produced in unstimulated cultures, or cultures stimulated with anti-CD40 antibodies and no cytokines. These results can be explained by "de novo" production of IgE by sequential switching of IgG1 cells to IgE in the in vitro cultures. The results are the first demonstration that IL-21 can inhibit the sequential switching of GC $IgG1^+$ B lymphocytes to IgE.

3.5 Conclusion

In this manuscript we proposed the hypothesis that high-affinity and low-affinity IgE antibodies are generated through different pathways (Fig. 3.2). High-affinity antibodies can be generated through sequential switching, whereas low-affinity antibodies are generated through direct switching, not involving a GC phase (Fig. 3.2). The existence of different pathways for IgE generation predicts that inhibitors of each of the pathways could be developed to bias the response toward high- or low-affinity IgE. For cancer immunotherapy, the generation of high-affinity antibodies is advantageous; therefore, a selective inhibition of the low-affinity IgE pathway could be beneficial.

Acknowledgments The Lafaille laboratory is supported by the NIH/NIAID, the National Multiple Sclerosis Society, the Strategic Program for Asthma Research, and the Crohn's and Colitis Foundation of America.

References

1. K. D. McCoy, N. L. Harris, P. Diener, S. Hatak, B. Odermatt, L. Hangartner, B. M. Senn, B. J. Marsland, M. B. Geuking, H. Hengartner, A. J. Macpherson, R. M. Zinkernagel. Natural IgE production in the absence of MHC Class II cognate help. *Immunity* 24: 329–339, 2006.
2. M. A. Curotto de Lafaille, S. Muriglan, M. J. Sunshine, Y. Lei, N. Kutchukhidze, G. C. Furtado, A. K. Wensky, D. Olivares-Villagomez, J. J. Lafaille. Hyper immunoglobulin E response in mice with monoclonal populations of B and T lymphocytes. *J Exp Med* 194: 1349–1359, 2001.
3. C. Gonzalez-Espinosa, S. Odom, A. Olivera, J. P. Hobson, M. E. Martinez, A. Oliveira-Dos-Santos, L. Barra, S. Spiegel, J. M. Penninger, J. Rivera. Preferential signaling and induction of allergy-promoting lymphokines upon weak stimulation of the high affinity IgE receptor on mast cells. *J Exp Med* 197: 1453–1465, 2003.

4. S. Yamasaki, E. Ishikawa, M. Kohno, T. Saito. The quantity and duration of FcRgamma signals determine mast cell degranulation and survival. *Blood* 103: 3093–3101, 2004.
5. H. C. Oettgen, R. S. Geha. IgE regulation and roles in asthma pathogenesis. *J Allergy Clin Immunol* 107: 429–440, 2001.
6. R. S. Geha, H. H. Jabara, S. R. Brodeur. The regulation of immunoglobulin E class-switch recombination. *Nat Rev Immunol* 3: 721–732, 2003.
7. L. Xu, B. Gorham, S. C. Li, A. Bottaro, F. W. Alt, P. Rothman. Replacement of germ-line epsilon promoter by gene targeting alters control of immunoglobulin heavy chain class switching. *Proc Natl Acad Sci USA* 90: 3705–3709, 1993.
8. L. Xu, P. Rothman. IFN-gamma represses epsilon germline transcription and subsequently down-regulates switch recombination to epsilon. *Int Immunol* 6: 515–521, 1994.
9. M. Sugai, H. Gonda, T. Kusunoki, T. Katakai, Y. Yokota, A. Shimizu. Essential role of Id2 in negative regulation of IgE class switching. *Nat Immunol* 4: 25–30, 2003.
10. J. P. Manis, M. Tian, F. W. Alt. Mechanism and control of class-switch recombination. *Trends Immunol* 23: 31–39, 2002.
11. K. Kinoshita, T. Honjo. Linking class-switch recombination with somatic hypermutation. *Nat Rev Mol Cell Biol* 2: 493–503, 2001.
12. J. A. Fenton, G. Pratt, A. C. Rawstron, G. J. Morgan. Isotype class switching and the pathogenesis of multiple myeloma. *Hematol Oncol* 20: 75–85, 2002.
13. T. Yoshimoto, H. Okamura, Y. I. Tagawa, Y. Iwakura, K. Nakanishi. Interleukin 18 together with interleukin 12 inhibits IgE production by induction of interferon-gamma production from activated B cells. *Proc Natl Acad Sci USA* 94: 3948–3953, 1997.
14. E. Severinson, C. Fernandez, J. Stavnezer. Induction of germ-line immunoglobulin heavy chain transcripts by mitogens and interleukins prior to switch recombination. *Eur J Immunol* 20: 1079–1084, 1990.
15. N. Liu, N. Ohnishi, L. Ni, S. Akira, K. B. Bacon. CpG directly induces T-bet expression and inhibits IgG1 and IgE switching in B cells. *Nat Immunol* 4: 687–693, 2003.
16. M. B. Harris, C. C. Chang, M. T. Berton, N. N. Danial, J. Zhang, D. Kuehner, B. H. Ye, M. Kvatyuk, P. P. Pandolfi, G. Cattoretti, R. Dalla-Favera, P. B. Rothman. Transcriptional repression of Stat6-dependent interleukin-4-induced genes by BCL-6: specific regulation of iepsilon transcription and immunoglobulin E switching. *Mol Cell Biol* 19: 7264–7275, 1999.
17. G. Perona-Wright, K. Mohrs, J. Taylor, C. Zaph, D. Artis, E. J. Pearce, M. Mohrs. Cutting edge: Helminth infection induces IgE in the absence of mu- or delta-chain expression. *J Immunol* 181: 6697–6701, 2008.
18. Z. Orinska, A. Osiak, J. Lohler, E. Bulanova, V. Budagian, I. Horak, S. Bulfone-Paus. Novel B cell population producing functional IgG in the absence of membrane IgM expression. *Eur J Immunol* 32: 3472–3480, 2002.
19. M. Hasan, B. Polic, M. Bralic, S. Jonjic, K. Rajewsky. Incomplete block of B cell development and immunoglobulin production in mice carrying the muMT mutation on the BALB/c background. *Eur J Immunol* 32: 3463–3471, 2002.
20. K. Yoshida, M. Matsuoka, S. Usuda, A. Mori, K. Ishizaka, H. Sakano. Immunoglobulin switch circular DNA in the mouse infected with Nippostrongylus brasiliensis: evidence for successive class switching from mu to epsilon via gamma 1. *Proc Natl Acad Sci USA* 87: 7829–7833, 1990.
21. F. C. Mills, G. Thyphronitis, F. D. Finkelman, E. E. Max. Ig mu-epsilon isotype switch in IL-4-treated human B lymphoblastoid cells. Evidence for a sequential switch. *J Immunol* 149: 1075–1085, 1992.
22. R. Mandler, F. D. Finkelman, A. D. Levine, C. M. Snapper. IL-4 induction of IgE class switching by lipopolysaccharide-activated murine B cells occurs predominantly through sequential switching. *J Immunol* 150: 407–418, 1993.
23. G. Siebenkotten, C. Esser, M. Wabl, A. Radbruch. The murine IgG1/IgE class switch program. *Eur J Immunol* 22: 1827–1834, 1992.

24. H. H. Jabara, R. Loh, N. Ramesh, D. Vercelli, R. S. Geha. Sequential switching from mu to epsilon via gamma 4 in human B cells stimulated with IL-4 and hydrocortisone. *J Immunol* 151: 4528–4533, 1993.
25. F. C. Mills, M. P. Mitchell, N. Harindranath, E. E. Max. Human Ig S gamma regions and their participation in sequential switching to IgE. *J Immunol* 155: 3021–3036, 1995.
26. B. Baskin, K. B. Islam, B. Evengard, L. Emtestam, C. I. Smith. Direct and sequential switching from mu to epsilon in patients with Schistosoma mansoni infection and atopic dermatitis. *Eur J Immunol* 27: 130–135, 1997.
27. K. Zhang, F. C. Mills, A. Saxon. Switch circles from IL-4-directed epsilon class switching from human B lymphocytes. Evidence for direct, sequential, and multiple step sequential switch from mu to epsilon Ig heavy chain gene. *J Immunol* 152: 3427–3435, 1994.
28. A. Erazo, N. Kutchukhidze, M. Leung, A. P. Christ, J. F. Urban, Jr., M. A. Curotto de Lafaille, J. J. Lafaille. Unique maturation program of the IgE response in vivo. *Immunity* 26: 191–203, 2007.
29. I. M. Katona, J. F. Urban, Jr., F. D. Finkelman. The role of L3T4+ and Lyt-2+ T cells in the IgE response and immunity to Nippostrongylus brasiliensis. *J Immunol* 140: 3206–3211, 1988.
30. F. D. Finkelman, J. Holmes, I. M. Katona, J. F. Urban, Jr., M. P. Beckmann, L. S. Park, K. A. Schooley, R. L. Coffman, T. R. Mosmann, W. E. Paul. Lymphokine control of in vivo immunoglobulin isotype selection. *Annu Rev Immunol* 8: 303–333, 1990.
31. S. Jung, G. Siebenkotten, A. Radbruch. Frequency of immunoglobulin E class switching is autonomously determined and independent of prior switching to other classes. *J Exp Med* 179: 2023–2026, 1994.
32. C. G. Vinuesa, S. G. Tangye, B. Moser, C. R. Mackay. Follicular B helper T cells in antibody responses and autoimmunity. *Nat Rev Immunol* 5: 853–865, 2005.
33. P. Schaerli, K. Willimann, A. B. Lang, M. Lipp, P. Loetscher, B. Moser. CXC chemokine receptor 5 expression defines follicular homing T cells with B cell helper function. *J Exp Med* 192: 1553–1562, 2000.
34. D. Breitfeld, L. Ohl, E. Kremmer, J. Ellwart, F. Sallusto, M. Lipp, R. Forster. Follicular B helper T cells express CXC chemokine receptor 5, localize to B cell follicles, and support immunoglobulin production. *J Exp Med* 192: 1545–1552, 2000.
35. T. Chtanova, S. G. Tangye, R. Newton, N. Frank, M. R. Hodge, M. S. Rolph, C. R. Mackay. T follicular helper cells express a distinctive transcriptional profile, reflecting their role as non-Th1/Th2 effector cells that provide help for B cells. *J Immunol* 173: 68–78, 2004.
36. A. U. Rasheed, H. P. Rahn, F. Sallusto, M. Lipp, G. Muller. Follicular B helper T cell activity is confined to CXCR5(hi)ICOS(hi) CD4 T cells and is independent of CD57 expression. *Eur J Immunol* 36: 1892–1903, 2006.
37. A. Suto, H. Nakajima, K. Hirose, K. Suzuki, S. Kagami, Y. Seto, A. Hoshimoto, Y. Saito, D. C. Foster, I. Iwamoto. Interleukin 21 prevents antigen-induced IgE production by inhibiting germ line C(epsilon) transcription of IL-4-stimulated B cells. *Blood* 100: 4565–4573, 2002.
38. K. Ozaki, R. Spolski, C. G. Feng, C. F. Qi, J. Cheng, A. Sher, H. C. Morse, 3rd, C. Liu, P. L. Schwartzberg, W. J. Leonard. A critical role for IL-21 in regulating immunoglobulin production. *Science* 298: 1630–1634, 2002.

Chapter 4
Epidemiological Evidence: IgE, Atopy, and Solid Tumors

Michelle C. Turner

Abstract Epidemiological investigation into a potential relation between a history of allergic disorders, typically characterized by high levels of IgE, and cancer occurrence has been conducted for at least the past five decades. Recently, there is renewed interest in the field, and the literature is expanding rapidly. This chapter summarizes the epidemiological literature examining the potential relation between allergy and cancer, with a particular focus on the most recent contributions to the field. Although the majority of new and previously published studies evaluated self-reported history of specific allergic disorders (asthma, hay fever, eczema), there were also several new studies examining total or allergen-specific IgE antibodies, hospital discharges for allergic conditions, skin prick tested patients, and allergy-related gene polymorphisms in relation to cancer risk. Although there are a number of inverse relations reported, particularly with pancreatic cancer and glioma, there remain a number of methodological considerations. Further research is recommended in order to better understand the nature of a possible inverse relation and possible mechanisms of action with implications for cancer treatment and prevention. Multidisciplinary collaborations between the population and laboratory-based sciences would be particularly useful.

4.1 Introduction

Epidemiological investigation into a potential relation between a history of allergic disorders and cancer occurrence has been conducted for at least the past five decades [1]. Allergic disorders are typically characterized as an abnormal or hyperactive immune response in reaction to exposure to environmental agents or allergens [2]. High levels of immunoglobulin E (IgE) are defining characteristics of such a response [2, 3]. Although allergic disorders are associated with substantial

---

M.C. Turner (✉)
McLaughlin Centre for Population Health Risk Assessment, Institute of Population Health, Faculty of Graduate and Post-Graduate Studies, University of Ottawa, Ottawa, ONT, Canada
e-mail: mturner@uottawa.ca

M.L. Penichet, E. Jensen-Jarolim (eds.), *Cancer and IgE*,
DOI 10.1007/978-1-60761-451-7_4, © Springer Science+Business Media, LLC 2010

morbidity and mortality, a prevailing theory exists to suggest that the presence of allergic disorders may in fact represent a manifestation of an enhanced capacity for immunosurveillance [4, 5].

Recently, there has been renewed interest in the field. Immunosuppressed patients have been found to experience greater cancer rates [6]. Concerns regarding the safety of anti-IgE therapy in the treatment of allergic asthma have also been raised. Due to suggestions of a possible increased cancer risk, it was recently suggested that omalizumab, the therapeutic anti-IgE antibody, not be used in asthma patients with a personal or family history of cancer [3]. Jensen-Jarolim et al. [7] have recently called for a role of IgE antibodies in cancer therapy and prevention. Fu et al. [8] have also suggested a potential therapeutic role for IgE in pancreatic cancer.

Although previous review articles have summarized the state of the epidemiological evidence [1, 9], the literature is expanding rapidly, and an updated synthesis is needed. The purpose of this chapter is to summarize the epidemiological literature examining the potential relation between allergy and cancer, with a particular focus on the most recent contributions to the field. Hematopoietic malignancies are examined separately in Chapter 5.

4.2 Methods

The search strategy was developed to identify previous observational epidemiological studies examining the relation between a personal history of allergic disorders and cancer (excluding hematopoietic malignancies). The search strategy used here served to update our previous review [1]. The OVID MEDLINE (2005 to September week 2 2008) database was searched using the following MeSH headings: exp Hypersensitivity, Immediate/, exp IgE/, exp Neoplasms by Histologic Type/, exp Neoplasms by Site/, and key words: allerg$, atop$, hypersensitiv$, asthma$, hay fever, rhinitis, conjunctivitis, eczema, dermatitis, hives, skin test$, IgE, cancer, tumor, tumour, malignan$, neoplasm$, carcinoma, glioma, meningioma, neuroma, and risk. The search was restricted to human studies and papers written in English. The reference lists of all included original studies were also handsearched in order to identify additional studies not captured by the search strategy. A summary of previous epidemiological studies is presented below ordered by cancer site and study design.

4.3 Results

A total of 32 original epidemiological studies [10–41] and two meta-analyses [5, 42] were identified that were published since our previous review [1]. A total of eight original studies [43–50] were also identified here through handsearching the reference lists of new papers that were not captured previously. Although the majority of newly published studies were case–control studies, there were nine cohort studies [10, 12, 16, 17, 20, 22, 23, 25, 29] with most of size of approximately 20,000 participants or less. Studies were mainly conducted in North America and Europe, with

several publications from each of the United States, Germany, the United Kingdom, and Sweden. Although the majority of new and previously published studies evaluated self-reported history of specific allergic disorders (asthma, hay fever, eczema), there were also three new studies examining total or allergen-specific IgE antibodies [23, 28, 38], two new record linkage studies examining hospital discharges for allergic conditions [20, 25], one study extending follow-up of a cohort of skin prick tested patients [16], and five studies examining allergy-related gene polymorphisms [11, 26, 36, 37, 39] in relation to cancer risk.

4.3.1 All Cancer

Although early case–control and cross-sectional studies tended to report inverse associations between a history of allergy and the occurrence of all cancer combined [51–65], there are a number of potential limitations that limit the strength of their findings [1]. A summary of cohort studies is presented in Table 4.1.

Results from several large record linkage studies of discharge diagnoses databases have reported conflicting results. A Swedish study linking 64,346 people discharged from hospital with asthma to the Swedish Cancer Registry reported 4,520 incident cancer cases [66]. A significant inverse association between asthma and all cancers was observed with a standardized incidence ratio (SIR)[1] of 66 (95% confidence interval $(CI)^2 = 64–68$) reported. More recently, Hagstromer et al. [20] linked 15,666 people with a discharge diagnosis of atopic dermatitis with the Swedish Cancer Registry. Over a mean follow-up period of 15.4 years, a total of 331 incident cancers were identified. Overall, a significant positive association was observed for all cancers (SIR = 113, 95% CI 101–125), particularly among men (SIR = 130, 95% CI 110–154) and those diagnosed in the first 9 years of follow-up (SIR = 119, 95% CI 101–140). Upon further examination, it was revealed, however, that the association was driven mainly by several smoking- and alcohol-related cancers. In a similar study of 2,030 hospitalized in Denmark for atopic dermatitis, an excess of cancer cases were also observed (SIR = 150, 95% CI 120–190), driven mainly by keratinocyte carcinomas of the skin (see Section 4.3.7) [25].

Vesterinen et al. [67] linked 77,952 asthmatics from the Finnish Social Insurance Institution register with the Finnish Cancer Registry. A total of 3,842 incident cases were observed. Overall, a significant excess of incident cancers was observed among men (SIR = 112, 95% CI 107–117), driven mainly by excesses in lung cancer. No

---

[1] The ratio of the number of new cancer cases observed in the population of interest (here subjects with a history of allergy) over a specified time period compared to that of a reference population, usually national cancer rates. An SIR of 100 indicates similar cancer incidence rates were observed in both the population of interest and in the reference population. SIRs above or below 100 indicate a higher than or lower than expected rate of cancer incidence respectively.

[2] The 95% confidence interval provides a range of values where the true value is found 95% of the time. 95% confidence intervals which exclude the null value of 1.0 (100 for standardized incidence/mortality ratios) indicate the result is "statistically significant", and the null hypothesis can be rejected with less than a 5% chance that the association observed was due to chance.

Table 4.1 Previous cohort studies evaluating the association between a history of allergy and all cancer

References (country)	Study population (number of cancer cases)	Allergy indicator	Relative risk (95% CI)
Alderson [115] (England)	1,892 from asthma clinic, 63 all cancer deaths	PD asthma	**71 (p< 0.01)**
Polednak [116] (USA)	12,098 *men* from Harvard, 1,074 all cancer deaths	SR asthma	8.3 deaths per 100 asthma, 8.9 without (NS)
Kaaber [50] (Denmark)	326 atopic dermatitis patients, 9 incident cancer cases	PD atopic dermatitis (M,F)	23, 132 (p > 0.05)
Robinette and Fraumeni [117] (USA)	9,550 *men* with asthma in army hospitals, 328 all cancer deaths	PD asthma	**128 (p< 0.01)**
Hughes and Raitz [118] (USA)	500 allergic and 421 non-allergic patients, 26 incident cancer cases	Atopy (scratch test or intradermal skin test)	No association
Markowe et al. [119] (England)	2,547 asthmatic and non-asthmatic patients, 34 all cancer deaths	PD asthma	0.9 (0.5–1.5)
Reynolds and Kaplan [120] (USA)	6,848 in California, 472 incident cancer cases, 277 all cancer deaths	SR asthma (incidence M,F)	**2.1 (p< 0.05),** 1.1 (p > 0.05)
		(mortality M,F)	**2.4 (p< 0.05),** 0.5 (p > 0.05)
Mills et al. [69] (USA)	34,198 Seventh-Day Adventists, 1,102 incident cancer cases	SR PT any allergy (M,F)	1.13 (0.92–1.39), 1.00 (0.85–1.17)
		SR PT asthma	0.78 (0.48–1.27), 0.96 (0.69–1.34)
		SR PT hay fever	1.06 (0.79–1.41), 1.15 (0.94–1.41)
		SR PT reaction to medication	**1.33 (1.02–1.74), 0.79 (0.65–0.98)**
		SR PT reaction to chemicals	0.67 (0.32–1.41), 0.80 (0.53–1.21)
		SR PT reaction to bee sting	0.67 (0.40–1.11), 1.06 (0.77–1.47)
		SR PT reaction to poisonous plants	1.13 (0.87–1.45), 0.98 (0.81–1.20)
Kallen et al. [66] (Sweden)	64,346 discharged from hospital with asthma, 4,520 incident cancer cases	PD asthma	**66 (64–68)**
Vesterinen et al. [67] (Finland)	77,952 asthmatics on Social Insurance Register, 3,842 incident cancer cases	PD asthma (M,F)	**112 (107–117),** 103 (98–107)
Lange et al. [121] (Denmark)	13,540 from Copenhagen Heart Study, 1,338 all cancer deaths	SR asthma	1.0 (0.7–1.4)
Knuiman et al. [122] (Australia)	4,277 in Busselton Health Study, 372 all cancer deaths	PT asthma (M,F)	1.26 (0.68–2.34), 0.88 (0.38–2.02)

Table 4.1 (continued)

References (country)	Study population (number of cancer cases)	Allergy indicator	Relative risk (95% CI)
Gergen et al. [123] (USA)	9,252 from NHANES II – Mortality Study, 998 all cancer deaths	Atopy (skin prick test)	0.89 (0.33–2.43) 30-to 44-year olds 0.78 (0.42–1.44) 45- to 59-year olds 1.13 (0.84–1.53) 60- to 75-year olds
Margolis et al. [101] (USA)	3,869 on Medicaid database, 165 incident cancer cases	PD severe eczema	1.04 (0.85–1.28)
Vandentorren et al. [74] (France)	14,267 in PAARC Study, 932 all cancer deaths	SR asthma	1.06 (0.81–1.40)
Eriksson et al. [16] (Sweden)	13,811 patients from allergy clinic, 401 incident cancer cases	Atopy (skin prick test)	100 (83–120)
Hagstromer et al. [20] (Sweden)	15,666 discharged from hospital with atopic dermatitis, 331 incident cancer cases	PD atopic dermatitis (M,F)	**130 (110–154),** 102 (88–188)
Lindelof et al. [23] (Sweden)	127,951 tested for total serum IgE or Phadiatop, 1,915 incident cancer cases	IgE highly elevated Positive Phadiatop	107 (82–137) 97 (82–114)
Olesen et al. [25] (Denmark)	2,030 discharged from hospital with atopic dermatitis, 67 incident cancer cases	PD atopic dermatitis	**150 (120–190)**
Turner et al. [70] (USA)	1,102,247 from CPS-II cohort, 81,114 all cancer deaths	SR PD asthma SR PD hay fever SR PD asthma and hay fever	**1.06 (1.02–1.11)** **0.92 (0.89–0.94)** **0.88 (0.83–0.93)**
Bellia et al. [10] (Italy)	1,233 elderly ambulatory patients, 59 all cancer deaths	PD asthma	17.3% of deaths with asthma versus 29.8% of deaths without (NS)

Eriksson et al. [16] extend cohort and follow-up from a previous publication [68]; standardized incidence ratios converted to base 100; NHANES II = Second National Health and Nutrition Examination Survey; PAARC = Air Pollution and Chronic Respiratory Diseases Study; CPS-II = Cancer Prevention Study – II; PD = physician diagnosed; SR = self-reported; M = male; F = female; PT = physician treated; IgE = immunoglobulin E; CI = confidence interval; NS = non-significant. See text for description of the various indicators of relative risk reported in individual studies. Statistically significant relative risk estimates are indicated by boldface type.

significant association with all incident cancers was observed in women. Recently, in an extended follow-up to a previous prospective study [68], Eriksson et al. [16] linked 13,811 skin prick tested patients to the Swedish Cancer Registry. A total of 119 incident cancer cases were observed among those with allergy with the same number expected (SIR = 100, 95% CI 83–120). Finally, in another recent prospective study, 70,136 patients for whom data on total serum IgE levels were known and 57,815 patients for whom data on allergen-specific IgE levels were known were followed up for cancer diagnosis according to the Swedish Cancer Registry [23]. No association with overall cancer incidence was reported for either measure (SIR IgE highly elevated = 107, 95% CI 82–137; SIR-positive Phadiatop = 97, 95% CI 82–114) among adults. Although an elevated SIR was observed among children with either a positive Phadiatop or elevated levels of total IgE (SIR = 262, 95% CI 131–469), these findings were based on only 11 childhood cancer cases.

There have also been several large cohort studies with data on individual level covariates. Mills et al. [69] evaluated the association between a history of allergy and cancer incidence in a cohort of 34,198 Seventh-Day Adventists. A total of 1,102 incident cases of cancer were observed over a 6-year follow-up period. No association was reported between a history of self-reported allergy, asthma, or hay fever, of sufficient severity to require treatment from a physician, and the occurrence of any type of cancer. In the largest prospective study conducted to date, over 1.1 million Cancer Prevention Study (CPS) – II study participants were followed up for 18 years with a total of 81,114 cancer deaths observed [70]. Overall, a significant inverse association was observed between a history of self-reported physician-diagnosed asthma and hay fever and all cancer mortality (hazard ratio (HR)[3] = 0.88, 95% CI 0.83–0.93), driven mainly by lung and colorectal cancer mortality, with a similar, although slightly attenuated, relation observed with restriction to never smokers only (HR = 0.91, 95% CI 0.83–1.00). Although this study provides some of the strongest evidence for a potential relation between a history of allergy and cancer overall, the strength of the evidence remains limited.

4.3.2 Lung Cancer

A meta-analysis of studies published up to the year 2002 reported a combined odds ratio (OR)[4] of 1.8 (95% CI 1.3–2.3) from previous case–control studies that evaluated the relation between asthma and lung cancer in never smokers [71].

---

[3] Here the survival experience of subjects in cohort studies with a history of allergy to those without is compared. Hazard ratios above 1.0 imply higher rates of cancer incidence (or death) in subjects with a history of allergy and hazard ratios below 1.0 imply lower rates of cancer incidence (or death) over the study follow-up period.

[4] Here an odds ratio denotes how much more likely cancer (or cancer death) occurs among study subjects with a history of allergy compared to those without in case-control studies. Odds ratios above 1.0 imply that cancer (or cancer death) was more likely to occur among study subjects with a history of allergy while odds ratios below 1.0 imply that cancer (or cancer death) was less likely to occur.

Similar findings were reported when combining the results for all previous studies that controlled for smoking history in the analysis. In contrast to the postulated protective effect of enhanced immunosurveillance among those with allergy, here it is thought that local mechanisms of inflammation and repair due to asthma may be responsible for a potential positive relation. Among the potential methodological limitations identified are misclassification and differential recall bias.

A number of subsequent studies have recently been published. Among case–control studies adjusting for smoking status, Schabath et al. [72] reported a positive association between self-reported physician-diagnosed asthma and lung cancer overall (OR = 1.25, 95% CI 0.99–1.57); however, upon exclusion of subjects with asthma diagnosis in the recent past (within 10 years of interview), the positive finding disappeared (OR = 1.06, 95% CI 0.80–1.40). An analysis of two large population-based case–control studies conducted in Montreal, Canada, reported no clear association between self-reported asthma and lung cancer overall, although there were some positive findings for specific lung cancer subtypes (below) [30]. In a case–control study nested in a cohort of asthmatic patients and the general population, a positive relation was observed (adjusted OR = 1.35, 95% CI 1.15–1.59) that weakened somewhat with the exclusion of asthma cases diagnosed within 1 year of lung cancer diagnosis (OR = 1.22, 95% CI 1.03–1.44) [18]. A positive, non-significant association was observed between allergen-specific IgE positivity and lung cancer (OR = 1.29, 95% CI 0.87–1.92) as well as self-reported physician-diagnosed asthma (OR = 1.40, 95% CI 0.71–2.77) in a case–control study nested in the ESTHER-I and -II prospective study by Wang et al. [38].

Two recent hospital-based case–control studies were conducted in never smokers (Table 4.2). In an extended analysis of the data collected as part of Schabath et al. [72], Gorlova et al. [19] reported a positive association between self-reported physician-diagnosed asthma and lung cancer overall (OR = 1.82, 95% CI 1.05–3.15); however, upon restriction to asthma only (and no hay fever), no association was reported (OR = 0.92, 95% CI 0.41–2.06). Seow et al. [37], in a study of never smoking Chinese women, reported a positive association between self-reported ever asthma/allergic rhinitis/atopic dermatitis and lung cancer overall (OR = 1.5, 95% CI 0.8–2.6) increasing to OR = 3.1 (95% CI 1.2–8.3) among those with an interleukin (IL) –6 CG/GG genotype, suggesting a role for inflammation in lung cancer. Brown et al. [13], in a case–control study nested in the Adverse Childhood Experiences (ACE) Study, reported an OR of 2.1 (95% CI 0.9–5.1) among non-smokers (including never and former smokers) with self-reported asthma.

Recent prospective studies controlling for smoking history reported mixed results [17, 73, 74]. In an analysis of 70 lung cancer deaths among the 6,144 non-smokers (including never and former smokers) in the second National Health and Nutrition Examination Survey (NHANES II) Mortality Study, Brown et al. [12] reported a positive relation between a history of self-reported physician-diagnosed asthma and lung cancer (HR = 1.69, 95% CI 0.94–3.04), increasing with exclusion of those with a history of physician-diagnosed emphysema and/or chronic bronchitis. In the CPS-II cohort, no clear relation was observed between a history of self-reported

Table 4.2 Previous studies evaluating the association between a history of allergy and lung cancer in non-smokers

References (country)	Population (number of cancer cases or cases/controls)	Allergy indicator	Relative risk (95% CI)
Cohort Studies			
Brown et al. [12] (USA)	6,144 NHANES II, *non-smokers*, 70 lung cancer deaths	SR PD asthma	1.69 (0.94–3.04)
Turner et al. [70] (USA)	448,613 CPS-II *never smokers*, 1,539 lung cancer deaths	SR PD asthma	1.11 (0.79–1.56)
		SR PD hay fever	1.02 (0.86–1.21)
		SR PD asthma and hay fever	0.83 (0.56–1.22)
Koh et al. [22] (China)	42,588 Singapore Chinese Health Study *never smokers*, 265 incident lung cancer cases	SR PD rhinitis or sinusitis	1.84 (0.97–3.47)
		SR PD asthma/hay fever/atopy	1.04 (0.70–1.54)
Case–Control Studies			
Samet et al. [124] (USA)	Population-based, *never smokers* (26/285)	SR PD asthma	0.77 (0.10–6.13)
Alavanja et al. [76] (USA)	Population-based, *women*, *never smokers* (154/1,166)	SR PD asthma	**2.7 (1.4–5.4)**
Wu et al. [77] (USA)	Population-based, *women*, *never smokers* (412/1,253)	SR PD asthma	1.48 (1.0–2.2)
Mayne et al. [125] (USA)	Population-based, *non-smokers* (437/437)	SR PD asthma	1.97 (0.90–4.32)
Brenner et al. [81] (China)	Population-based, *never smokers* (253/540)	SR PD asthma	2.0 (0.9–4.2)
Castaing et al. [14] (Europe and UK)	Hospital-based, *never smokers* (223/1,039)	SR eczema	0.55 (0.28–1.08)
Brown et al. [13] (USA)	Nested in ACE Study, *non-smokers* (35/8,236)	SR asthma	2.1 (0.9–5.1)
Gorlova et al. [19] (USA)	Hospital-based, *never smokers* (280/242)	SR PD asthma	0.92 (0.41–2.06)
		SR PD hay fever	**0.50 (0.30–0.83)**
Seow et al. [37] (Singapore)	Hospital-based, *women*, *never smokers* (132/163)	SR asthma/allergic rhinitis/atopic dermatitis	1.5 (0.8–2.6)

Results for never smokers are presented where available; Gorlova et al. [19] re-analyze data in Schabath et al. [72] focussing on never smokers only; NHANES II = Second National Health and Nutrition Examination Survey; CPS-II = Cancer Prevention Study – II; ACE = Adverse Childhood Experiences Study; PD = physician diagnosed; SR = self-reported; CI = confidence interval; odds ratio and 95% CI for Samet et al. [124] calculated. See text for description of the various indicators of relative risk reported in individual studies. Statistically significant relative risk estimates are indicated by boldface type.

physician-diagnosed asthma and lung cancer mortality among nearly 450,000 never smoker participants (HR = 1.11, 95% CI 0.79–1.56) [70].

There are no consistent results for asthma associated with lung cancer subtypes. In case–control studies, Wu et al. [75] found that the risk of adenocarcinoma was not associated with self-reported physician-diagnosed asthma in women (OR = 1.0, 95% CI 0.5–2.1). Elevated ORs were reported for adenocarcinoma and other histological types of lung cancer in non-smoking women with a history of asthma by both Alavanja et al. [76] and Wu et al. [77]. Osann et al. [78] reported a positive relation between self-reported physician-diagnosed asthma and small cell lung cancer (OR = 4.8, 95% CI 1.0–22.8) in women. Ramanakumar et al. [30] reported an elevated, although imprecise, OR for the relation between a self-reported asthma history and adenocarcinoma (OR population controls = 2.0, 95% CI 0.8–4.8) but not squamous cell carcinoma (OR population controls = 1.2, 95% CI 0.6–2.5) in one study, with no positive findings in the other study.

In a cohort of 92,986 asthmatics in Sweden, a significant positive association was noted in both males and females for squamous cell carcinoma (SIR = 206, 95% CI 184–230) and small cell carcinoma (SIR = 234, 95% CI 160–331), but not for adenocarcinoma (SIR = 106, 95% CI 87–127) [79]. In a Finnish record linkage study, a significant positive association was noted for adenocarcinoma (SIR = 146) and squamous cell carcinoma (SIR = 117), but not for small cell carcinoma (SIR = 103), among individuals with a history of asthma [67]. Both of these studies were unable to control for individual-level variables. Lastly, no clear association was reported in heavy smokers with a self-reported physician-diagnosed asthma history and any lung cancer subtype [80].

Age at and timing of diagnosis of asthma may affect the association between asthma and lung cancer. One study showed a significant positive association among those with an asthma diagnosis at or prior to 20 years of age (OR = 1.95, 95% CI 1.1–3.6), and with a lapse of 11–20 years since first diagnosis of asthma (OR = 2.99, 95% CI 1.1–8.3) [77]. Both Brenner et al. [81] and Kallen et al. [66], however, reported significant positive associations for lung cancer within 1–5 years of an asthma diagnosis only.

In terms of other allergic disorders, Schabath et al. [72] reported an inverse association between self-reported physician-diagnosed hay fever and lung cancer overall (OR = 0.58, 95% CI 0.48–0.70) that was attenuated in never smokers (OR = 0.81, 95% CI 0.53–1.23). In a further examination of the never smokers [19] the inverse relation, however, was found to be fairly robust across categories of timing of diagnosis, duration of disease, and a history of hay fever only (with no asthma). Schabath et al. [72] also evaluated the influence of polymorphisms of matrix metalloproteinase-1 (MMP-1) and myeloperoxidase (MPO) genes and reported increasingly inverse associations between hay fever and lung cancer with increasing number of protective genotypes. A subsequent publication reported that cases with hay fever exhibited lower mutagen sensitivity in bleomycin and benzo[a]pyrene diol epoxide (BPDE) assays [41]. Another large case–control study by Castaing et al. [14] reported an inverse association between a history of self-reported eczema and lung cancer (OR = 0.61, 95% CI 0.48–0.76) that remained following stratification

by current age, sex, and smoking status (OR never smokers = 0.55, 95% CI 0.28–1.08) but was no longer significant. The OR was also seen to lower when cases with eczema further reported a history of asthma (OR = 0.45, 95% CI 0.19–1.08) or use of eczema medication (OR = 0.55, 95% CI 0.41–0.72). Upon stratification by histologic subtype, ORs tended to be lower for squamous cell carcinoma (OR = 0.51, 95% CI 0.36–0.73) and small cell carcinoma (OR = 0.54, 95% CI 0.34–0.85) (OR adenocarcinoma = 0.83, 95% CI 0.58–1.19). Wang et al. [38] reported an inverse association with self-reported physician-diagnosed hay fever (OR = 0.34, 95% CI 0.11–1.10), but not atopic dermatitis, in a nested case–control study.

No clear association between a positive skin prick test and lung cancer incidence was reported in three prospective studies [16, 73, 82]. Hagstromer et al. [20] reported a significant excess of lung cancer cases among females discharged from hospital with atopic dermatitis. Koh et al. [22], in a large Chinese prospective study, reported a positive association between self-reported physician-diagnosed allergic rhinitis/nonallergic rhinitis/sinusitis and lung cancer (HR = 1.59, 95% CI 1.06–2.37) that increased for females (HR = 2.32, 95% CI 1.23–4.39), adenocarcinoma cases (HR = 1.91, 95% CI 1.07–3.42), and never smokers (HR = 1.84, 95% CI 0.97–3.47). However, no association was reported between physician-diagnosed asthma, hay fever, allergic dermatitis, food allergy, or other allergy and lung cancer (HR = 1.11, 95% CI 0.90–1.36). Lindelof et al. [23] reported no association in participants who underwent testing for total and allergen-specific IgE levels in Sweden, although the precise SIR was not provided. In the CPS-II cohort, no clear relation was observed between a history of self-reported physician-diagnosed hay fever and lung cancer mortality among never smokers (HR = 1.02, 95% CI 0.86–1.21), although there was a non-significant inverse relation with a history of both asthma and hay fever (HR = 0.83, 95% CI 0.56–1.22) [70].

4.3.3 Pancreatic Cancer

A meta-analysis of studies published up to the year 2004 by Gandini et al. [4] reported significant inverse associations between pancreatic cancer and a history of any allergy (relative risk (RR)[5] = 0.82, 95% CI 0.68–0.99) or atopy (RR = 0.71, 95% CI 0.64–0.80). Although a significant inverse association was also observed for respiratory allergy (RR = 0.63, 95% CI 0.52–0.76), no association was observed for asthma (RR = 1.01, 95% CI 0.77–1.31). Since then, at least six additional studies have been published with some similar findings reported [15, 16, 20, 24, 26, 70] (Table 4.3).

[5] Here the relative risk is the ratio of cancer risk (or death) among study subjects with a history of allergy to those without. Since most cancers are considered rare diseases, the various ratio measures (such as odds ratios and rate ratios) reported in individual studies approximate each other.

Table 4.3 Previous studies evaluating the association between a history of allergy and pancreatic cancer

References (country)	Population (number of cases or cases/controls)	Allergy indicator	Relative risk (95% CI)
Cohort Studies			
Robinette and Fraumeni [117] (USA)	9,550 *men* with asthma in army hospitals, 17 pancreatic cancer deaths	PD asthma	17 deaths among asthmatics versus 5 for nasopharyngitis patients ($p \leq 0.05$)
Mills et al. [126] (USA)	34,198 Seventh-Day Adventists, 40 pancreatic cancer deaths	SR PT asthma	0.87 (0.21–3.63)
		SR PT hay fever	0.66 (0.23–1.87)
		SR PT reaction to plants	0.99 (0.44–2.27)
		SR PT reaction to bee sting	0.43 (0.06–3.16)
		SR PT reaction to medication	0.67 (0.07–5.98)
		SR PT reaction to chemicals	1.53 (0.37–6.30)
Kallen et al. [66] (Sweden)	64,346 discharged from hospital with asthma, 160 incident pancreatic cancer cases	PD asthma	**64 (55–75)**
Vesterinen et al. [67] (Finland)	77,952 asthmatics on Social Insurance Register, 142 incident pancreatic cancer cases	PD asthma (M,F)	88 (67–113), 101 (80–124)
Stolzenberg-Solomen et al. [127] (Finland)	29,048 *male smokers* in ATBC study, 172 pancreatic cancer deaths	SR asthma	**2.16 (1.17–3.98)**
		SR allergic skin lesions	0.59 (0.29–1.20)
Eriksson et al. [16] (Sweden)	13,811 patients from allergy clinic, two incident pancreatic cancer cases	Atopy (skin prick test)	72 (9–260)
Hagstromer et al. [20] (Sweden)	15,666 discharged from hospital with atopic dermatitis, 11 incident pancreatic cancer cases	PD atopic dermatitis	190 (100–340)
Lindelof et al. [23] (Sweden)	70,136 tested for total serum IgE and 57,815 tested with Phadiatop	IgE highly elevated	No association
		Positive Phadiatop	No association
Turner et al. [70] (USA)	1,102,247 from CPS-II cohort, 5,159 pancreatic cancer deaths	SR PD asthma	1.02 (0.85–1.23)
		SR PD hay fever	**0.85 (0.77–0.95)**
		SR PD asthma and hay fever	1.14 (0.94–1.38)
Case–Control Studies			
Lin and Kessler [128] (USA)	Hospital-based (109/109)	SR allergy/eczema/ dermatitis	**2.56 (1.33–4.93)**

Table 4.3 (continued)

References (country)	Population (number of cases or cases/controls)	Allergy indicator	Relative risk (95% CI)
Gold et al. [129] (USA)	Hospital and population-based (201/201/201)	SR allergic disorders (HB, PB)	**0.39 (0.22–0.71),** 0.97 (0.50–1.90)
Mack et al. [130] (USA)	Population-based (490/490)	SR asthma	0.7 (0.4–1.1)
		SR allergic skin reactions	**0.2 (0.1–0.5)**
		SR allergy to natural antigens	**0.5 (0.3–0.9)**
		SR allergy to commercial	0.9 (0.5–1.6)
		products	**0.6 (0.4–0.8)**
		SR any allergic disease	
Farrow and Davis [131] (USA)	Population-based, *men* (148/188)	SR asthma	1.1 (0.4–3.2)
		SR allergy to medication	1.7 (1.0–3.0)
		SR food allergy	2.1 (0.8–5.5)
		SR plant allergy	0.7 (0.3–1.8)
		SR animal allergy	1.2 (0.4–3.4)
La Vecchia et al. [132] (Italy)	Hospital-based (247/1,089)	SR drug allergy	0.94 (0.56–1.57)
Jain et al. [133] (Canada)	Population-based (249/505)	SR hay fever	0.47 (0.18–1.27)
		SR eczema	0.68 (0.30–1.51)
		SR asthma	0.52 (0.16–1.70)
		SR other allergies	1.26 (0.70–2.28)
Bueno de Mesquita et al. [134] (Netherlands)	Population-based (176 cases of exocrine cancer/487)	SR PT any allergy	**0.57 (0.36–0.90)**
		SR PT eczema	0.75 (0.42–1.32)
		SR PT other allergies	**0.41 (0.21–0.82)**
Kalapothaki et al. [135] (Greece)	Hospital-based (181/362)	SR allergic asthma	0.33 ($p = 0.28$)
		SR skin allergies	No association
Dai et al. [136] (China)	Population-based (108/275)	SR PD any allergic condition	0.7 (0.4–1.1)
		SR PD drug allergy	1.1 (0.5–2.4)
		SR PD food allergy	0.3 (0.0–2.6)
		SR PD contact dermatitis	0.5 (0.1–1.7)
		SR PD urticaria	0.5 (0.2–1.3)
		SR PD asthma	1.0 (0.3–3.2)
		SR PD allergic rhinitis	0.3 (0.1–1.4)
		SR moderate reaction to	0.7 (0.1–1.1)
		mosquito	1.0 (0.3–3.1)
		SR strong reaction to mosquito	
Silverman et al. [137] (USA)	Population-based (484/2,099)	SR PD any allergic condition	**0.7 (0.5–0.9)**
		SR PD hay fever	**0.6 (0.5–0.9)**
		SR PD asthma	1.0 (0.6–1.5)
		SR PD eczema	1.1 (0.7–1.9)
		SR PD animal allergy	0.5 (0.2–1.1)
		SR PD insect bite/sting allergy	0.8 (0.6–1.2)
		SR PD dust or mold allergy	0.6 (0.3–1.1)
		SR PD drug allergy	**1.4 (1.1–1.9)**
		SR PD household products allergy	1.5 (0.8–2.9)

Table 4.3 (continued)

References (country)	Population (number of cases or cases/controls)	Allergy indicator	Relative risk (95% CI)
Holly et al. [138] (USA)	Population-based (532/1,701)	SR any allergy	**0.77 (0.63–0.95)**
		SR runny nose	0.84 (0.67–1.00)
		SR burning or watery eyes	0.80 (0.64–1.00)
		SR sneezing or congestion	**0.75 (0.60–0.93)**
		SR wheezing or asthma	**0.53 (0.37–0.75)**
		SR hives	0.92 (0.62–1.40)
		SR severe swelling	0.82 (0.54–1.20)
		SR anaphylactic shock	0.38 (0.11–1.30)
		SR PD eczema	**0.66 (0.46–0.93)**
Lo et al. [24] (Egypt)	Hospital-based (194/194)	SR allergy	0.8 (0.3–1.9)
Olson et al. [26] (USA)	Hospital-based (405/212)	SR any allergy	**0.58 (0.40–0.84)**
		SR hay fever	**0.45 (0.29–0.70)**
		SR medication	0.75 (0.46–1.19)
		SR animals	**0.43 (0.23–0.80)**
		SR any food	0.74 (0.39–1.40)
		SR dust	0.57 (0.29–1.12)
		SR mold	0.71 (0.31–1.65)
Eppel et al. [15] (Canada)	Population-based (276/378)	SR allergies/hay fever	**0.43 (0.29–0.63)**
		SR PD asthma	0.60 (0.31–1.16)

Eriksson et al. [16] extend cohort and follow-up from a previous publication [68]; standardized incidence ratios converted to base 100; ATBC = Alpha-Tocopherol, Beta-Carotene Cancer Prevention Study; IgE = immunoglobulin E; CPS-II = Cancer Prevention Study – II; PD = physician diagnosed; SR = self-reported; PT = physician treated; M = male; F = female; HB = hospital-based; PB = population-based; CI = confidence interval; odds ratio and 95% CI for Lin and Kessler [128] calculated. See text for description of the various indicators of relative risk reported in individual studies. Statistically significant relative risk estimates are indicated by boldface type.

Olson et al. [26] reported significant inverse associations between pancreatic cancer and a history of self-reported allergy (OR = 0.58, 95% CI 0.40–0.84), hay fever (OR = 0.45, 95% CI 0.29–0.70), and allergy to animals (OR = 0.43, 95% CI 0.23–0.80) in a US hospital-based case–control study. However, no exposure–response relationship was observed with increasing number of allergies reported. Olson et al. [26] also examined variants in IL-4 and IL-4Rα genes with no overall association with pancreatic cancer reported. Eppel et al. [15] reported a significant 60% reduction in risk for pancreatic cancer associated with self-reported allergies or hay fever. The magnitude of the association was found to increase, however, with increasing age at onset. Lo et al. [24] reported no association between self-reported allergy and pancreatic cancer in a small hospital-based case–control study conducted in Egypt.

Among recent prospective studies, Turner et al. [70] reported a significant inverse association between a history of self-reported physician-diagnosed hay fever and pancreatic cancer mortality in the CPS-II cohort (HR = 0.85, 95% CI 0.77–0.95),

with a similar finding in never smokers (HR = 0.86, 95% CI 0.60–1.22). No association was found with asthma (HR = 1.02, 95% CI 0.85–1.23). Lindelof et al. [23] reported no association with total or allergen-specific IgE levels, although the precise SIR was not provided. An imprecise association among skin prick tested patients was reported by Eriksson et al. [16] with only two incident cases of pancreatic cancer observed. Hagstromer et al. [20] reported an excess of pancreatic cancer cases among patients discharged from hospital with atopic dermatitis.

4.3.4 Tumors of the Brain and Nervous System

A meta-analysis combining results from previous studies published up to the beginning of the year 2007, including 3,450 glioma patients and 1,070 meningioma patients, reported significant inverse associations between a history of allergy (RR = 0.61, 95% CI 0.55–0.67), asthma (RR = 0.68, 95% CI 0.58–0.80), eczema (RR = 0.69, 95% CI 0.5–0.82), and glioma [5]. No overall association was observed between allergy and meningioma (RR = 0.93, 95% CI 0.72–1.19). See Table 4.4 for a summary of previous studies. A subsequent case–control study combining data from five INTERPHONE study countries (UK and the Nordic countries) examined the relation between self-reported allergic status and glioma and meningioma [40]. Significant inverse associations were reported between a history of physician-diagnosed asthma, hay fever, eczema, and glioma of approximately 35%. Although, little change was observed with increasing duration of asthma, or age at onset, there was a significant trend with increasing number of allergies. Little change was observed with the exclusion of proxy respondents (a closest relative) where the case had died. A significant inverse association was observed between self-reported physician-diagnosed eczema and meningioma (OR = 0.74, 95% CI 0.60–0.91) but not asthma or hay fever. The inverse association was found to remain, however, only for current (OR = 0.61, 95% CI 0.47–0.79) as opposed to past (OR = 1.05, 95% CI 0.78–1.43) eczema.

In follow-up to epidemiological studies examining the potential relation between self-reported allergic status and glioma, recently, there have been some studies examining potential biological indicators of allergic status or polymorphisms in selected allergy-related genes. In 2004, significant inverse associations were reported by Wiemels et al. [83] between elevated total (OR = 0.37, 95% CI 0.22–0.64) and food-specific IgE (OR = 0.12, 95% CI 0.04–0.41) and glioma. The OR for respiratory-specific IgE was 0.76 (95% CI 0.52–1.10). IgE levels, however, were not found to be strongly related with allergic status based on self-report. In 2005, Schwartzbaum et al. [49] reported associations between IL-4RA and IL-13 polymorphisms and glioblastoma risk in Sweden. A subsequent follow-up study using data from the United Kingdom, Denmark, and Finland, however, failed to confirm these findings [36]. Wiemels et al. [39], in a California study, provided some evidence for a role of IL-4, IL-4R, and IL-13 polymorphisms in glioma risk. Finally, Brenner et al. [11], pooling data from two US studies, reported associations between IL-4 and IL-6 polymorphisms and risk of glioma.

Table 4.4 Previous studies evaluating the association between a history of allergy and glioma, meningioma, or acoustic neuroma

References (country)	Population (number of cases or cases/controls)	Allergy indicator	Relative risk (95% CI)
GLIOMA			
Cohort Studies			
Schwartzbaum et al. [139] (Sweden)	14,535 (C1) and 29,573 (C2) in Swedish Twin Registry (37 and 42 incident gliomas)	SR hay fever (C1)	0.74 (0.26–2.08)
		SR eczema (C1)	0.52 (0.19–1.48)
		SR allergic conditions (C1)	0.45 (0.19–1.07)
		SR allergic conditions (C2)	1.09 (0.48–2.48)
Case–Control Studies			
Hochberg et al. [140] (USA)	Hospital-based (160 glioblastoma cases/128)	SR PT allergies	0.6 (0.4–1.0)
Schlehofer et al. [141] (International)	Population-based (1,178/1,987)	SR PD allergy	**0.59 (0.49–0.71)**
		SR PD asthma	0.75 (0.55–1.03)
		SR PD eczema	**0.64 (0.47–0.86)**
		SR PD other allergies	**0.59 (0.48–0.73)**
Brenner et al. [84] (USA)	Hospital-based (489/799)	SR any allergy	**0.67 (0.52–0.86)**
		SR PD asthma	**0.63 (0.43–0.92)**
		SR PD eczema	0.76 (0.45–1.27)
		SR PD hay fever	0.97 (0.69–1.37)
		SR allergy to medicine	0.79 (0.49–1.27)
		SR allergy to insects	0.61 (0.36–1.05)
		SR allergy to food	0.66 (0.25–1.74)
		SR chemical allergy	**0.23 (0.07–0.79)**
		SR other allergy	0.79 (0.32–1.96)
Wiemels et al. [83, 142] (USA)	Population-based (405/402)	SR any allergy	**0.47 (0.33–0.67)**
		SR runny nose	**0.66 (0.49–0.88)**
		SR watery eyes	**0.66 (0.49–0.88)**
		SR sneezing	**0.60 (0.45–0.80)**
		SR wheezing	**0.57 (0.38–0.86)**
		SR rash/hives	0.85 (0.64–1.12)
		SR swelling	**0.61 (0.45–0.83)**
		SR anaphylactic shock	**0.24 (0.08–0.73)**
		Elevated total IgE	**0.37 (0.22–0.64)**
		Elevated respiratory IgE	0.76 (0.52–1.10)
		Elevated food IgE	**0.12 (0.04–0.41)**
Schwartzbaum et al. [49] (Sweden)	Population-based (111/422)	SR PD asthma	0.64 (0.33–1.25)
		SR PD hay fever	0.98 (0.62–1.57)
		SR PD eczema	0.67 (0.43–1.05)
		SR PD contact allergy	1.02 (0.53–2.00)
		SR PD food allergy	1.23 (0.61–2.49)
Schoemaker et al. [33] (SE/N UK)	Population-based INTERPHONE study (965/1,716)	SR PD asthma	**0.71 (0.54–0.92)**
		SR PD hay fever	**0.73 (0.59–0.90)**
		SR PD eczema	**0.74 (0.56–0.97)**
		SR PD any allergy	**0.63 (0.53–0.76)**
Wigertz et al. [40] (SE UK and Nordic)	Population-based INTERPHONE study (1,527/3,309)	SR PD asthma	**0.65 (0.51–0.82)**
		SR PD hay fever	**0.66 (0.56–0.78)**
		SR PD eczema	**0.65 (0.54–0.79)**
		SR PD any allergy	**0.70 (0.61–0.80)**

Table 4.4 (continued)

References (country)	Population (number of cases or cases/controls)	Allergy indicator	Relative risk (95% CI)
Harding et al. [21] (UK)	Population-based, *children* (326/6,292)	PR asthma	0.90 (0.66–1.23)
		PR eczema	0.89 (0.65–1.21)
		PR early-onset flexural rash	1.17 (0.77–1.79)
		PR asthma and eczema	0.55 (0.28–1.06)
MENINGIOMA			
Cohort Studies			
Schwartzbaum et al. [139] (Sweden)	14,535 (C1) and 29,573 (C2) in Swedish Twin Registry (41 and 42 incident meningiomas)	SR hay fever (C1)	0.85 (0.33–2.17)
		SR eczema (C1)	0.72 (0.30–1.70)
		SR allergic conditions (C1)	0.84 (0.42–1.68)
		SR allergic conditions (C2)	**2.44 (1.08–5.51)**
Case–Control Studies			
Schlehofer et al. [141] (International)	Population-based (331/1,123)	SR PD allergy	0.89 (0.65–1.22)
		SR PD asthma	0.82 (0.46–1.44)
		SR PD eczema	0.68 (0.42–1.08)
		SR PD other allergies	0.97 (0.67–1.41)
Brenner et al. [84] (USA)	Hospital-based (197/799)	SR any allergy	0.98 (0.70–1.38)
		SR PD asthma	0.86 (0.53–1.40)
		SR PD eczema	0.80 (0.42–1.53)
		SR PD hay fever	0.93 (0.58–1.50)
		SR allergy to medicine	0.76 (0.40–1.46)
		SR allergy to insects	1.32 (0.72–2.43)
		SR allergy to food	1.18 (0.40–3.48)
		SR chemical allergy	0.26 (0.06–1.16)
		SR other allergy	1.19 (0.41–3.42)
Schneider et al. [32] (Germany)	Population-based (118/7,466)	SR asthma	No association
Schoemaker et al. [35] (UK)	Population-based INTERPHONE study (475/1,716)	SR PD asthma	0.85 (0.61–1.18)
		SR PD hay fever	0.81 (0.62–1.06)
		SR PD eczema	0.72 (0.51–1.02)
		SR PD any allergy	**0.76 (0.61–0.96)**
Wigertz et al. [40] (SE UK and Nordic)	Population-based INTERPHONE study (1,120/3,309)	SR PD asthma	0.94 (0.74–1.20)
		SR PD hay fever	0.93 (0.77–1.12)
		SR PD eczema	**0.74 (0.60–0.91)**
		SR PD any allergy	0.95 (0.82–1.10)
ACOUSTIC NEUROMA			
Case–Control Studies			
Brenner et al. [84] (USA)	Hospital-based (96/799)	SR any allergy	1.02 (0.64–1.63)
		SR PD asthma	1.34 (0.73–2.46)
		SR PD eczema	0.92 (0.34–2.48)
		SR PD hay fever	**2.36 (1.38–4.03)**
		SR allergy to medicine	0.53 (0.20-1.42)
		SR allergy to insects	1.12 (0.49–2.54)
		SR allergy to food	**3.01 (1.06–8.53)**
		SR chemical allergy	0.79 (0.22–2.84)
		SR other allergy	**3.81 (1.45–9.99)**

Table 4.4 (continued)

References (country)	Population (number of cases or cases/controls)	Allergy indicator	Relative risk (95% CI)
Schoemaker et al. [34] (UK and Nordic)	Population-based INTERPHONE study (563/2,703)	SR PD asthma	1.1 (0.8–1.5)
		SR PD hay fever	0.9 (0.7–1.1)
		R PD Eczema	1.0 (0.8–1.3)
		SR PD any allergy	0.9 (0.8–1.1)
Schlehofer et al. [31] (Germany)	Population-based INTERPHONE study (97/194)	SR PD asthma	1.06 (0.40–2.82)
		SR PD hay fever	**2.20 (1.09–4.45)**
		SR PD eczema	1.11 (0.51–2.38)

Studies by Ryan et al. [143], Schlehofer et al. [144], and Cicuttini et al. [145] present preliminary findings from the international study of Schlehofer et al. [141] and are not presented here; results of studies examining allergy-related gene polymorphisms not presented here, but described in text [11, 36, 39, 49]; PD = physician diagnosed; SR = self-reported; PT = physician treated; PR = parental reported; C1 = cohort 1; C2 = cohort 2; IgE = immunoglobulin E; CI = confidence interval. See text for description of the various indicators of relative risk reported in individual studies. Statistically significant relative risk estimates are indicated by boldface type.

Recent cohort studies examining broader outcome categories have reported no clear findings. Two previous record linkage studies were conducted in Sweden with that of Kallen et al. [66] reporting an inverse association for incident tumors of the "eye and nervous system" among asthmatics (SIR = 75, 95% CI 64–88) while that of Hagstromer et al. [20] reported a positive association for incident brain tumors among men (SIR = 150, 95% CI 70–270) and women (SIR = 170, 95% CI 100–280) with atopic dermatitis. No association was observed between atopy defined by skin prick testing and incident brain tumors by Eriksson et al. [16], although the number of brain cancer cases observed was small. No association between a history of self-reported physician-diagnosed asthma or hay fever and brain cancer mortality was reported in the CPS-II cohort (HRs ranging from 0.96 to 0.97 overall) [70].

Three studies have examined the relation between allergic status and acoustic neuroma. Significant positive associations were noted by Brenner et al. [84] for self-reported physician-diagnosed hay fever (OR = 2.36, 95% CI 1.38–4.03), and self-reported allergy to food (OR = 3.01, 95% CI 1.06–8.53), or other substances (OR = 3.81, 95% CI 1.45–9.99). Schlehofer et al. [31] also reported a significant positive association between self-reported physician-diagnosed hay fever and acoustic neuroma (OR = 2.20, 95% CI 1.09–4.45) but not with asthma or eczema in the German arm of the INTERPHONE study. Findings from the UK and Nordic INTERPHONE case–control studies combined revealed no association between acoustic neuroma and any previous diagnosis of allergic disease (asthma, hay fever, eczema) nor with increasing duration or increasing number of allergic conditions ($p = 0.6$) [34].

There have also been four case–control studies in children. An early case–control study reported an inverse relation between asthma or allergy and childhood brain tumors [85]. In 2001, a population-based case–control study suggested an inverse

relation between a history of allergy and neuroblastoma in children less than 8 years of age (OR = 0.20, 95% CI 0.06–0.65), although there were only three cases with allergy [48]. A subsequent case–control study of neuroblastoma in patients under the age of 19 years conducted by the Children's Oncology Group reported inverse associations between neuroblastoma and asthma, hay fever, and eczema ranging in magnitude from approximately 20–60% [45]. Finally, a UK study examining risk factors for childhood (less than 15 years of age) central nervous system (CNS) tumors reported a significant inverse association between parental-reported asthma and all CNS tumors (OR = 0.75, 95% CI 0.58–0.97) but no association with eczema [21]. Some inverse, non-significant, associations were reported for glioma and a significant inverse association reported between asthma and PNET/medulloblastoma of nearly 60%. Interestingly, when using physician notes to ascertain asthma status (as opposed to parental report) for a small subset of participants, no association with CNS tumors was observed (OR = 1.20, 95% CI 0.74–1.94).

4.3.5 Colorectal Cancer

A large hospital-based case–control study reported significant inverse associations between self-reported physician-diagnosed allergy and colon (OR = 0.76, 95% CI 0.59–0.97) and rectal (OR = 0.54, 95% CI 0.37–0.77) cancer [86]. Lower ORs were observed, however, with an age of diagnosis of at least 30 years (OR colon cancer = 0.71, 95% CI 0.52–0.96; OR rectal cancer = 0.42, 95% CI 0.26–0.68). Upon stratification by gender, the inverse association between allergy and colon cancer remained for males only (OR = 0.57, 95% CI 0.39–0.85). The remaining case–control studies report no significant findings [65, 87], although some inverse relations were noted [88–90]. Recently, Gonzalez-Perez et al. [18] reported an OR of 0.86 (95% CI 0.70–1.06) for colorectal cancer associated with asthma in a nested case–control study in the United Kingdom. However, in a nested case–control study in Germany, no association between allergen-specific IgE positivity and colorectal cancer (OR = 1.03, 95% CI 0.80–1.34) was observed [38].

In cohort studies, Talbot-Smith et al. [73] recently reported some imprecise inverse associations between a history of self-reported physician-diagnosed asthma or hay fever and colorectal cancer occurrence. For atopy, as defined by skin prick testing, ORs of 0.32 (95% CI 0.03–2.84) and 1.42 (95% CI 0.41–4.95) were reported for males and females, respectively. An analysis of 21,292 participants followed prospectively in the Iowa Women's Health Study reported a significant 26% reduction in risk of colorectal cancer associated with self-reported physician-diagnosed allergy [29]. Similar findings were reported with examination of colon and rectal cancer separately (ORs = 0.77, 95% CI 0.60–0.99 and 0.63, 95% CI 0.36–1.12, respectively) and in never smokers (OR = 0.74, 95% CI 0.56–0.98). A significant exposure–response association was also observed with increasing number of allergies. In an analysis of the CPS-II cohort, a significant inverse association was observed between a history of both self-reported physician-diagnosed asthma and

hay fever and colorectal cancer mortality overall (HR = 0.76, 95% CI 0.64–0.91) [70]. The inverse association persisted, although was no longer significant, among never smokers (HR = 0.78, 95% CI 0.60–1.02).

The remaining cohort studies evaluated colon and rectal cancer separately with no clear findings [16, 20, 66–69]. Although a significant inverse association was reported by Kallen et al. [66] for both colon (SIR = 72, 95% CI 65–79) and rectal cancer (SIR = 59, 95% CI 52–68) in asthmatics, Vesterinen et al. [67] reported a significant positive association for rectal cancer among women with asthma (SIR = 142, 95% CI 117–169). Finally, imprecise inverse associations of approximately 30% were observed for colon cancer occurrence in studies by Hagstromer et al. [20] and Eriksson et al. [16], with no association reported for rectal cancer.

4.3.6 Reproductive Cancers

It is difficult to draw any conclusions regarding the potential association between a history of allergy and reproductive cancers with few significant and largely inconsistent findings. Several of the large cohort studies described above have evaluated cancer outcomes at multiple sites. In the study of Seventh-Day Adventists, Mills et al. [69] reported a significant inverse relation between an allergic reaction to poisonous plants requiring treatment by a physician and ovarian cancer (RR = 0.13, 95% CI 0.02–0.95). A significant trend was also observed with risk of ovarian cancer decreasing with increasing number of allergies reported. No other significant associations were found between any other allergy measure in this study and any of ovarian, uterine, cervical, breast, or prostate cancer, although there were some positive, non-significant associations observed. In the Swedish record linkage study of asthmatics by Kallen et al. [66], significant inverse associations were reported for ovarian cancer (SIR 52, 95% CI 42–63), cancer of the corpus uterus (SIR = 36, 95% CI 28–46) and uterus, not otherwise specified (NOS) (SIR = 58, 95% CI 32–104), as well as for cervical (SIR = 52, 95% CI 39–69), breast (SIR = 53, 95% CI 47–58), prostate (SIR = 72, 95% CI 67–78), and testicular cancer (SIR = 37, 95% CI 16–85). In contrast, the Finnish record linkage study by Vesterinen et al. [67] reported no significant findings with the exception of an inverse relation reported between asthma and cancer of the corpus uterus (SIR = 76, 95% CI 61–92). In an extended follow-up of a cohort of skin prick tested patients in Sweden, Eriksson et al. [16] reported no clear findings. Although in a previous analysis, an SIR of 250 (95% CI 101–516) was reported for breast cancer among atopic subjects [68], in the extended analysis, no association was found (SIR = 106, 95% CI 65–162) [16]. In an evaluation of the association between both self-reported physician-diagnosed allergy and atopy as defined by skin prick testing in the 1981 Busselton cohort, Talbot-Smith et al. [73] reported no association between asthma or hay fever and breast or prostate cancer, although there was a significant positive relation observed for prostate cancer in those with allergy to house dust mites (HR = 2.90, 95% CI

1.26–6.68). A recent Danish record linkage study following 2,030 adults hospitalized for atopic dermatitis tended to report an excess of male (SIR = 230, 95% CI 80–500) and female (SIR = 220, 95% CI 100–400) genital cancers, although the number of incident cancers was small [25]. No clear relation was reported for breast cancer. In a Swedish study of patients discharged with atopic dermatitis, no association was reported with endometrial, cervical, breast, or prostate cancer, although again the number of new cancer cases was also small [20]. Lindelof et al. [23] reported no association between total or allergen-specific IgE levels and cervical cancer occurrence. In two small, cancer site-specific prospective studies, significant positive associations were observed between non-atopic eczema and cervical cancer (OR = 3.27, 95% CI 1.95–5.49) [91] as well as asthma and prostate cancer (RR = 22.8, 95% CI 5.48–94.7) [92]. Finally, in an analysis of the CPS-II cohort, some inverse, although non-significant, findings were reported between a history of self-reported physician-diagnosed asthma and ovarian cancer mortality (HR = 0.79, 95% CI 0.56–1.11) as well as a history of both asthma and hay fever and uterine (HR = 0.59, 95% CI 0.33–1.05) and breast cancer mortality (HR = 0.86, 95% CI 0.71–1.05), with no clear relation reported between any indicator of allergic status and prostate cancer mortality [70].

Case–control studies also reported few significant findings. Vena et al. [65] reported a significant inverse relation between a history of self-reported physician-diagnosed hives and cervical (OR = 0.73), breast (OR = 0.75), and cancer of the corpus uterus (OR = 0.63) but no relation with other specific allergic disorders. A hospital-based case–control study reported significant positive relations between a history of atopy (OR = 1.8, 95% CI 1.1–3.1) and hay fever (OR = 2.6, 95% CI 1.2–5.6) and testicular cancer [93]. No relation was reported between a history of self-reported physician-diagnosed allergy and breast or prostate cancer in a case–control study nested in the first NHANES cohort [94]. Among more recent studies, Hedderson et al. [95] reported an OR of 0.77 (95% CI 0.60–0.99) for breast cancer among women aged older than 35 years with a history of self-reported physician-diagnosed allergies. Although no association was observed among women diagnosed with breast cancer less than 35 years of age (OR = 1.30, 95% CI 0.94–1.81), it was suggested that this finding may be due to the strong genetic aspect of the disease among younger women. A positive association was reported between allergen-specific IgE and breast cancer by Petridou et al. [28] (OR = 1.73, 95% CI 0.95–3.14) with no clear relation reported in the nested case–control study by Wang et al. [38]. Wang et al. [38] also reported a positive relation between allergen-specific IgE positivity and prostate cancer (OR = 1.35, 95% CI 1.00–1.83) with no clear relation observed for several self-reported physician-diagnosed allergic diseases. Recently, a population-based case–control study in Ontario, Canada, reported an inverse association between a history of self-reported physician-diagnosed allergies and prostate cancer (OR = 0.78, 95% CI 0.60–1.00) [44]. A UK-based nested case–control study reported some inverse, non-significant, findings between a history of asthma and breast (OR = 0.91, 95% CI 0.78–1.06) and prostate cancer (OR = 0.86, 95% CI 0.69–1.07) occurrence [18].

4.3.7 Other Cancer Sites

Few other specific cancer sites have received much study. Some inverse relations were reported between a history of allergies and esophageal cancer [63, 96]. More recently, an OR of 0.86 (95% CI 0.65–1.12) for gastro-esophageal cancer was reported in a nested case–control study of asthmatics in the United Kingdom [18]. Bosetti et al. [86] reported a non-significant inverse association between a history of self-reported physician-diagnosed allergy and esophageal cancer in an Italian case–control study (OR = 0.80, 95% CI 0.46–1.39). Although a Swedish record linkage study reported a greater than threefold increase in risk for esophageal cancer among those discharged from hospital with atopic dermatitis, this finding was based on only six incident cases and confounding by cigarette smoking and other factors could not be ruled out [20]. Conflicting results were reported in remaining cohort studies [66, 97].

No clear relation was reported between a history of allergy and stomach cancer in several prospective studies with few cases [16, 20, 68, 69] and in a prior hospital-based case–control study [65]. Although Ye et al. [97] reported an excess of gastric cardia adenocarcinomas among asthma patients (SIR = 140, 95% CI 100–190), Vesterinen et al. [67] reported an SIR of 85 (95% CI 71–100) for stomach cancer in men and 91 (95% CI 77–107) in women with asthma, and Kallen et al. [66] reported a 50% reduction in risk for stomach cancer in asthmatics. Although an inverse association was observed between a history of self-reported physician-diagnosed asthma and stomach cancer in the CPS-II cohort overall (HR = 0.72, 95% CI 0.51–1.01), it was not found to persist among never smokers (HR = 0.95, 95% CI 0.55–1.65) [70].

Several significant positive relations were observed between a history of asthma or allergy and bladder cancer. Urothelial cancer was positively associated with a history of allergic asthma (OR = 3.1, 95% CI 1.4–6.8) but not allergic dermatitis (OR = 0.8, 95% CI 0.4–1.6) or allergic rhinitis (OR = 0.9, 95% CI 0.5–1.6) in a Swedish case–control study [98]. Kim et al. [99] reported an OR of 4.15 (95% CI 1.61–10.75) for the relation between asthma and bladder cancer with risk increasing severalfold in those with glutathione *S*-transferase-[mu] (GSTM1) and glutathione *S*-transferase-[theta] (GSTT1) null genotypes in a hospital-based case–control study. Imprecise relations were reported in previous prospective studies [16, 68, 69], although an excess of male bladder cancer cases was reported in Finnish asthma patients (SIR = 125, 95% CI 100–150) [67].

A case–control study nested in the Finnish Adult Twin Cohort Study reported some imprecise positive associations between a history of atopic eczema (OR males = 1.10, 95% CI 0.47–2.59; OR females = 1.80, 95% CI 0.83–3.90) and urticaria (OR males = 3.00, 95% CI 0.31–28.8; OR females = 2.00, 95% CI 0.68–5.85) and basal cell carcinoma among 333 twin pairs discordant for the disease [46]. In a hospital-based case–control study in Italy, with 528 cases and 512 controls hospitalized for unrelated acute conditions, a significant inverse association was reported between self-reported physician-diagnosed asthma and basal cell carcinoma (OR = 0.45, 95% CI 0.24–0.82) [27]. Ming et al. [47] observed an inverse association between the UK Working Party diagnostic criteria for atopic dermatitis

(OR = 0.78, 95% CI 0.61–0.98) and nonmelanoma skin cancer, although ORs for self-reported history of dermatitis, atopic dermatitis, and eczema were 1.00 (95% CI 0.80–1.26), 0.92 (95% CI 0.68–1.26), and 0.85 (95% CI 0.67–1.08), respectively. No relation between allergy and malignant melanoma was reported in two early hospital-based case–control studies [65, 100].

Although no clear association between hospitalization for atopic dermatitis and melanoma (SIR = 60; 95% CI 30–120) or nonmelanoma (SIR = 150, 95% CI 80–260) skin cancer was reported by Hagstromer et al. [20] and Olesen et al. [25] reported a significant excess of keratinocyte carcinomas (SIR = 240, 95% CI 140–390) among hospitalized atopic dermatitis patients in Denmark, although the positive relation was observed only among those diagnosed in either the first four (SIR = 250, 95% CI 90–550) or five to nine (SIR = 380, 95% CI 160–740) years of follow-up and not those diagnosed with at least 10 years of follow-up (SIR = 90, 95% CI 10–340), suggesting that at least part of the observed association may be due to a potential detection bias. A US cohort study based on the Medicaid database reported a significant relation between a history of severe eczema and nonmelanoma skin cancer (RR = 2.14, 95% CI 1.50–3.05) [101]. No association between total or allergen-specific IgE levels and nonmelanoma skin cancer was reported by Lindelof et al. [23], although details regarding the precise nature of the association were not provided. Finally, no clear association between atopy defined through skin prick testing and melanoma was reported in two other recent prospective studies [16, 73].

An international case–control study reported an OR of 2.19 (95% CI 1.01–4.74) for the relation between a history of allergies and medullary thyroid carcinoma [102], although the authors suggested that reverse causality may be responsible for the association observed.

Finally, a small case–control study examining risk factors for juvenile bone tumors reported inverse associations with skin allergy (unadjusted OR = 0.76, 95% CI 0.37–1.55) and asthma/bronchitis (OR = 0.61, 95% CI 0.29–1.28) but not hay fever (OR = 1.49, 95% CI 0.65–3.43) [43]. This study examined incident and prevalent cases combined and recruited controls from the hospital, neighborhood, and family members.

4.4 Discussion

This chapter has summarized the epidemiological literature examining the potential relation between allergy and cancer, focusing on solid tumors. Although there are a number of inverse relations reported, particularly with pancreatic cancer and glioma, there remain a number of methodological considerations. Previous studies were largely based on self-reported allergy history. Although little is known regarding the reporting of allergic disorders throughout the life course, questionnaires ascertaining previous physician-diagnosed allergies may be preferred [1]. Recently, there have also been a number of studies that have attempted to improve on the predominance of self-reported exposure assessment in prior research by assessing biological indicators of allergic status including total or allergen-specific IgE antibodies, skin prick

tested patients, or allergy-related gene polymorphisms described above. Although it is unclear to what extent results of previous case–control studies examining current levels of IgE may be affected by either the developing tumor or its treatment, case–control studies examining allergy-related gene polymorphisms do not suffer the same potential limitation [49]. Although several associations have been observed between specific polymorphisms and glioma risk, additional research is needed to further clarify these findings [49]. Although there were some recent prospective studies following cohorts of either skin prick tested patients [16, 68, 73] or patients with data on total and allergen-specific IgE levels [23], few relations were observed, and there were small numbers of cancer cases. There are also several early studies (not described here) examining such indicators in cases and controls with no clear findings [52, 103–108].

Another key consideration relates to the timing of allergy diagnosis. As noted above, in the cohort study of patients hospitalized for atopic dermatitis by Olesen et al. [25], an excess of incident keratinocyte carcinomas was observed among patients diagnosed with cancer in the first several years of follow-up only, suggesting that a detection bias may have influenced study findings, whereby there may be enhanced monitoring of skin disorders among such patients. It is also possible that reverse causality may explain some positive associations between allergy and cancer, whereby the allergic symptoms or conditions reported may simply be a manifest of the developing cancer [102]. Indeed, in several studies, the positive association between asthma and lung cancer was found to weaken or disappear upon exclusion of those with a recent diagnosis [18, 66, 72, 81]. There were also some inverse relations at other cancer sites that were found to strengthen with increasing age at allergy diagnosis, possibly suggesting some non-atopic factor may be at play [1, 15, 86].

Similar to prior research, there are several recent studies that have reported significant trends with the strength of the inverse relation increasing with number of allergies reported [29, 40]. Although it is possible that this finding may be due to improvements in exposure ascertainment, whereby participants with multiple allergic disorders are more likely to truly be allergic, the possibility of some form of reporting bias remains.

There may also be a screening bias in studies of cancer mortality whereby, due to frequent contact with the medical profession, allergy patients may be diagnosed earlier, thereby improving cancer survival [70]. Some studies have also examined the possibility for differential cancer survival due to the presence or absence of asthma with mixed findings [109–112]. Recently, two studies have reported improved prognosis among those with allergic disorders [113], although subject selection is uncertain, as well as improved glioma survival associated with elevated IgE levels [114].

Confounding may also represent an important issue in such studies. Indeed, a variety of factors, including cigarette smoking and socio-economic status in particular, have been widely associated with both allergic status and cancer occurrence [1]. Although several large record linkage studies have been conducted, primarily in the Nordic countries, the strength of the evidence from such studies remains

limited due to the absence of data on such potentially confounding factors. Patients hospitalized for such disorders, and other clinic-based studies, may also represent a selected subsample of all allergy sufferers. Although studies with detailed data on sociodemographic and lifestyle variables, and studies in never smokers, particularly for smoking-related cancers, are preferred, residual confounding remains a possibility. In our analysis of the CPS-II cohort, there were differences in these and other variables, including diet, multivitamin use, and use of oral contraceptives or estrogen replacement therapy, among those with and without a self-report of physician-diagnosed asthma or hay fever [70]. Bellia et al., [10] in a prospective study of elderly asthmatics, recently, reported a clustering of mortality risk factors among asthmatics.

4.5 Conclusion

In conclusion, although there are a number of important methodological considerations, there remain a number of high-quality epidemiological studies that have pointed to a possible role of allergy in the occurrence of cancer, with potential implications for cancer treatment and prevention. Further research is recommended in order to better understand the nature of a possible inverse relation, and mechanisms of action, including further prospective studies using biological indicators of allergic status, studies validating allergic status based on self-report, and further examination of potential roles for IgE and Th2 cytokines in cancer treatment and prevention [1, 5, 7, 49]. Multidisciplinary collaborations between the population and the laboratory-based sciences would be particularly useful.

Acknowledgments Michelle C. Turner holds a Canada Graduate Scholarship from the Canadian Institutes of Health Research.

References

1. Turner MC, Chen Y, Krewski D, Ghadirian P (2006) An overview of the association between allergy and cancer. Int J Cancer 118:3124–3132
2. Galli SJ, Tsai M, Piliponsky AM (2008) The development of allergic inflammation. Nature 454:445–454
3. Struck R, Bloomberg G (2006) Omalizumab for asthma. N Engl J Med 354(2689):2695
4. Gandini S, Lowenfels AB, Jaffee EM, Armstrong TD, Maisonneuve P (2005) Allergies and the risk of pancreatic cancer: a meta-analysis with review of epidemiology and biological mechanisms. Cancer Epidemiol Biomarkers Prev 14:1908–1916
5. Linos E, Raine T, Alosno A, Michaud D (2007) Atopy and risk of brain tumors: a meta-analysis. J Natl Cancer Inst 99:1544–1550
6. Grulich AE, van Leeuwen MT, Falster MO, Vajdic CM (2007) Incidence of cancers in people with HIV/AIDS compared with immunosuppressed transplant recipients: a meta-analysis. Lancet 370:59–67
7. Jensen-Jarolim E, Achatz G, Turner MC, Karagiannis S, Legrand F, Capron M, Penichet ML, Rodriguez JA, Siccardi AG, Vangelista L, Riemer AB, Gould H (2008) AllergoOncology: the role of IgE-mediated allergy in cancer. Allergy 63:1255–1266

8. Fu SL, Pierre J, Smith-Norowitz TA, Hagler M, Bowne W, Pincus MR, Mueller CM, Zenilman ME, Bluth MH (2008) Immunoglobulin E antibodies from pancreatic cancer patients mediate antibody-dependent cell-mediated cytotoxicity against pancreatic cancer cells. Clin Exp Immunol 153:401–409
9. Wang H, Diepgen T (2005) Is atopy a protective or a risk factor for cancer? A review of epidemiological studies. Allergy 60:1098–1111
10. Bellia V, Pedone C, Catalano F, Zito A, Davi E, Palange S, Forastiere F, Incalzi RA (2007) Asthma in the elderly. Mortality rate and associated risk factors for mortality. Chest 132:1175–1182
11. Brenner AV, Butler MA, Wang SS, Ruder AM, Rothman N, Schulte PA, Chanock SJ, Fine HA, Linet MS, Inskip PD (2007) Single-nucleotide polymorphisms in selected cytokine genes and risk of adult glioma. Carcinogenesis 28:2543–2547
12. Brown DB, Young KE, Anda RF, Giles WH (2005). Asthma and risk of death from lung cancer: NHANES II Mortality Study. J Asthma 42:597–600
13. Brown DB, Young KE, Anda RF, Felitti VJ, Giles WH (2006) Re: Asthma and the risk of lung cancer. Findings from the Adverse Childhood Experiences (ACE). Cancer Causes Control 17:349–350
14. Castaing M, Youngson J, Zaridze D, Szeszenia-Dabrowska N, Rudnai P, Lissowska J, Fabianova E, Mates D, Bencko V, Foretova L, Navratilova M, Janout V, Fletcher T, Brennan P, Boffetta P (2005) Is the risk of lung cancer reduced among eczema patients? Am J Epidemiol 162:542–547
15. Eppel A, Cotterchio M, Gallinger S (2007) Allergies are associated with reduced pancreas cancer risk: A population-based case-control study in Ontario, Canada. Int J Cancer 121:2241–2245
16. Eriksson N, Mikoczy Z, Hagmar L (2005) Cancer incidence in 13811 patients skin tested for allergy. J Invest Allergol Clin Immunol 15:161–166
17. Frostad A, Soyseth V, Haldorsen T, Andersen A, Gulsvik A (2008) Impact of respiratory symptoms on lung cancer: 30-year follow-up of an urban population. Lung Cancer 60:22–30
18. Gonzalez-Perez A, Fernandez-Vidaurre C, Rueda A, Rivero E, Garcia Rodriguez LA (2006) Cancer incidence in a general population of asthma patients. Pharmacoepidemiol Drug Saf 15:131–138
19. Gorlova OY, Zhang Y, Schabath MB, Lei L, Zhang Q, Amos CI, Spitz MR (2006) Never smokers and lung cancer risk: a case-control study of epidemiological factors. Int J Cancer 118:1798–1804
20. Hagstromer L, Ye W, Nyren O, Emtestam L (2005) Incidence of cancer among patients with atopic dermatitis. Arch Dermatol 141:1123–1127
21. Harding NJ, Birch JM, Hepworth SJ, McKinney PA, on behalf of the UKCCS investigators (2008) Atopic dysfunction and risk of central nervous system tumours in children. Eur J Cancer 44:92–99
22. Koh W-P, Yuan J-M, Wang R, Seow A, Lee H-P, Yu MC (2008) Chronic rhinosinusitis and risk of lung cancer in the Singapore Chinese Health Study. Int J Cancer 123:1398–1402
23. Lindelof B, Granath F, Tengvall-Linder M, Ekbom A (2005) Allergy and cancer. Allergy 60:1116–1120
24. Lo A-C, Soliman AS, El-Ghawalby N, Abdel-Wahab M, Fathy O, Khaled HM, Omar S, Hamilton SR, Greenson JK, Abbruzzese JL (2007) Lifestyle, occupational, and reproductive factors in relation to pancreatic cancer risk. Pancreas 35:120–129
25. Olesen AB, Engholm G, Storm HH, Thestrup-Pedersen K (2005) The risk of cancer among patients previously hospitalized for atopic dermatitis. J Invest Dermatol 125:445–449
26. Olson SH, Orlow I, Simon J, Tommasi D, Roy P, Bayuga S, Ludwig E, Zauber AG, Kurtz RC (2007) Allergies, variants in IL-4 and IL-4Rα genes, and risk of pancreatic cancer. Cancer Detect Prev 31:345–351
27. Pelucchi C, Naldi L, Di Landro A, La Vecchia C, on behalf of the Oncology Study Group of the Italian Group for Epidemiologic Research in Dermatology (GISED) (2008)

Anthropometric measures, medical history and risk of basal cell carcinoma in an Italian case-control study. Dermatology 216:271–276
28. Petridou ET, Chavelas C, Dikalioti SK, Dessypris N, Terzidis A, Nikoulis DI, Markopoulos C, PapadiamantisY, Germenis AE (2007) Breast cancer risk in relation to most prevalent IgE specific antibodies: a case-control study in Greece. Anticancer Res 27:1709–1714
29. Prizment AE, Folsom AR, Cerhan JR, Flood A, Ross JA, Anderson KE (2007) History of allergy and reduced incidence of colorectal cancer, Iowa Women's Health Study. Cancer Epidemiol Biomarkers Prev 16:2357–2362
30. Ramanakumar A, Parent M-E, Menzies D, Siemiatycki J (2006) Risk of lung cancer following nonmalignant respiratory conditions: Evidence from two case-control studies in Montreal, Canada. Lung Cancer 53:5–12
31. Schlehofer B, Schlaefer K, Blettner M, Berg G, Bohler E, Hettinger I, Kunna-Grass K, Wahrendorf J, Schuz J (2007) Environmental risk factors for sporadic acoustic neuroma (Interphone Study Group, Germany). Eur J Cancer 43:1741–1747
32. Schneider B, Pulhorn H, Rohrig B, Rainov NG (2005) Predisposing conditions and risk factors for development of symptomatic meningioma in adults. Cancer Detect Prev 29: 440–447
33. Schoemaker MJ, Swerdlow AJ, Hepworth SJ, McKinney PA, van Tongeren M, Muir KR (2006) History of allergies and risk of glioma in adults. Int J Cancer 119:2165–2172
34. Schoemaker MJ, Swerdlow AJ, Auvinen A, Christensen HC, Feychting M, Johansen C, Klaeboe L, Lonn S, Salminen T, Tynes T (2006) Medical history, cigarette smoking and risk of acoustic neuroma: an international case-control study. Int J Cancer 120:103–110
35. Schoemaker MJ, Swerdlow AJ, Hepworth SJ, van Tongeren M, Muir KR, McKinney PA (2007) History of allergic disease and risk of meningioma. Am J Epidemiol 165: 477–485
36. Schwartzbaum JA, Ahlbom A, Lonn S, Malmer B, Wigertz A, Auvinen A, Brookes AJ, Christensen HC, Henriksson R, Johansen C, Salminen T, Schoemaker MJ, Swerdlow AJ, Debinski W, Feychting M (2007) An international case-control study of interleukin-4Rα, interleukin-13, and cyclooxygenase-2 polymorphisms and glioblastoma risk. Cancer Epidemiol Biomarkers Prev 16:2448–2454
37. Seow A, Ng DPK, Choo S, Eng P, Poh W-T, Ming T, Wang Y-T (2006) Joint effect of asthma/atopy and an IL-6 gene polymorphism on lung cancer risk among lifetime non-smoking Chinese women. Carcinogenesis 27:1240–1244
38. Wang H, Rothenbacher D, Low M, Stegmaier C, Brenner H, Diepgen TL (2006) Atopic diseases, immunoglobulin E and risk of cancer of the prostate, breast, lung and colorectum. Int J Cancer 119:695–701
39. Wiemels JL, Wiencke JK, Kelsey KT, Moghadassi M, Rice T, Urayama KY, Miike R, Wrensch M (2007) Allergy-related polymorphisms influence glioma status and serum IgE levels. Cancer Epidemiol Biomarkers Prev 16:1229–1235
40. Wigertz A, Lonn S, Schwartzbaum J, Hall P, Auvinen A, Christensen HC, Johansen C, Klaeboe L, Salminen T, Schoemaker MJ, Swerdlow AJ, Tynes T, Feychting M (2007) Allergic conditions and brain tumor risk. Am J Epidemiol 166:941–950
41. Wu X, Lin J, Etzel C, Dong Q, Gorlova OY, Zhang Q, Amos CI, Spitz MR (2007) Interplay between mutagen sensitivity and epidemiological factors in modulating lung cancer risk. Int J Cancer 120:2687–2695
42. Tennis P, Sherrill D, Fernandez C, Dolan C (2005) Cancer risk in asthmatic populations. Ann Allergy Asthma Immunol 95:354–360
43. Frentzel-Beyme R, Becher H, Salzer-Kuntschik M, Kotz R, Salzer M (2004) Factors affecting the incident juvenile bone tumors in an Austrian case-control study. Cancer Detect Prev 28:159–169
44. Lightfoot N, Conlon M, Kreiger N, Sass-Kartsak A, Purdham J, Darlington G (2004) Medical history, sexual, and maturational factors and prostate cancer risk. Ann Epidemiol 14:655–662

45. Menegaux F, Olshan AF, Neglia JP, Pollock BH, Bondy ML (2004) Day care, childhood infections, and risk of neuroblastoma. Am J Epidemiol 159:843–851
46. Milan T, Verkasalo PK, Kaprio J, Koskenvuo M (2003) Lifestyle differences in twin pairs discordant for basal cell carcinoma of the skin. Br J Dermatol 149:115–123
47. Ming ME, Levy R, Hoffstad O, Filip J, Abrams BB, Fernandez C, Margolis DJ (2004) The lack of a relationship between atopic dermatitis and nonmelanoma skin cancers. J Am Acad Dermatol 50:357–362
48. Schuz J, Kaletsch U, Meinert R, Kaatsch P, Spix C, Michaelis J (2001) Risk factors for neuroblastoma at different stages of disease. Results from a population-based case-control study in Germany. J Clin Epidemiol 54:702–709
49. Schwartzbaum J, Ahlbom A, Malmer B, Lonn S, Brookes AJ, Doss H, Debinshi W, Henriksson R, Feychting M (2005) Polymorphisms associated with asthma are inversely related to glioblastoma multiforme. Cancer Res 65:6459–6465
50. Kaaber K (1976) Occurrence of malignant neoplasms in patients with atopic dermatitis. Acta Derm Venereol 56:445–447
51. Allegra J, Lipton A, Harvey H, Luderer J, Brenner D, Mortel R, Demers L, Gillin M, White D, Trautlein J (1976) Decreased prevalence of immediate hypersensitivity (atopy) in a cancer population. Cancer Res 36:3225–3226
52. Augustin R, Chandradasa KD (1971) IgE levels and allergic skin reactions in cancer and non-cancer patients. Int Arch Allergy Immunol 41:141–143
53. Chilvers C, Johnson B, Leach S, Taylor C, Vigar E (1986) The common cold, allergy, and cancer. Br J Cancer 54:123–126
54. Cockroft DW, Klein GJ, Dovevan RE, Copland GM (1979) Is there a negative correlation between malignancy and respiratory atopy? Ann Allergy 43:345–347
55. Fisherman EW (1960) Does the allergic diathesis influence malignancy? J Allergy Clin Immunol 31:74–78
56. Henderson BE, Bogdanoff E, Gerkins VR, SooHoo J, Arthur M (1974) Evaluation of cancer risk in a retirement community. Cancer Res 34:1045–1048
57. Johnson KJ (1979) Cancer and allergy. Ann Allergy 43:375
58. Logan J, Saker D (1953) The incidence of allergic disorders in cancer. N Z Med J 52: 210–212
59. Mackay WD (1966) The incidence of allergic disorders and cancer. Br J Cancer 20:434–437
60. McKee WD, Arnold CA, Perlman MD (1967) A double blind study of the comparative incidence of malignancy and allergy. J Allergy 39:294–301
61. Meers PD (1973) Allergy and cancer. Lancet 1:884–885
62. Moussa MAA, Karnik AM, Omar YT, Fenech FF (1985) On the analysis of three-dimensional contingency tables – application to the influence of allergy and age on cancer. Methods Inf Med 24:35–36
63. Petroianu A, Chaves DNB, De Oliveira O Jr (1995) Comparative incidence of allergy in the presence or absence of cancer. J Int Med Res 23:358–363
64. Shapiro S, Heinonen OP, Siskind V (1971) Cancer and allergy. Cancer 28:396
65. Vena JE, Bona JR, Byers TE, Middleton E Jr, Swanson MK, Graham S (1985) Allergy-related diseases and cancer: an inverse association. Am J Epidemiol 122:66–74
66. Kallen B, Gunnarskog J, Conradson T-B (1993) Cancer risk in asthmatic subjects selected from hospital discharge registry. Eur Respir J 6:694–697
67. Vesterinen E, Pukkala E, Timonon T, Aromaa A (1993) Cancer incidence among 78 000 asthmatic patients. Int J Epidemiol 22:976–982
68. Eriksson NE, Holmen A, Hogstedt B, Mikoczy Z, Hagmar L (1995) A prospective study of cancer incidence in a cohort examined for allergy. Allergy 50:718–722
69. Mills PK, Beeson WL, Fraser GE, Phillips RL (1992) Allergy and cancer: organ site-specific results from the Adventist Health Study. Am J Epidemiol 136:287–295
70. Turner M, Chen Y, Krewski D, Ghadirian P, Thun MJ, Calle EE (2005) Cancer mortality among US men and women with asthma and hay fever. Am J Epidemiol 162:212–221

71. Santillan A, Camargo C Jr, Colditz G (2003) A meta-analysis of asthma and risk of lung cancer (United States). Cancer Causes Control 14:327–334
72. Schabath MB, Delclos GL, Martynowicz MM, Greisinger AJ, Lu C, Wu X, Spitz MR (2005) Opposing effects of emphysema, hay fever, and select genetic variants on lung cancer risk. Am J Epidemiol 161:412–422
73. Talbot-Smith A, Fritschi L, Divitini ML, Mallon DFJ, Knuiman MW (2003) Allergy, atopy, and cancer: a prospective study of the 1981 Busselton Cohort. Am J Epidemiol 157: 606–612
74. Vandentorren S, Baldi I, Annesi-Maesano I, Charpin D, Neukirch F, Filleul L, Cantagrel A, Tessier JF (2003) Long-term mortality among adults with or without asthma in the PAARC study. Eur Respir J 21:462–467
75. Wu AH, Yu MC, Thomas DC, Pike MC, Henderson BE (1988) Personal and family history of lung disease as risk factors for adenocarcinoma of the lung. Cancer Res 48:7279–7284
76. Alavanja MCR, Brownson RC, Boice JD Jr, Hock E (1992) Preexisting lung disease and lung cancer among nonsmoking women. Am J Epidemiol 136:623–632
77. Wu AH, Fontham ETH, Reynolds P, Greenberg RS, Buffler P, Liff J, Boyd P, Henderson BE (1995) Previous lung disease and risk of lung cancer among lifetime nonsmoking women in the United States. Am J Epidemiol 141:1023–1032
78. Osann KE, Lowery JT, Schell MJ (2000) Small cell lung cancer in women: risk associated with smoking, prior respiratory disease, and occupation. Lung Cancer 28:1–10
79. Boffetta P, Ye W, Boman G, Nyren O (2002) Lung cancer risk in a population-based cohort of patients hospitalized for asthma in Sweden. Eur Respir J 19:127–133
80. Littman AJ, Thornquist MD, White E, Jackson LA, Goodman GE, Vaughan TL (2004) Prior lung disease and risk of lung cancer in a large prospective study. Cancer Causes Control 15:819–827
81. Brenner AV, Wang Z, Kleinerman RA, Wang Longde, Zhang S, Metayer C, Chen K, Lei S, Cui H, Lubin, JH (2001) Previous pulmonary diseases and risk of lung cancer in Gansu Province, China. Int J Epidemiol 30:118–124
82. Hospers JJ, Postma DS, Rigcken B, Weiss ST, Schouten JP (2000) Histamine airway hyper-responsiveness and mortality from chronic obstructive pulmonary disease: a cohort study. Lancet 356:1313–1317
83. Wiemels JL, Wiencke JK, Patoka J, Moghadassi M, Chew T, McMillan A, Miike R, Barger G, Wrensch M (2004) Reduced immunoglobulin E and allergy among adults with glioma compared with controls. Cancer Res 64:8468–8473
84. Brenner AV, Linet MS, Fine HA, Shapiro WR, Selker RG, Black PM, Inskip PD (2002) History of allergies and autoimmune diseases and risk of brain tumors in adults. Int J Cancer 99:252–259
85. Giuffre R, Liccardo G, Pastore FS, Spallone A, Vagnozzi R (1990) Potential risk factors for brain tumors in children. Childs Nerv Syst 6:8–12
86. Bosetti C, Talamini R, Franceschi S, Negri E, Giacosa A, La Vecchia C (2004) Allergy and the risk of selected digestive and laryngeal neoplasms. Eur J Cancer Prev 13:173–176
87. Vobecky J, Caro J, Devroede G (1983) A case-control study of risk factors for large bowel carcinoma. Cancer 51:1958–1963
88. Ghadirian P, Maisonneuve P, Perret C, Lacroix A, Boyle P (1998) Epidemiology of sociodemographic characteristics, lifestyle, medical history, and colon cancer: a case-control study among French Canadians in Montreal. Cancer Detect Prev 22:396–404
89. Kune GA, Kune S, Watson LF (1988) Colorectal cancer risk, chronic illnesses, operations, and medications: case control results from the Melbourne Colorectal Cancer Study. Cancer Res 48:4399–4404
90. La Vecchia C, D'Avanzo B, Negri E, Franceschi S (1991) History of selected diseases and the risk of colorectal cancer. Eur J Cancer 27:582–586
91. Montgomery S, Ehlin A, Sparen P, Franceschi S (2002) Childhood indicators of susceptibility to subsequent cervical cancer. Br J Cancer 87:989–993

92. Ohrui T, Yamaya M, Sato T, Matsui T, Sasaki H, Namina T (2002) Risk of prostate cancer in older Japanese asthmatics. J Am Geriatr Soc 50:202
93. Swerdlow AJ, Huttly SRA, Smith PG (1987) Testicular cancer and antecedent diseases. Br J Cancer 55:97–103
94. McWhorter WP (1988) Allergy and risk of cancer. Cancer 62:451–455
95. Hedderson MM, Malone KE, Daling JR, White E (2003) Allergy and risk of breast cancer among young women (United States). Cancer Causes Control 14:619–626
96. Dai Q, Zheng W, Ji B-T, Shu X-O, Jin F, Cheng H-X, Gao Y-T (1997) Prior immunity-related medical conditions and oesophageal cancer risk: a population-based case-control study in Shanghai. Eur J Cancer Prev 6:152–157
97. Ye W, Chow W-H, Lagergren J, Boffetta P, Boman G, Adami H-O, Nyren O (2001) Risk of adenocarcinomas of the oesophagus and gastric cardia in patients hospitalized for asthma. Br J Cancer 85:1317–1321
98. Steineck G, Wiholm BE, Gerhardsson de Verder M (1995) Acetaminophen, some other drugs, some diseases and the risk of transitional cell carcinoma. Acta Oncol 34: 741–748
99. Kim W-J, Lee H-L, Lee S-C, Kim Y-T, Kim H (2000) Polymorphisms of n-acetyltransferase 2, glutathione s-transferase mu and theta genes as risk factors of bladder cancer in relation to asthma and tuberculosis. J Urol 164:209–213
100. Beral V, Evans S, Shaw H, Milton G (1983) Cutaneous factors related to the risk of malignant melanoma. Br J Dermatol 109:165–172
101. Margolis D, Bilker W, Hennessy S, Vittorio C, Santanna J, Strom BL (2001) The risk of malignancy associated with psoriasis. Arch Dermatol 137:778–783
102. Negri E, Ron E, Franceschi S, La Vecchia C, Preston-Martin S, Kolonel L, Kleinerman RA, Mabuchi K, Jin F, Wingren G, Hallquist A, Levi F, Linos A, Fraumeni JF Jr (2002) Risk factors for medullary thyroid carcinoma: a pooled analysis. Cancer Causes Control 13:365–372
103. Hallgren R, Arrendal H, Hiesche K, Lundquist G, Nou E, Zetterstrom O (1981) Elevated serum immunoglobulin E in bronchial carcinoma: its relation to the histology and prognosis of the cancer. J Allergy Clin Immunol 67:398–406
104. McDuffie HH, Cockroft DW, Talebi Z, Klaassen DJ, Dosman JA (1988) Lower prevalence of positive atopic skin tests in lung cancer patients. Chest 93:241–246
105. McDuffie HH (1991) Atopy and primary lung cancer. Chest 99:404–407
106. Michils A, Yernault J-C, Noel E, Gossart B, Servais G, Duchateau J (1992) Abnormal humoral immune response to mucosal antigenic stimulation in patients with lung cancer. Cancer 69:2252–2257
107. Sanchez-Borges M, De Orozco A, Arellano S, De Gallego V, Avila-Millian E, Suarez-Chacon R (1986) Preventive role of atopy in lung cancer. Clin Immunol Immunopathol 41:314–319
108. Van der Wal AM, Huizinga E, Orie NGM, Sluiter HJ, De Vries K (1966) Cancer and chronic non-specific lung disease (C.N.S.L.D.). Scand J Resp Dis 47:161–172
109. Tammemagi C, Neslund-Dudas C, Simoff M, Kvale P (2003) Impact of comorbidity on lung cancer survival. Int J Cancer 103:792–802
110. Vesterinen E, Karjalainen S, Timonen T, Pukkala E, Hakulinen T (1993) Survival rates in lung cancer patients with and without bronchial asthma. Acta Oncol 32:517–520
111. Yancik R, Wesley MN, Ries LAG, Havlik RJ, Long S, Edwards BK, Yates JW (1998) Comorbidity and age as predictors of risk for early mortality of male and female colon carcinoma patients: a population-based study. Cancer 82:2123–2134
112. Yancik R, Wesley MN, Ries LAG, Havlik RJ, Edwards BK, Yates JW (2001) Effect of age and comorbidity in postmenopausal breast cancer patients aged 55 and older. JAMA 285:885–892
113. Pompei R, Lampis G, Ingianni A, Nonnos D, Ionta MT, Massidda B (2004) Allergy and tumour outcome after primary cancer therapy. Int Arch Allergy Immunol 133:174–178

114. Wrensch M, Wiencke JK, Wiemels JL, Miike R, Patoka J, Moghadassi M, McMillan A, Kelsey KT, Aldape K, Lamborn KR, Parsa AT, Sison JD, Prados MD (2006) Serum IgE, tumor epidermal growth factor receptor expression, and inherited polymorphisms associated with glioma survival. Cancer Res 66:4531–4541
115. Alderson M (1974) Mortality from malignant disease in patients with asthma. Lancet 2:1475–1477
116. Polednak AP (1975) Asthma and cancer mortality. Lancet 2:1147–1148
117. Robinette CD, Fraumeni JF Jr (1978) Asthma and subsequent mortality in world war II veterans. J Chron Dis 31:619–624
118. Hughes W, Raitz R (1979) A comparison of cancer occurrence in allergic and nonallergic populations. Ann Allergy 43:163–164
119. Markowe HLJ, Bulpitt CJ, Shipley MJ, Rose G, Crombie DL, Fleming DM (1987) Prognosis in adult asthma: a national study. BMJ 295:949–952
120. Reynolds P, Kaplan GA (1987) Asthma and cancer. Am J Epidemiol 125:539–540
121. Lange P, Ulrik CS, Vestbo J, for the Copenhagen City Health Study Group (1996) Mortality in adults with self-reported asthma. Lancet 347:1285–1289
122. Knuiman MW, James AL, Divitini ML, Ryan G, Bartholomew HC, Musk AW (1999) Lung function, respiratory symptoms, and mortality: results from the Busselton Health Study. Ann Epidemiol 9:297–306
123. Gergen PJ, Turkeltaub PC, Sempos CT (2000) Is allergen skin test reactivity a predictor of mortality? Findings from a national cohort. Clin Exp Allergy 30:1717–1723
124. Samet JM, Humble CG, Pathak DR (1986) Personal and family history of respiratory disease and lung cancer risk. Am Rev Respir Dis 134:466–470
125. Mayne ST, Buenconsejo J, Janerich DT (1999) Previous lung disease and risk of lung cancer among men and women nonsmokers. Am J Epidemiol 149:13–20
126. Mills PK, Beeson WL, Abbey DE, Fraser GE, Phillips RL (1988) Dietary habits and past medical history as related to fatal pancreas cancer risk among Adventists. Cancer 61: 2578–2585
127. Stolzenberg-Solomon RZ, Pietinen P, Taylor PR, Virtamo J, Albanes D (2002) A prospective study of medical conditions, anthropometry, physical activity, and pancreatic cancer in male smokers (Finland). Cancer Causes Control 13:417–426
128. Lin RS, Kessler II (1981) A multifactorial model for pancreatic cancer in man: epidemiologic evidence. JAMA 245:147–152
129. Gold EB, Gordis L, Diener MD, Seltser R, Boitnott JK, Bynum TE, Hutcheon DF (1985) Diet and other risk factors for cancer of the pancreas. Cancer 55:460–467
130. Mack TM, Yu MC, Hanisch R, Henderson BE (1986) Pancreas cancer and smoking, beverage consumption, and past medical history. JCNI 76:49–60
131. Farrow DC, Davis S (1990) Risk of pancreatic cancer in relation to medical history and the use of tobacco, alcohol and coffee. Int J Cancer 45:816–820
132. La Vecchia C, Negri E, D'Avanzo B, Ferraroni M, Gramenzi A, Savoldelli R, Boyle P, Franceschi S (1990) Medical history, diet and pancreatic cancer. Oncology 47:463–466
133. Jain M, Howe GR, St. Louis P, Miller AB (1991) Coffee and alcohol as determinants of risk of pancreas cancer: a case-control study from Toronto. Int J Cancer 47:384–389
134. Bueno de Mesquita HB, Maisonneuve P, Moerman CJ, Walker AM (1992) Aspects of medical history and exocrine carcinoma of the pancreas: a population-based case-control study in the Netherlands. Int J Cancer 52:17–23
135. Kalapothaki V, Tzonou A, Hsieh C-C, Toupaadaki N, Karakatsani A, Trichopoulos D (1993) Tobacco, ethanol, coffee, pancreatitis, diabetes mellitus, and cholelithiasis as risk factors for pancreatic carcinoma. Cancer Causes Control 4:375–382
136. Dai Q, Zheng W, Ji B-T, Shu X-O, Jin F, Zhu J-L, Gao Y-T (1995) Prior immunity-related medical conditions and pancreatic cancer risk in Shanghai. Int J Cancer 63:337–340
137. Silverman DT, Schiffman M, Everhart J, Goldstein A, Lillemoe KD, Swanson GM, Schwartz AG, Brown LM, Greenberg RS, Schoenberg JB, Pottern LM, Hoover RN, Fraumeni JF Jr

(1999) Diabetes mellitus, other medical conditions and familial history of cancer as risk factors for pancreatic cancer. Br J Cancer 80:1830–1837
138. Holly EA, Eberle CA, Bracci PM (2003) Prior history of allergies and pancreatic cancer in the San Francisco Bay Area. Am J Epidemiol 158:432–441
139. Schwartzbaum J, Jonsson F, Ahlbom A, Preston-Martin S, Lonn S, Soderberg KC, Feychting M (2003) Cohort studies of association between self-reported allergic conditions, immune-related diagnoses and glioma and meningioma risk. Int J Cancer 106:423–428
140. Hochberg F, Toniolo P, Cole P (1990) Nonoccupational risk indicators of glioblastoma in adults. J Neurooncol 8:55–60
141. Schlehofer B, Blettner M, Preston-Martin S, Niehoff D, Wahrendorf J, Arslan A, Alhbom A, Choi WN, Giles GG, Howe GR, Little J, Menegoz F, Ryan P (1999) Role of medical history in brain tumor development. Results from the International Adult Brain Tumor Study. Int J Cancer 82:155–160
142. Wiemels JL, Wiencke JK, Sison JD, Miike R, McMillan A, Wrensch M (2002) History of allergies among adults with glioma and controls. Int J Cancer 98:609–615
143. Ryan P, Lee MW, North B, McMichael AJ (1992) Risk factors for tumors of the brain and meninges: results from the Adelaide Adult Brain Tumor Study. Int J Cancer 51:20–27
144. Schlehofer B, Blettner M, Becker N, Martinsohn C, Wahrendorf J (1992) Medical risk factors and the development of brain tumors. Cancer 69:2541–2547
145. Cicuttini FM, Hurley SF, Forbes A, Donnan GA, Salzberg M, Giles GG, McNeil JJ (1997) Association of adult glioma with medical conditions, family and reproductive history. Int J Cancer 71:203–207

Chapter 5
Epidemiological Evidence: IgE, Allergies, and Hematopoietic Malignancies

Otoniel Martínez-Maza, Alan Duane Moreno, and Wendy Cozen

Abstract This chapter presents an overview of recent epidemiologic studies that address the association between atopic diseases and IgE and the risk of hematopoietic cancers, including a discussion of potential biological mechanisms. The strongest and most consistent (inverse) associations have been observed between allergic conditions and childhood leukemia, especially acute lymphoblastic leukemia. The cumulative evidence for an inverse association between atopy and non-Hodgkin lymphoma is suggestive, but the inconsistency of the associations with specific types of atopic conditions, the lack of any associations observed in most cohort studies, and the correlation between timing of diagnosis and decreasing IgE levels warrant further clarification. No consistent evidence has been found supporting an association between atopy and either plasma cell neoplasms or Hodgkin lymphoma.

There are several potential mechanisms by which allergic conditions could contribute to the risk of hematopoietic cancers. These include features of allergic responses (IgE, mast cell products) that may mediate enhanced antitumor immune responses, as well as allergy-associated changes in immune responses that inhibit immune cell activation, resulting in less exposure to DNA mutating and potentially oncogenic activities.

5.1 Introduction

This chapter presents an overview of recent epidemiologic studies that address the association between atopic (e.g., allergic) conditions and IgE and the risk of hematopoietic cancers, as well as a discussion of potential biological mechanisms. Since many hematopoietic cancers are malignancies that originate from cells of the immune system, including B and T cells, there are unique potential interactions

---

W. Cozen (✉)
Departments of Preventive Medicine and Pathology, Keck School of Medicine, University of Southern California, Los Angeles, CA, USA
e-mail: wcozen@usc.edu

M.L. Penichet, E. Jensen-Jarolim (eds.), *Cancer and IgE*,
DOI 10.1007/978-1-60761-451-7_5,

within the immune system environment present in allergic individuals that may contribute to the etiology of these cancers.

Hematopoietic cancers, or cancers that arise from blood cells, include myeloid and lymphoid leukemias and Hodgkin and non-Hodgkin lymphomas (NHLs), as well as plasma cell malignancies (Table 5.1). These cancers reflect and parallel the entire developmental spectrum of the cells of the hematopoietic system. For example, most leukemias are cancers that arise from progenitor cells for lymphocytes, monocytes, and other white blood cells; lymphomas represent cancers that arise from mature lymphocytes; and plasma cell malignancies represent cancers that correspond to terminally differentiated B lymphocytes. A brief description

Table 5.1 Incidence and incidence rates of the major hematological cancers, 2000–2005, SEER[a]

	Males		Females		Total	
	No. cases	AAIR[b]	No. cases	AAIR[b]	No. cases	AAIR[b]
Leukemias						
Acute lymphocytic (ALL)[c]	3,937	1.74	3,060	1.35	6,997	1.55
ALL < 14 years at diagnosis	2,107	4.18	1,696	3.53	3,803	3.86
Chronic lymphocytic (CLL)[d]	10,175	5.64	6,890	2.85	17,065	4.04
Acute myeloid (AML)[e]	9,287	4.94	7,763	3.27	17,050	3.97
Chronic myeloid (CML)[f]	2,827	1.43	2,180	0.92	5,007	1.15
Non-Hodgkin lymphoma (NHL)[g]	38,609	20.07	33,237	14.04	71,846	16.73
Hodgkin lymphoma (HL)[h]	6,683	3.06	5,588	2.43	12,271	2.72
<15 years at diagnosis	332	0.66	217	0.45	549	0.56
15–45 years at diagnosis	3,703	3.62	3,387	3.42	7,090	3.52
45+ years at diagnosis	2,648	3.83	1,984	2.41	4,632	3.06
Multiple myeloma and plasmacytoma[i]	12,969	7.05	11,035	4.62	24,004	5.66

Software: Surveillance Research Program, National Cancer Institute SEER*Stat software (www.seer.cancer.gov/seerstat) version 6.4.4.

[a]Surveillance, Epidemiology and End-Results Program of the National Cancer Institute (www.SEER.gov).

[b]Age-adjusted incidence rates/100,000 population at risk, age-adjusted to the 2000 US standard population age distribution standard (United States Census P25–1130).

[c]International Classification for Diseases for Oncology Third Edition morphology codes 9835–9837.

[d]International Classification for Diseases for Oncology Third Edition morphology codes 9823.

[e]International Classification for Diseases for Oncology Third Edition morphology codes 9840, 9861,9866, 9867, 9870–9874, 9891, 9895–9897, 9910, 9920, 9930–9931.

[f]International Classification for Diseases for Oncology Third Edition morphology codes 9863, 9875–9876.

[g]International Classification for Diseases for Oncology Third Edition morphology codes 9670–9719, 9727–9729.

[h]International Classification for Diseases for Oncology Third Edition morphology codes 9650–9667.

[i]International Classification for Diseases for Oncology Third Edition morphology codes 9731–9732, 9734.

of the biological origin is included, along with a review of the epidemiology relevant to atopic conditions, for each of the major types of hematopoietic neoplasms.

Hematopoietic cancers are unique in that the cell of origin for many of these cancers are the cells that make up the immune system—the same cells involved in immunoregulation, mediation of allergic responses, and antitumor immunity. Therefore, the link between allergy and hematopoietic cancers may be significantly more complex than that seen between allergy and other forms of cancer because the immunoregulatory mechanisms that promote, or inhibit, allergic responses may also induce immune cell activities that protect from, or promote, the development of hematopoietic cancers.

5.2 Methods of Review

We used a wide range of search terms in our review of papers to identify all epidemiologic studies that examined the association between the following conditions and the risk of hematopoietic cancer: atopy, allergy, asthma, hay fever, eczema, atopic dermatitis, and IgE. All of these conditions are associated (to varying degrees) with a Th2-skewed immune response and elevated IgE levels. However, it is important to note that certain conditions are heterogeneous, notably asthma, and include non-allergic subtypes that may not be associated with elevated IgE levels. Only a handful of studies measured IgE or other objective indicators of atopy [1–4]. Most epidemiological studies have not focused solely on allergy and IgE, and the exposures are thus usually assessed as one in a long series of questions such as "Have you ever been diagnosed with..." or "Have you ever experienced [symptoms of allergy]," therefore misclassification due to imprecise exposure measurement is common. We generally excluded studies that used hospital-based controls since bias due to control selection would be likely in such studies, except when these studies were included in larger pooled analyses in combination with studies that used population controls. We also excluded case–control studies with less than 100 cases, and cohort studies with less than 10 expected cases, since these would be unlikely to have adequate power to detect a reasonable association. Finally, because acquired immune deficiency syndrome (AIDS) is not representative of the normal immune response, we have excluded studies of patients with AIDS-related hematopoietic malignancies except for those that were included in a comprehensive population-based study (e.g., [5]).

Epidemiologic studies included in this review fall into two main categories—cohort and case–control studies. In cohort studies, a sample of subjects is chosen based on exposure status and is followed over time for observance of outcomes. The measure of risk is the relative risk (RR), also known as the rate ratio; it is simply the proportion of subjects who develop the outcome among the exposed divided by the proportion of subjects who develop the outcome among the unexposed. Other measures of effect used in cohort studies include the standardized mortality (SMR)

or incidence (SIR) ratios, in which the number of deaths or new cases occurring in the sample of subjects is compared to that expected in the general population of the same demographic composition. Cohort studies are less subject to recall bias since the exposures are documented prior to the onset of disease, but they are expensive to conduct, they may be less powerful for the study of rare diseases such as hematopoietic malignancies, and the exposure may change during the follow-up period.

Case–control studies are the other major type of etiologic study. Here, cases are selected and controls for comparison are chosen, ideally from the same source population as the cases; they may or may not be matched to the cases on age, sex, and various demographic or other factors. The exposure is then measured retrospectively in the cases and controls by self-report, medical record review, and/or physiological measurement, and the prevalence of the exposure between the groups is compared. The measure of risk in case–control studies is the odds ratio (OR), which is the close approximation to the RR when certain assumptions are met (e.g., the outcome is rare). The OR measures the likelihood that cases were exposed relative to the likelihood that controls were exposed. An OR or RR of 1.0 signifies no association at all between the exposure and the outcome; an OR or RR greater than 1.0 indicates that the exposure is more common among those affected and is compatible with an increased risk of developing the outcome, and an OR or RR less than 1.0 indicates that the exposure is less common among those affected by the disease and therefore is consistent with a protective effect. By convention, estimates representing SIRs and SMRs are multiplied by 100, and thus 100 signifies no link between exposure and outcome.

The preferred measure of statistical significance for epidemiological studies is the 95% confidence interval (CI), which is the range of values that would include the true risk estimate (e.g., OR or RR) 95 times, were the same study to be repeated 100 times. Another way to interpret the 95% CI is that there is 95% certainty that the true risk estimate falls within the interval. If 1.0 falls within the 95% CI range, then a 1.0 OR or RR signifying a null association cannot be ruled out. The advantage of using the 95% CI over a simple p-value is that more information is provided, especially when no link is demonstrated. When the 95% CI range is very wide, the decrease in precision may be due to a small sample size. Conversely, when the sample size is very large, the range becomes very narrow providing more confidence in a positive finding (when 1.0 is outside the range) or a negative finding (when 95% of the possible values are all close to 1.0). Throughout the tables, any 95% CI that excludes the null hypothesis (therefore consistent with a finding of statistical significance of $p > 0.05$) is indicated by boldface type.

5.3 Leukemias

Leukemias are cancers that are characterized by the abnormal proliferation of white blood cells in blood and bone marrow. They are a heterogeneous group with

different pathologic and cellular characteristics, etiology, age of onset, and clinical outcome. Acute leukemias are distinguished by increased numbers of immature blood cells, while chronic leukemias are characterized by elevated numbers of more mature abnormal blood cells. Leukemias also can be categorized by the normal type of blood cell that they correspond to, with lymphocytic leukemias corresponding to lymphocytes and myelogenous leukemias to cells that form granulocytes. Broad classifications are usually made for use in epidemiologic studies according to the cell of origin (myeloid or lymphoid) and the clinical course (acute or chronic), each of which has distinct epidemiologic and etiologic risk patterns [6]. There are numerous clinical subclassifications based on cell-surface markers and chromosomal rearrangements, many of which are correlated with prognosis but not necessarily etiology. Many early studies conducted prior to the availability of the technology to distinguish these subtypes simply combined all types of leukemia under one heading, obscuring any subtype-specific effects. Where subtypes have been examined separately, some general patterns emerge (Tables 5.2 and 5.3).

Childhood acute lymphoblastic leukemia (ALL) has been inversely linked to various atopic conditions in four questionnaire-based studies (from parent interviews) [7–10]. Two studies based on Swedish and British national medical record databases found a decreased risk linked to asthma [11, 12] and a number of other atopic conditions [12]. One medical record-based study [13] found a positive association between allergic and atopic conditions and childhood ALL based on a small number of cases relative to the other studies.

Hay fever specifically was linked to a decreased risk of childhood ALL in all four studies that examined this exposure [8–10, 12]. Eczema was inversely associated with risk in two [9, 10] out of the five [8–10, 12, 13] studies. Note that risk estimates were below 1.0 but the 95% CI did not exclude 1.0 [8, 12]. Only one of seven studies found that asthma was negatively associated with ALL [7], and six found no association [8–13].

Allergies to specific substances have not been consistently associated with ALL [8–10, 13]. Two groups examined the much less common childhood acute myelogenous leukemia (AML) and reported no association with any type of atopy [9, 12]. In summary, some forms of atopy were consistently associated with a decreased risk of childhood ALL, but not AML.

The evidence on adult leukemia subtypes is mixed. Adult ALL, which is quite rare, (Table 5.1), has generally not been linked to allergic conditions (Table 5.3), excepting penicillin allergy [14]. AML was inversely associated with an increasing number of allergies in a small case–control study [15]. Hay fever has been inversely linked to AML in one study [16]; a borderline increased risk was found in another [17]. No association has been found between asthma [11, 16] or unspecified allergies [16] and adult leukemias. Only one study has examined chronic myelogenous leukemia (CML) with null results for asthma [11].

Table 5.2 Cohort studies examining atopic conditions and risk of hematopoietic cancers

Author	Type of study	Source of subjects	Measure of risk	Exposure validation	Disease validation	Cancer type and subtype	Exposure	Relative risk (95% CI[a])
Bourget et al. [58]	Prospective cohort (14,407 individuals)	National Health and Nutrition Examination Survey (NHANES)	Rate ratio	Questionnaire	Hospital records and death certificates	Multiple myeloma ($n = 18$)	1 Atopic condition	1.7 (0.3, 10.6)
							2+ Atopic conditions	3.4 (0.0, 285.8)
Kallen et al. [31]	Retrospective linkage study $n = (64,346$ individuals)	Swedish National Hospital Discharge Registry, 1969–1983	Standardized mortality ratio	Hospital record	Swedish National Death Index	NHL ($n = 104$)	Asthma	**61 (50.6, 74.0)**
						Hodgkin lymphoma ($n = 23$)		68 (45.5, 102.5)
						Multiple myeloma ($n = 39$)		**38 (28.3, 51.8)**
Mills et al. [59]	Prospective cohort ($n = 34,000$ individuals followed for 6 years)	Seventh-Day Adventists (California)	Rate ratio	Questionnaire and medical record if hospitalized	Cancer registry linkage or hospital record	Multiple myeloma ($n = 23$)	Asthma	0.8 (0.1, 6.1)
							Hay fever	1.5 (0.5, 4.6)
							Allergic reaction to:	
							Medications	1.2 (0.4, 3.6)
							Chemicals	1.3 (0.2, 10.1)
							Bee sting	1.8 (0.4, 7.7)
							Poisonous plants	1.1 (0.4, 3.4)
							History of any allergy	1.7 (0.7, 4.0)
Soderberg et al. [22]	Prospective cohort of Swedish twins ($n = 16,539$ individuals followed for mean of 23 years)	Birth records in Sweden	Rate ratio	Questionnaire	Cancer registry linkage and death registry linkage	Multiple myeloma ($n = 78$)	Asthma, hay fever or hives	0.7 (0.4, 1.4)
							Hay fever	0.9 (0.5, 1.7)
							Eczema	0.6 (0.2, 2.0)
							Childhood eczema	0.5 (0.1, 3.9)
						NHL ($n = 112$)	Asthma, hay fever or hives	1.1 (0.7, 1.8)
							Hay fever	1.3 (0.8, 2.2)
							Eczema	1.3 (0.6, 2.6)
							Childhood eczema	2.3 (1.0, 5.3)

Table 5.2 (continued)

Author	Type of study	Source of subjects	Measure of risk	Exposure validation	Disease validation	Cancer type and subtype	Exposure	Relative risk (95% CI[a])
						CLL ($n = 67$)	Asthma, hay fever or hives	0.8 (0.4, 1.6)
							Hay fever	0.7 (0.3, 1.6)
							Eczema	1.2 (0.5, 3.1)
							Childhood eczema	-
Turner et al. [32]	Prospective cohort of healthy volunteers ($n = 1,102,247$)	ACS cohort	Relative risk	Questionnaire	National Death Index	Multiple myeloma ($n = 2,162$)	Asthma	1.0 (0.7, 1.4)
							Hay fever	0.9 (0.8, 1.1)
							Asthma + hay fever	1.0 (0.7, 1.4)
							Asthma or hay fever	1.0 (0.8, 1.1)
						NHL ($n = 4,2780$)	Asthma	1.1 (0.9, 1.3)
							Hay fever	1.0 (0.9, 1.1)
							Asthma + hay fever	0.9 (0.7, 1.2)
							Asthma or hay fever	1.0 (0.9, 1.1)
						Leukemia ($n = 3,782$)	Asthma	0.8 (0.6, 1.0)
							Hay fever	1.0 (0.9, 1.1)
							Asthma + hay fever	0.8 (0.6, 1.1)
							Asthma or hay fever	0.9 (0.8, 1.0)
Vesterinen et al. [33]	Retrospective cohort ($n = 77,952$) (Sweden)	National database linkage	Standardized incidence ratio	National Pharmacy Database	National Cancer Registry	Males: Multiple myeloma ($n = 22$)	Asthma medications	1.1 (0.7, 1.6)
						NHL ($n = 28$)		0.9 (0.6, 1.4)
						Leukemia ($n = 31$)		0.8 (0.5, 1.1)
						Females: Multiple myeloma ($n = 16$)	Asthma medications	**0.5 (0.3, 0.9)**
						NHL ($n = 37$)		1.0 (0.7, 1.4)
						Leukemia ($n = 39$)		0.9 (0.6, 1.2)

[a]95% confidence interval.

Table 5.3 Case–control studies examining atopic conditions and risk of leukemia

Author	Design	Sample size cases/controls	Response rate	Source of subjects/criteria	Disease validation	Exposure validation	Leukemia subtype	Exposure	Exposed cases/ exposed controls	Odds ratio (95% CI[a])
Becker et al. [19]	Frequency-matched multi-center European study	Cases: 414 Controls: 2,458	Cases: 87.7% Controls: 68.5%	Cases: identified from hospitals and physicians Controls: population-based in 2 studies; hospital-based in 5 studies.	Pathology reports	Questionnaire	CLL[b] ($n = 414$)	Respiratory allergy	60/375	1.0 (0.8, 1.4)
								Food allergy	17/171	0.6 (0.4, 1.1)
								Medicine allergy	52/322	1.0 (0.7, 1.4)
Cooper et al. [14]	Frequency matched	Cases: 748 Controls: 637	Cases: 83% in first recruitment 95% in second recruitment Controls: 80%	Cases: age 18–79 participants in trials Controls: population-based	Pathology reports	Questionnaire	Adult AML[c] ($n = 624$)	Hay fever	94/96	1.0 (0.7, 1.4)
								Allergies to: bee or wasp	31/32	1.0 (0.6, 1.7)
								Penicillin	38/39	1.0 (0.6, 1.7)
								No. of allergies:		
								1	141/155	0.9 (0.7, 1.2)
								2	76/58	1.3 (0.9, 2.0)
								Asthma	38/54	0.7 (0.5, 1.2)
								Eczema	27/26	1.1 (0.6, 2.0)
							Adult ALL[d]	Hay fever	23/96	1.0 (0.6, 1.8)
								Allergies to: bee or wasp	5/32	0.8 (0.3, 2.1)
								Penicillin	12/39	**2.2 (1.04, 4.40)**
								No. of allergies:		
								1	28/155	0.9 (0.6, 1.5)

Table 5.3 (continued)

Author	Design	Sample size cases/controls	Response rate	Source of subjects/criteria	Disease validation	Exposure validation	Leukemia subtype	Exposure	Exposed cases/ exposed controls	Odds ratio (95% CI[a])
								2	15/58	1.1 (0.6, 2.2)
								Asthma	10/54	0.9 (0.4, 1.9)
								Eczema	9/26	1.7 (0.7, 4.2)
Doody et al. [17]	Individually matched	Cases: 133 Controls: 162	NA	Kaiser Permanente (HMO)	Medical record	Medical record	AML[c] 15+ years	Hay fever	17/8	2.5 (1.0, 6.1)
								Eczema	9/15	0.6 (0.3, 1.4)
Hughes et al. [12]	Individually matched	Cases: 940 Controls: 1,337	NA	Cases: all regional hospitals, national clinical trials and cancer registries Controls: general practice rolls, matched to case by practice	Medical record	Questionnaire by mother, validated by medical record	ALL[d] (< 14 years) ($n = 839$)	Probable asthma	69/135	1.0 (0.7, 1.3)
								Use of asthma medications	65/129	1.0 (0.7, 1.3)
								Probable hay fever	15/60	**0.5 (0.3, 0.8)**
								Use of hay fever medications	15/58	**0.5 (0.3, 0.9)**
								Probable eczema	217/433	0.9 (0.7, 1.1)
								Use of eczema medications	60/156	**0.7 (0.51, 0.97)**
								At least one atopic condition	260/523	0.9 (0.7, 1.1)
								Use of medication for at least one atopic condition	125/288	0.8 (0.6, 1.0)
							AML[c] (< 14 years) ($n = 101$)	Probable asthma	13/135	1.1 (0.6, 2.2)
								Use of asthma medications	13/129	1.2 (0.6, 2.2)

Table 5.3 (continued)

Author	Design	Sample size cases/controls	Response rate	Source of subjects/criteria	Disease validation	Exposure validation	Leukemia subtype	Exposure	Exposed cases/ exposed controls	Odds ratio (95% CI[a])
								Probable hay fever	8/60	1.2 (0.5, 2.8)
								Use of hay fever medications	8/58	1.3 (0.6, 2.9)
								Probable eczema	28/433	0.8 (0.5, 1.2)
								Use of eczema medications	12/156	1.0 (0.5, 1.9)
								At least one atopic condition	38/523	0.8 (0.5, 1.3)
								Use of medication for at least one atopic condition	23/288	0.9 (0.6, 1.5)
Jourdan-Da Silva et al. [7]	Frequency matched	Cases: 473 Controls: 805	Cases: 73.2% Controls: 71%	Cases: National Registry of Childhood Leukemia and Lymphoma Controls: population-based	Medical records	Questionnaire by mother	ALL[d] < 15 years	Asthma	17/44	**0.5 (0.3, 0.9)**
								Asthma or bron-chodilators	25/31	1.0 (0.6, 1.8)
								Asthma and bron-chodilators	6/29	**0.3 (0.1, 0.7)**

Table 5.3 (continued)

Author	Design	Sample size cases/controls	Response rate	Source of subjects/criteria	Disease validation	Exposure validation	Leukemia subtype	Exposure	Exposed cases/ exposed controls	Odds ratio (95% CI[a])
Melbye et al. [20]	Frequency matched	Cases: 3,055 Controls: 3,187	Eligible cases: 81% Eligible controls: 71%	Cases: hospitals and cancer registry Controls: population registers	Histopathology review and/or pathology report	Questionnaire	CLL[b]	Allergic rhinitis or hay fever	161/815	0.9 (0.8, 1.1)
								Childhood eczema	37/202	1.1 (0.70, 1.6)
								Asthma	60/275	0.9 (0.7, 1.2)
								Elevated IgE	43/372	**0.4 (0.3, 0.5)**
Rosenbaum et al. [8]	Frequency matched	Cases: 255 Controls: 760	Case: 71% Control: 55%	Cases: tumor registry at multi center medical center Controls: birth certificate registry	Pathology report	Questionnaire	ALL[d] < 15 years	Any allergy	34/153	**0.6 (0.4, 0.9)**
								Asthma	7/31	0.6 (0.3, 1.4)
								Pollen, dust, dander	8/47	**0.5 (0.21, 0.97)**
								Food, drug, bee	11/72	**0.4 (0.2, 0.8)**
								Eczema	16/58	0.7 (0.4, 1.3)
Schulz et al. [9]	Population-based individually matched case–control study (3 centers)	Cases: 1,294 Controls: 2,957	Cases: 80.5–83.6% Controls: 68.1–71.0%	Cases: German Childhood Cancer Registry Controls: census-based	Cancer registry	Questionnaire	ALL[d] < 14 years (n = 1,130)	Hay fever	36/208	**0.5 (0.3, 0.7)**
								Neuro-dermatitis	38/192	**0.5 (0.3, 0.7)**
								Asthma	7/35	0.6 (0.3, 1.4)
								Eczema	25/97	**0.6 (0.39, 0.99)**
								Hives	9/19	1.3 (0.6, 2.9)
								Food or drug allergy	40/123	0.8 (0.6, 1.2)
								Allergic reaction to insects and other unspecified substances	13/46	0.6 (0.3, 1.1)

Table 5.3 (continued)

Author	Design	Sample size cases/controls	Response rate	Source of subjects/criteria	Disease validation	Exposure validation	Leukemia subtype	Exposure	Exposed cases/ exposed controls	Odds ratio (95% CI[a])
							AML ($n = 164$)	Hay fever	11/208	1.0 (0.5, 2.1)
								Neuro-dermatitis	9/192	0.8 (0.4, 1.7)
								Asthma	0/35	-
								Eczema	5/97	0.8 (0.3, 2.1)
								Hives	0/19	-
								Food or drug allergy	3/123	0.6 (0.2, 1.9)
								Allergic reaction to insects and other unspecified substances	3/46	0.9 (0.3, 3.3)
Severson et al. [15]	Frequency matched	Cases: 164 Controls: 133	Cases: 69.5% Controls: 65.2%	Cases: acute non-lymphocytic leukemia from Cancer Surveillance System (SEER), Age 20–79 Controls: group matched by sex and 5-year age group.	Pathology report	In person interview	Adult AML[c]	Any allergy	31/79	**0.4 (0.2, 0.6)**
								Penicillin	8/16	0.4 (0.2, 1.1)
								Sulfa drugs	3/6	0.4 (0.1, 1.8)
								Other antibiotics	3/9	0.3 (0.1, 1.1)
								Other drugs	6/18	**0.3 (0.1, 0.8)**
								Dust	10/35	**0.3 (0.1, 0.5)**
								Eggs/feathers	3/15	**0.2 (0.1. 0.6)**
								Foods	5/30	**0.2 (0.1, 0.4)**
								Pollen	12/44	**0.2 (0.1, 0.5)**
								Bee/insect stings	3/15	**0.2 (0.1, 0.6)**
								Dogs/cats	15/2	**0.1 (0.1, 0.4)**
								Other allergies	39/10	**0.2 (0.1, 0.5)**

Table 5.3 (continued)

Author	Design	Sample size cases/controls	Response rate	Source of subjects/criteria	Disease validation	Exposure validation	Leukemia subtype	Exposure	Exposed cases/ exposed controls	Odds ratio (95% CI[a])
								No. of allergies:		
								1	19/15	0.7 (0.3, 1.6)
								2	17/6	0.4 (0.1, 1.1)
								3	43/10	**0.2 (0.1, 0.5)**
Spector et al. [13]	Individually matched	Cases: 180 Controls: 718	N/A	Kaiser Permanente (HMO)	Pathology reports	Medical records	ALL[d] < 6 years	Allergy Dx > 1-year prior	48/173	1.2 (0.8, 1.9)
								Allergy Dx < 1-year prior	21/53	**1.8 (1.02, 3.33)**
								No. of allergies Dx > 1-year prior:		
								1	34/132	1.1 (0.7, 1.8)
								2	9/33	1.4 (0.6, 3.2)
								3	5/8	2.9 (0.9, 2.6)
								No. of allergies Dx < 1-year prior:		
								1	20/48	**1.9 (1.1, 3.6)**
								2	1/5	0.6 (0.1, 5.9)
								Asthma Dx> 1-year prior	18/57	1.6 (0.9, 2.9)
								Asthma Dx < 1-year prior	13/21	**3.1 (1.4, 7.0)**
								Atopy	19/45	**2.2 (1.2, 4.2)**

Table 5.3 (continued)

Author	Design	Sample size cases/controls	Response rate	Source of subjects/criteria	Disease validation	Exposure validation	Leukemia subtype	Exposure	Exposed cases/ exposed controls	Odds ratio (95% CI[a])
								Dx > 1-year prior		
								Atopy Dx < 1-year prior	5/9	3.8 (1.0, 14.3)
								Eczema Dx > 1year prior	20/62	1.1 (0.6, 2.0)
								Eczema Dx < 1-year prior	0/14	∞
								Food, drug, bee allergy Dx > 1-year prior	8/44	0.7 (0.3, 1.5)
								Food, drug, bee allergy Dx < 1-year prior	4/14	1.2 (0.4, 4.4)
								Pollen, dust, dander Dx > 1-year prior	3/10	1.1 (0.3, 5.2)
								Pollen, dust, dander Dx < 1year prior	0/0	-
							B-cell ALL[d]	Allergy Dx > 1-year prior	44/158	1.2 (0.8, 1.9)

Table 5.3 (continued)

Author	Design	Sample size cases/controls	Response rate	Source of subjects/criteria	Disease validation	Exposure validation	Leukemia subtype	Exposure	Exposed cases/ exposed controls	Odds ratio (95% CI[a])
								Allergy Dx < 1-year prior	15/39	1.7 (0.9, 3.3)
								No. allergies Dx > 1-year prior:		
								1	31/121	1.1 (0.7, 1.8)
								2	9/29	1.5 (0.7, 3.5)
								3	4/8	2.4 (0.7, 8.5)
								No. allergies Dx < 1-year prior:		
								1	14/35	1.7 (0.9, 3.5)
								2	1/4	0.7 (0.1, 7.3)
								Asthma Dx > 1-year prior	18/57	1.6 (0.9, 3.0)
								Asthma Dx < 1-year prior	10/16	**3.4 (1.3, 8.7)**
								Atopy Dx > 1-year prior	16/41	**2.0 (1.03, 3.96)**
								Atopy Dx < 1-year prior	4/7	3.7 (0.9, 16.2)
								Eczema Dx > 1-year prior	19/62	1.1 (0.6, 2.0)

Table 5.3 (continued)

Author	Design	Sample size cases/controls	Response rate	Source of subjects/criteria	Disease validation	Exposure validation	Leukemia subtype	Exposure	Exposed cases/ exposed controls	Odds ratio (95% CI[a])
								Eczema Dx < 1-year prior	0/12	∞
								Food, drug, bee allergy Dx > 1-year prior	8/41	0.7 (0.3, 1.7)
								Food, drug, bee allergy Dx < 1-year prior	2/8	0.9 (0.2, 4.8)
								Pollen, dust, dander Dx > 1-year prior	3/10	1.1 (0.2, 5.2)
								Pollen, dust dander Dx < 1-year prior	0/0	-
Soderberg et al. [11]	Swedish National Database Study; randomly selected controls	Cases: 12,397 Controls: 149,344	N/A	Swedish Cancer Registry, Population Registry and Hospital Discharge Database	Cancer Registry	National Hospital Discharge Database	ALL[d] ($n = 1446$)	Asthma	10/2,176	0.6 (0.3, 1.0)
							CLL[b] ($n = 4744$)	Asthma	70/2,176	0.9 (0.7, 1.1)
							AML[c] ($n = 3490$)	Asthma	46/2,176	0.8 (0.6, 1.1)
							CML[e] ($n = 1164$)	Asthma	16/2,176	1.0 (0.6, 1.6)
Vineis et al. [16]	Population based cases;	Cases: 574 Controls:1,718	Cases: 90% Controls: 81%	Cases: all hospitals in	Hospital record	Questionnaire	Adult lymphoid	Eczema Allergies	Not given	1.2 (0.7, 2.1) 1.0 (0.6, 1.6)

Table 5.3 (continued)

Author	Design	Sample size cases/controls	Response rate	Source of subjects/criteria	Disease validation	Exposure validation	Leukemia subtype	Exposure	Exposed cases/ exposed controls	Odds ratio (95% CI[a])
	randomly selected controls			catchment area Controls: randomly selected from census and health system			(n = 261) Adult myeloid (n = 313)	Hay fever	Not given	1.1 (0.6, 1.9)
								Eczema		0.8 (0.4, 1.4)
								Allergies		0.7 (0.4, 1.2)
								Hay fever		**0.5 (0.2, 0.9)**
Wen et al. [10]	Individually matched	Cases: 1,842 Control:,1,986	Case: 92% Controls: 76.5%	Cases: Children's Cancer Study Controls: RDD[f]	Medical record, slide review	Telephone interview with mother of case	ALL[d] < 15 years	Asthma	135/176	0.8 (0.6, 1.0)
								Hay fever	86/150	**0.6 (0.5, 0.8)**
								Food, drug allergies	327/487	**0.7 (0.6, 0.8)**
								Eczema	91/145	**0.7 (0.5, 0.9)**
								Hives	136/166	0.9 (0.7, 1.2)
								Any condition	545/746	**0.7 (0.6, 0.8)**
								No, of atopic conditions		
								1	Not given	**0.8 (0.7, 0.9)**
								2+	Not given	**0.6 (0.5, 0.7)**
Zhang et al. [21]	Frequency matched; females only	Cases: 601 Controls: 717	Cases: 54% of total cases; 72% of eligible cases Controls: 69% 47% for Medicare/ Medicaid	Cases: Connecticut Tumor Registry (population-based) Controls: RDD[f] and Medicare/ Medicaid	Histologically confirmed by registry	Questionnaire	CLL[b]	Eczema	5/62	1.0 (0.4, 2.6)

[a]95% confidence interval; [b]chronic lymphocytic leukemia; [c]acute myelogenous leukemia; [d]acute lymphocytic leukemia; [e]chronic myelogenous leukemia; [f]random digit dial.

The most common adult-onset leukemia is chronic lymphocytic leukemia (CLL), which has been recently reclassified together with small lymphocytic NHL based on the common origin from a mature, but naïve (no antigen contact), B-lymphocyte [18]. Prior to this reclassification, when considered as a separate entity apart from NHL, CLL risk was not found to be associated with allergy, eczema, or asthma in either case–control [11, 19–21] or cohort [22] studies. However, when physiological measures were used (IgE levels), a decreased risk was reported [20].

5.4 Non-Hodgkin Lymphoma

Lymphomas are solid collectively tumors of lymphocyte origin and are the most common hematopoietic cancers, representing the fifth most common cancer, in terms of incidence rate, and the sixth in terms of cancer deaths, among both men and women in the United States {http://apps.nccd.cdc.gov/uscs} (Table 5.1). Most lymphomas originate from mature B lymphocytes, cells that have undergone the initial developmental stages and somatic DNA changes that result in the formation and expression of cell-surface Ig molecules, (the B-cell receptor for antigen). However, this broad classification represents epidemiologically, pathologically, clinically, and etiologically heterogeneous groups of cancers, consisting of Hodgkin lymphoma and plasma cell tumors (see sections below), T cell and natural killer cell lymphoma, and various types of B-cell NHL, including follicular lymphoma, diffuse large B-cell lymphoma (DLBCL), mantle cell lymphoma, and Burkitt lymphoma [23, 24]. While some NHLs are infected with Epstein–Barr virus (EBV), the great majority of the B-cell NHL seen in immunocompetent persons are EBV-negative.

Several types of B-cell NHL reflect different stages of B-cell differentiation, originating from naïve B cells, as well as B cells that have undergone various molecular changes that occur after initial encounter with antigen and exposure to helper T cells in secondary lymphoid organs [18]. As these activation-promoting interactions occur in the germinal centers of lymph nodes and other lymphoid organs, these cells are referred to as post-germinal center B cells. The germinal center reaction, which occurs in lymph nodes and other secondary lymphoid organs after initial encounter of B cells with antigen, involves rapid B-cell proliferation and somatic DNA changes that result in both changes in the isotype of the Ig that is produced by these cells (from IgM to IgG or other isotypes), as well as enhanced antigen-binding affinity. These DNA-modifying processes consist of Ig class switch recombination (CSR), which involves the recombination of the Ig variable region segment in Ig heavy chain genes (*IgH*) from IgM to another isotype (i.e., IgG), with the looping out and excision of intervening DNA; and somatic hypermutation (SHM), the active mutation of the variable region of Ig genes, which, when combined with selection by antigen, results in the production of antibodies with enhanced antigen-binding affinity. Errors in both *IgH* CSR and SHM are believed to lead to the seminal molecular lesions for many forms of B-cell lymphoma, as well as other mature B-cell cancers. Translocations/mutations involving other oncogenes, such as *BCL6*, are involved in

other forms of NHL (diffuse large B-cell lymphoma) and are thought to result from errors in SHM.

The association between atopy and NHL has been examined in 14 case–control studies and four cohort studies meeting our criteria, some with [19–21] and some without [5, 11, 16, 17, 22, 25–33] the inclusion of CLL patients (Tables 5.2 and 5.4). The majority used self-reported history as a measure of exposure. Nine case–control studies and one cohort study found a decreased risk of NHL linked to at least one allergic condition [5, 19, 20, 25, 27–31, 34], but the specificity of the exposure was not consistent across the studies. Hay fever or allergic rhinitis was inversely associated in three studies [20, 27, 34], but no association was observed in seven studies [16, 17, 19, 21, 22, 26, 32]. Two general population-based studies [19, 29] and one study of human immunodeficiency virus (HIV) sero-negative homosexual men [5] found food allergies to be inversely linked, but no such link was reported in five other studies (in men and women generally [25–27, 30] and in HIV sero-positive homosexual men [5]). Eczema was inversely associated with NHL in two studies [25, 28], positively associated in one [22], and no statistically significant association was observed in five others [16, 17, 20, 21, 27]. Inconsistent results have also been reported for allergies to specific antigenic substances [5, 26, 27, 29, 30], allergy shots, and asthma [11, 20, 21, 27, 28] (Tables 5.2 and 5.4).

As described above, NHL constitutes a heterogeneous and sometimes progressive group of lymphoid malignancies with subtypes corresponding to the stage of B- or T-cell development of the neoplastic clone. Major subtypes may have different descriptive risk patterns, which would suggest different etiological pathways [23, 24]. Thus examination by subtype is desirable, although often limited by power. Using cases classified by the World Health Organization (WHO)/Revised European-American Classification of Lymphoid Neoplasms (REAL) classification system [18], we [27] found that a history of any allergy, excluding allergy to medications, was inversely linked to DLBCL but not to follicular lymphoma. Conversely, eczema was associated with an increased risk of follicular but not DLBCL [27]. No link between self-reported allergic conditions and these common NHL subtypes was seen in two other studies using the same classification system [20, 21]. However, in an earlier study based on the Working Formulation, reclassified into the WHO/REAL classification, Holly and Bracci [35] reported a negative association between plant allergy and both DLBCL and small lymphocytic subtypes, and between animal allergy and DLBCL. These investigators also reported an increased risk of small lymphocytic and follicular lymphoma linked to hives [35]. T-cell lymphoma (mycosis fungoides) was assessed in a single small study and found to be inversely linked to metal, food allergy and to positive skin prick tests [36].

Two cohort studies attempting to assess the relationship between physiologic measures of atopy and NHL had insufficient power [1, 2]. In a large case–control study, Melbye et al. reported an inverse link between high serum IgE levels and total NHL and CLL subtypes in particular [20]. In a parallel analysis, they conducted a nested case–control study examining IgE levels measured from blood samples collected decades earlier as part of a national pregnancy cohort study [20]. An inverse

Table 5.4 Case–control studies examining atopic conditions and risk of non-Hodgkin lymphoma (NHL)

Author	Design	Sample size cases/controls	Response rate	Source of subjects/criteria	Disease validation	Exposure validation	NHL subtype	Exposure	Exposed cases/ exposed controls	Odds ratio (95% CI[a])
Becker et al. [19]	Frequency-matched multi-center European study	Cases: 2,480 NHL (excluding CLL[b]) Controls: 2,458	Cases: 87.7% Controls: 68.5%	Cases: identified from hospitals and physicians Controls: population-based in two studies and hospital-based in five studies	Pathology reports	Questionnaire	B-NHL ($n = 1879$)	Respiratory allergy	252/375	0.9 (0.7, 1.1)
								Food allergy	91/171	**0.7 (0.5, 0.9)**
								Medicine allergy	272/322	1.1 (0.9, 1.4)
							Diffuse large B cell ($n = 543$)	Respiratory allergy	65/375	0.8 (0.6, 1.0)
								Food allergy	29/171	0.8 (0.5, 1.1)
								Medicine allergy	73/322	1.1 (0.8, 1.4)
							Follicular ($n = 251$)	Respiratory allergy	36/375	0.9 (0.6, 1.2)
								Food allergy	21/171	1.0 (0.6, 1.6)
								Medicine allergy	42/322	1.2 (0.9, 1.7)
							Other B cells ($n = 671$)	Respiratory allergy	51/375	1.1 (0.8, 1.5)
								Food allergy	13/171	0.6 (0.3, 1.1)
								Medicine allergy	56 /322	**1.5 (1.1, 2.0)**
							T cell ($n = 137$)	Respiratory allergy	15/375	0.7 (0.4, 1.2)
								Food allergy	6/171	0.7 (0.3, 1.6)
								Medicine allergy	13/322	0.7 (0.4, 1.3)

Table 5.4 (continued)

Author	Design	Sample size cases/controls	Response rate	Source of subjects/criteria	Disease validation	Exposure validation	NHL subtype	Exposure	Exposed cases/ exposed controls	Odds ratio (95% CI[a])
Bernstein et al. [25]	Individually matched	Cases: 619 Controls: 619	Cases: 67% Controls: 72%	Cases: population-based cancer registry Controls: neighborhood controls	Pathology reports	Questionnaire	NHL (excluding leukemia)	Eczema	33/52	**0.6 (0.4, 0.96)**
								Allergy to nuts/ berries	44/61	0.7 (0.5, 1.1)
								Allergy to insect stings	47/64	0.7 (0.4, 1.0)
								Asthma, hay fever, allergies to: eggs, milk, other foods, animal furs, pollen/dust, fabric, soaps/ perfumes, jewelry/ metals, detergents, cleaning com- pounds, aerosol sprays, stain removers, other allergies	–	All non- significant ($p > 0.05$)

Table 5.4 (continued)

Author	Design	Sample size cases/controls	Response rate	Source of subjects/criteria	Disease validation	Exposure validation	NHL subtype	Exposure	Exposed cases/ exposed controls	Odds ratio (95% CI[a])
Bracci et al. [34]	Frequency matched	Cases: 1,593 Controls: 2,515	Cases: 72% Controls: 78%	Cases: Northern California Cancer Center rapid case ascertainment Controls: RDD[c] of Medicare, Medicaid, frequency matched by age (5year), sex, residence	Pathology report	Questionnaire	NHL (excluding leukemia)	Allergic rhinitis	276/691	**0.7 (0.6, 0.8)**
Briggs et al. [26]	Population based cases; Randomly selected controls	Cases: 952 Controls: 1,691	Cases: 88.1% Controls: 83.1%	Cases: 8 population cancer registries Controls: RDD[c], by age, region of cancer registry	Histopathological slide review	Questionnaire	NHL (excluding leukemia)	Any allergies	248/476	1.0 (0.8, 1.2)
								No. allergies:		
								1	133/271	0.9 (0.7, 1.2)
								2	60/121	0.9 (0.6, 1.2)
								3+	55/84	1.2 (0.9, 1.8)
								Plants	141/258	1.0 (0.8, 1.3)
								Dust	84 /166	0.9 (0.7, 1.2)
								Food	40/79	1.1 (0.7, 1.6)
								Animals	37/64	1.1 (0.7, 1.7)
								Medication	62/112	1.0 (0.7, 1.4)
								Insect bite or sting	8/13	1.1 (0.5, 2.8)
								Specific chemical	11/8	**2.7 (1.1, 7.0)**
								Class of compound	5/20	0.5 (0.2, 1.2)
								Tobacco smoke	6/7	1.6 (0.5, 4.8)
								Fabrics	7/11	1.2 (0.4, 3.1)
Cozen et al. [27]	Frequency matched	Cases: 1,321 Controls: 1,057	Cases: 59% Controls: 44%	Cases: population-based cancer registries	Pathology reports	Questionnaire	NHL (excluding leukemia)	Hay fever	**149/155**	**0.7 (0.5, 0.9)**

Table 5.4 (continued)

Author	Design	Sample size cases/controls	Response rate	Source of subjects/criteria	Disease validation	Exposure validation	NHL subtype	Exposure	Exposed cases/ exposed controls	Odds ratio (95% CI[a])
				Controls: RDD[c] and HCFA[d] <65 y/o				Food allergies	78/82	0.8 (0.5, 1.1)
								Animal allergies	74/63	0.9 (0.6, 1.3)
								Insect allergies	48/42	0.9 (0.6, 1.4)
								Dust allergies	119/105	0.9 (0.7, 1.2)
								Medication allergies	193/141	**1.4 (1.1, 1.8)**
								Any allergy	343/298	0.9 (0.7, 1.2)
								Any non-medication allergy	252/210	0.7 (0.6, 1.0)
								Asthma	60/48	1.0 (0.7, 1.5)
								Eczema	52/35	1.2 (0.8, 1.9)
							Diffuse large B cell ($n = 417$)	Hay fever	46/155	**0.6 (0.4, 0.9)**
								Food allergies	29/82	0.8 (0.5, 1.4)
								Animal allergies	21/63	0.7 (0.4, 1.2)
								Insect allergies	13/42	0.7 (0.3, 1.3)
								Dust allergies	36/105	0.7 (0.5, 1.1)
								Medication allergies	69/141	**1.6 (1.1, 2.4)**
								Any allergy	116/298	0.9 (0.6, 1.3)

Table 5.4 (continued)

Author	Design	Sample size cases/controls	Response rate	Source of subjects/criteria	Disease validation	Exposure validation	NHL subtype	Exposure	Exposed cases/ exposed controls	Odds ratio (95% CI[a])
								Any non-medication allergy	85/210	**0.6 (0.4, 0.9)**
								Asthma	17/48	0.9 (0.5, 1.6)
								Eczema	11/35	0.9 (0.4, 1.8)
							Follicular ($n = 319$)	Hay fever	38/155	0.7 (0.5, 1.1)
								Food allergies	19/82	0.7 (0.4, 1.3)
								Animal allergies	19/63	0.9 (0.5, 1.6)
								Insect allergies	9/42	0.6 (0.3, 1.3)
								Dust allergies	30/105	0.8 (0.5, 1.3)
								Medication allergies	46/141	1.3 (0.7, 1.2)
								Any allergy	86/298	0.8 (0.5, 1.2)
								Any non-medication allergy	67 /252	0.7 (0.5, 1.0)
								Asthma	19/48	1.5 (0.8, 2.7)
								Eczema	21/35	**2.3 (1.1, 4.2)**
								Hay fever	6/24	0.5 (0.2, 1.2)
Doody et al. [17]	Individually matched (two controls per case)	Cases: 100 Controls: 191	NA	Kaiser Permanente (HMO)	Medical record	Medical record	NHL (excluding leukemia)	Eczema	7/7	1.9 (0.6, 5.8)
Fabbro-Peray et al. [28]	Quasi population-based for cases; randomly selected controls	Cases: 445 Controls: 1,025	Cases: 82.5% Controls: 52.2%	Cases: Hospitals Controls: Election roles	Medical records	Questionnaire	NHL (excluding leukemia)	Eczema	36/168	**0.5 (0.3, 0.7)**
								Hives	120/208	**1.7 (1.2, 2.1)**
								Asthma	27/79	0.8 (0.5, 1.3)

Table 5.4 (continued)

Author	Design	Sample size cases/controls	Response rate	Source of subjects/criteria	Disease validation	Exposure validation	NHL subtype	Exposure	Exposed cases/ exposed controls	Odds ratio (95% CI[a])
Grulich et al. [29]	Frequency matched	Cases: 704 Controls: 694	Cases: 60% Controls: 41%	Cases: New South Wales Cancer Registry, age 20–74 Control: randomly selected from electoral rolls	Not mentioned	Questionnaire	NHL (excluding leukemia)	Allergic to:		
								Food or medicine	222/228	1.0 (0.8, 1.2)
								One or more foods	41/119	**0.3 (0.2, 0.4)**
								Seafood	8/30	**0.3 (0.1, 0.6)**
								Preservatives	6/6	1.0 (0.3, 3.3)
								Dairy foods	11/22	0.5 (0.2, 1.0)
								One or more medicines	184/178	1.0 (0.8, 1.3)
								Antibiotics	117/110	1.1 (0.8, 1.5)
								Penicillin	65/62	1.1 (0.7, 1.5)
								Sulfa drugs	39/34	1.1 (0.7, 1.8)
								Analgesics	46/36	1.3 (0.8, 2.0)
Holly et al. [35]	Frequency matched	Cases: 1,304 Controls: 2,515	Cases: 57% (including deceased) 72% excluding deceased Controls: 78%	Cases: population-based cancer registry Controls: RDD[c] and HCFA[d] (for > 65)	Cancer registry validation and pathology review	Questionnaire	Small lymphocytic ($n = 152$)	Animal dander	5/179	0.6 (0.2, 1.4)
								Plants	23/691	**0.5 (0.3, 0.8)**
								Hives	9/62	**2.2 (1.1, 4.5)**
								Childhood eczema	–	–
							Follicular ($n = 352$)	Animal dander	18/179	0.7 (0.4, 1.2)
								Plants	87/691	0.9 (0.7, 1.1)
								Hives	20/62	**2.1 (1.3, 3.6)**
								Childhood eczema	12/81	0.9 (0.5, 1.8)
							Diffuse small cleaved-cell ($n = 68$)	Animal dander	2/179	0.5 (0.1, 2.2)
								Plants	18/691	1.0 (0.6, 1.8)
								Hives	3/62	1.7 (0.5, 5.5)
								Childhood eczema	2/81	1.0 (0.2, 4.0)

Table 5.4 (continued)

Author	Design	Sample size cases/controls	Response rate	Source of subjects/criteria	Disease validation	Exposure validation	NHL subtype	Exposure	Exposed cases/exposed controls	Odds ratio (95% CI[a])
							Diffuse mixed small cleaved and large cell ($n = 75$)	Animal dander	5/179	1.0 (0.4, 2.7)
								Plants	24/691	1.3 (0.8, 2.1)
								Hives	4/62	2.0 (0.7, 5.7)
								Childhood eczema	2/81	0.8 (0.2, 3.2)
							Diffuse large B cell ($n = 510$)	Animal dander	13/179	**0.3 (0.2, 0.6)**
								Plants	100/691	**0.6 (0.5, 0.8)**
								Hives	23/62	1.7 (1.0, 2.8)
								Childhood eczema	29/81	**1.6 (1.1, 2.6)**
Holly et al. [5]	Frequency matched	Cases: 312 Controls: 412	Cases: 57% (including deceased) 72% excluding deceased Controls: 75%	Cases: population-based cancer registry Controls: RDD[c] and HCFA[d] (for > 65)	Cancer registry validation and pathology review	Questionnaire	NHL (excluding leukemia)	Any non-medication allergies	114/59	**0.5 (0.3, 0.8)**
							HIV-positive homosexual men ($n = 263$ cases, 97 controls)	Food allergies	26/11	0.9 (0.4, 1.8)
								Allergies to plants, pollen	35/30	**0.3 (0.2, 0.6)**
								Allergies to dust, chalk, mold	11/13	**0.3 (0.1, 0.7)**
								Allergy to animals	13/9	0.5 (0.2, 1.3)
								Antihistamine use for 4 weeks	46/28	**0.5 (0.3, 0.9)**

Table 5.4 (continued)

Author	Design	Sample size cases/controls	Response rate	Source of subjects/criteria	Disease validation	Exposure validation	NHL subtype	Exposure	Exposed cases/ exposed controls	Odds ratio (95% CI[a])
							NHL (excluding leukemia)	Any non-medication allergies	16/199	**0.3 (0.2, 0.6)**
							HIV negative homosexual men ($n = 48$ cases, 321 controls)	Food allergies	3/55	**0.3 (0.1, 0.9)**
								Allergies to plants, pollen	7/88	0.5 (0.2, 1.1)
								Allergies to dust, chalk, mold	2/38	0.4 (0.1, 1.6)
								Allergy to animals	2/40	0.4 (0.1, 1.5)
								Antihistamine use for 4 weeks	1/58	**0.1 (0.0, 0.7)**
Holly et al. [30]	Frequency matched	Cases: 1,281 Controls: 2,095	Cases: 57% (including deceased) 72% (excluding deceased) Controls: 78%	Cases from cancer registry, controls from RDD[c] and HCFA[d] (> 65-year old)	Cancer registry validation and pathology review	Questionnaire	NHL (excluding leukemia) Heterosexual Men (cases $n = 701$; controls $n = 1,257$)	Medication allergies	147/243	1.0 (0.8, 1.3)
								Any non-medication allergies	268/557	0.8 (0.7, 1.0)

Table 5.4 (continued)

Author	Design	Sample size cases/controls	Response rate	Source of subjects/criteria	Disease validation	Exposure validation	NHL subtype	Exposure	Exposed cases/exposed controls	Odds ratio (95% CI[a])
								Food allergies	80/149	1.0 (0.7, 1.3)
								Allergies to plants, pollen	70/211	**0.6 (0.4, 0.8)**
								Allergies to dust, chalk, mold	41/91	0.9 (0.6, 1.3)
								Allergy to animals	19/76	**0.5 (0.3, 0.8)**
								Hives	105/161	1.2 (0.9, 1.5)
								Asthma	50/104	0.9 (0.6, 1.2)
								Allergy shots	25/84	**0.5 (0.3, 0.9)**
							NHL (excluding leukemia) Women (cases = 580; controls = 838)	Medication allergies	176/307	**0.8 (0.6, 0.9)**
								Any non-medication allergies	271/452	**0.8 (0.6, 0.9)**
								Food allergies	96/169	0.8 (0.6, 1.0)
								Allergies to plants, pollen	65/159	**0.5 (0.4, 0.7)**
								Allergies to dust, chalk, mold	43/91	0.7 (0.5, 1.0)
								Allergy to animals	32/64	0.7 (0.5, 1.1)
								Hives	110/221	**0.7 (0.5, 0.8)**
								Asthma	39/68	0.8 (0.5, 1.2)

Table 5.4 (continued)

Author	Design	Sample size cases/controls	Response rate	Source of subjects/criteria	Disease validation	Exposure validation	NHL subtype	Exposure	Exposed cases/ exposed controls	Odds ratio (95% CI[a])
								Allergy shots	22/54	0.6 (0.3, 1.0)
Melbye et al. [20]	Frequency matched	Cases: 3,055 Controls: 3,187	Eligible cases: 81% Eligible Controls: 71%	Cases: hospitals and cancer registry Controls: population registers	Histopathology review and/or pathology report	Questionnaire	NHL	Allergic rhinitis or hay fever	658/815	**0.9 (0.77, 0.98)**
								Childhood eczema	151/202	0.9 (0.7, 1.2)
								Asthma	251/275	1.0 (0.8, 1.2)
								Elevated IgE	341/372	**0.7 (0.6, 0.8)**
							Diffuse large B cell (*n* = 796)	Allergic rhinitis or hay fever	170/815	0.8 (0.7, 1.0)
								Childhood eczema	39/202	0.9 (0.6, 1.3)
								Asthma	68/275	1.0 (0.8, 1.3)
								Elevated IgE	110/372	0.8 (0.7, 1.1)
							Follicular (*n* = 568)	Allergic rhinitis or hay fever	142 /815	1.0 (0.8, 1.2)
								Childhood eczema	32/202	1.0 (0.7, 1.5)
								Asthma	39/275	0.8 (0.6, 1.1)
								Elevated IgE	76/372	0.8 (0.6, 1.0)
							T cell (*n* = 204)	Allergic rhinitis or hay fever	42/815	0.8 (0.5, 1.1)
								Childhood eczema	14/202	1.0 (0.6, 1.8)
								Asthma	22/275	1.3 (0.7, 1.6)
								Elevated IgE	37/372	1.1 (0.7, 1.6)

Table 5.4 (continued)

Author	Design	Sample size cases/controls	Response rate	Source of subjects/criteria	Disease validation	Exposure validation	NHL subtype	Exposure	Exposed cases/ exposed controls	Odds ratio (95% CI[a])
							Mantle cell ($n = 148$)	Allergic rhinitis or hay fever	22/815	0.6 (0.4, 1.0)
								Childhood eczema	5/202	0.8 (0.3, 2.1)
								Asthma	11/275	0.9 (0.5, 1.7)
								Elevated IgE	19/372	0.8 (0.5, 1.4)
							Marginal zone ($n = 117$)	Allergic rhinitis or hay fever	22/815	0.7 (0.4, 1.2)
								Childhood eczema	3/202	0.5 (0.2, 1.7)
								Asthma	10/275	0.9 (0.5, 1.9)
								Elevated IgE	8/372	0.5 (0.2, 1.0)
							Lympho-Plasmacytic ($n = 116$)	Allergic rhinitis or hay fever	18/815	0.8 (0.3, 2.3)
								Childhood eczema	4/202	0.8 (0.3, 2.1)
								Asthma	14/275	1.3 (0.7, 2.4)
								Elevated IgE	11/372	0.6 (0.3, 1.2)
Melbye et al. [20]	Nested individually matched	Cases: 198 Controls: 594	98% for the cohort	Finnish Pregnancy Cohort	Cancer registry linkage	Serum antigen-specific IgE	NHL*	Detectable versus non-detectable serum IgE	34/127	0.7 (0.5, 1.2)
								< 1-year before dx	1/10	0.3 (0.0, 2.3)
								1–4 years before dx	4/27	0.3 (0.1, 1.0)
								5–9 years before dx	15/49	1.0 (0.5, 1.8)
								≥10 years before dx	14/41	1.0 (0.5, 2.1)

Table 5.4 (continued)

Author	Design	Sample size cases/controls	Response rate	Source of subjects/criteria	Disease validation	Exposure validation	NHL subtype	Exposure	Exposed cases/ exposed controls	Odds ratio (95% CI[a])
Soderberg et al. [11]	Swedish National Database Study; randomly selected controls	Cases: 18,186 Controls: 149,344	NA	Swedish Cancer Registry, Population Registry and Hospital Discharge Database	Cancer registry	National Hospital Discharge Database	NHL (excluding leukemia)	Asthma Asthma > 10 years prior to dx	254/2,176 101/not given	0.9 (0.8, 1.0) 0.9 (0.7, 1.1)
Vineis et al. [16]	Population based cases; randomly selected controls	Cases: 1,388 Controls: 1,718	Cases: 90% Controls: 81%	Cases: all hospitals in catchment area Controls: randomly selected from census data	Hospital record	Questionnaire	NHL (excluding leukemia)	Eczema Allergies Hay fever	Not given Not given Not given	1.2 (0.9, 1.6) 0.9 (0.7, 1.3) 0.7 (0.5, 1.0)

Table 5.4 (continued)

Author	Design	Sample size cases/controls	Response rate	Source of subjects/criteria	Disease validation	Exposure validation	NHL subtype	Exposure	Exposed cases/ exposed controls	Odds ratio (95% CI[a])
Whittemore et al. [36]	Frequency matched	Cases: 174 Controls: 294	Cases: 60% Controls: 76%	Cases: population-based cancer registries and hospitals Controls: RDD[c]	Pathology report and slide review (subset)	Questionnaire	Mycosis fungoides	Type of skin allergy:		
								Any	100/203	0.7 (0.5, 1.0)
								Plants	64/132	0.7 (0.4, 1.1)
								Metals	10/36	**0.3 (0.1, 0.8)**
								Cosmetics	30/63	0.7 (0.4, 1.2)
								Skin medications (men)	8/2	**5.9 (1.2, 29.9)**
								Skin medications (women)	6/12	0.5 (0.1, 1.6)
								Other drugs	30/44	0.9 (0.5, 1.6)
								Hair dyes (women)	7/6	1.2 (0.3, 4.4)
								Food (men)	12/12	1.5 (0.6, 3.8)
								Food (women)	6/22	**0.3 (0.1, 0.8)**
								Insect bites (men)	8/6	1.8 (0.6, 5.6)
								Insect bites (women)	5/17	0.3 (0.1, 1.1)
								Skin allergy prick test positive	12/39	**0.2 (0.1, 0.7)**
								Skin allergy patch test positive	24/29	0.5 (0.2, 1.4)

Table 5.4 (continued)

Author	Design	Sample size cases/controls	Response rate	Source of subjects/criteria	Disease validation	Exposure validation	NHL subtype	Exposure	Exposed cases/ exposed controls	Odds ratio (95% CI[a])
Zhang et al. [21]	Frequency matched; females only	Cases: 601 Controls: 717	Cases: 54% of total cases; 72% of eligible cases Controls: 69% 47% for Medicare/ Medicaid	Cases: Connecticut Tumor Registry (population-based) Controls: RDD[c] and Medicare/ Medicaid	Histologically confirmed by registry	Questionnaire	NHL	Eczema	60/62	1.3 (0.9, 1.9)
								Hay fever	96/112	1.0 (0.8, 1.4)
								Asthma	57/66	1.0 (0.7, 1.4)
							B cell	Eczema	40/62	1.1 (0.7, 1.6)
							T-cell	Eczema	8/62	**2.5 (1.1, 5.7)**
							Other	Eczema	12/62	2.0 (1.0. 3.9)
							Follicular	Eczema	10/62	0.9 (0.4, 1.7)
							Marginal zone	Eczema	3/62	1.1 (0.3, 3.9)
							Diffuse large B cell	Eczema	19/62	1.3 (0.7, 2.3)

[a]95% confidence interval; [b]chronic lymphocytic leukemia (CLL]) included in total NHL, but CLL results shown separately in Table 5.3; [c]random digit dial; [d]Health care financing administration.

association between high IgE levels and NHL was most evident within a year of diagnosis, but became progressively weaker as the time prior to diagnosis increased, leading the authors to suggest that the apparent protective effect of atopy was, in fact, due to downregulation of IgE production caused by the developing NHL [20]. This is a plausible interpretation since B-cell lymphoma might interfere with the ability to produce antibodies, including IgE. However this substudy was based on a relatively small sample of subjects, none of the CIs excluded 1.0 and no p-value was given, so the results need to be replicated before the conclusion can be generally accepted. De Sanjose and colleagues found that Ig levels of all classes were lower in patients with advanced relative to early stage NHL [4], evidence supporting a pathogenic effect of the cancer on IgE levels.

Overall, the cumulative data suggest a modest protective effect of atopic conditions, especially allergy and hay fever, on NHL risk. This conclusion is strengthened by a recent pooled analysis of 13 case–control studies (13,535 NHL cases, 16,388 controls) [37]. (Only some of the case–control studies incorporated into this pooled analysis are included in this review; the excluded studies did not meet the criteria to be considered individually). The pooled data showed that hay fever and food allergies were associated with a 30% statistically significant decreased risk of several NHL subtypes and of NHL overall. The protective effect persisted when allergies were reported 10 years or more prior to diagnosis, supporting an etiological effect. Thus there appears to be some evidence that decreased IgE levels and/or allergy could be both etiologically and pathogenically linked to NHL. Further cohort studies with objective measures of atopy and allergy are needed to clarify this issue. We (Martinez-Maza and colleagues) are currently conducting a nested case–control study among a cohort of US military recruits to measure indicators of atopy and B-cell activation years prior to diagnosis.

5.5 Hodgkin Lymphoma

Hodgkin lymphoma consists of several etiologically distinct entities defined by age at diagnosis, histologic subtype, and presence or absence of EBV in the genome of the neoplastic cells [38, 39], which have in common the neoplastic giant cell (Hodgkin–Reed Sternberg cell). Childhood (usually defined as diagnosed under 15 years of age) and older age Hodgkin lymphoma (usually defined as diagnosed over 44 years of age) occurs more often in males, is associated inversely with socioeconomic status, is usually EBV positive and consists mainly of the mixed cellularity subtype [38, 39]. Adolescent/young adult Hodgkin lymphoma, diagnosed from 15 to 44 years old, occurs equally among males and females, is more common among those of higher socioeconomic status and in developed countries, and consists primarily of the EBV-negative, nodular sclerosis subtype [38–40]. These etiologically distinct subtypes are often presented singly as one disease, which can obscure true associations if there is heterogeneity between subtypes.

Hodgkin lymphoma, especially adolescent/young adult nodular sclerosis, is associated with clinical and immunological abnormalities suggestive of a T-helper type 2 (Th2)-skewed pro-allergic immune response [41]. About 30–50% of untreated patients have elevated IgE levels [42, 43], and IgE bound to cell-associated CD23 is detected on the neoplastic Hodgkin–Reed Sternberg cells in most Hodgkin lymphoma tumors [44]. Amlot and colleagues reported similar increases in IgE level among both atopic and non-atopic Hodgkin lymphoma patients and in patients with both nodular sclerosis and mixed cellularity subtypes [45]. This group also suggested that clinical atopy was a favorable prognostic factor for Hodgkin lymphoma [45]. A corresponding decrease in T-helper type 1 (Th1) responses, including anergy to skin tests and decreased numbers of cytotoxic T cells and natural killer cells in lymph nodes, is a common occurrence in Hodgkin lymphoma patients [46]. Cohort studies have generally not considered Hodgkin lymphoma separately from NHL, and those that did identified only a small number of cases and thus had insufficient power with unstable risk estimates. Investigators using the Swedish National Death index (death certificates) to identify cases and the Swedish National Hospital Discharge Database to identify asthma hospitalizations found no effect of severe asthma (Table 5.2) [11, 31]; when incident cases were substituted for deaths, a decreased risk of any Hodgkin lymphoma was seen [11].

Null results for atopic conditions were reported from the majority of questionnaire-based studies (Table 5.5) [16, 19, 47–49]) with a few exceptions. Food allergy [19] and hay fever [16] were linked to a decreased risk in two studies. A roughly threefold increased risk associated with childhood eczema was found in twins discordant for adolescent/young adult Hodgkin lymphoma [51]. In a case–case study, asthma, but not allergy, was linked to a borderline increased risk of EBV-positive compared to EBV-negative Hodgkin lymphoma [48].

Thus, overall there has been no consistent evidence to support a relationship between Hodgkin lymphoma and atopy, although the number of studies is small and most combined all Hodgkin lymphoma etiological subtypes together, making interpretation difficult. The high IgE levels and atopic response observed clinically may be a result of pathogenesis; however, more well-designed studies are needed to rule out an etiological effect.

5.6 Plasma Cell Malignancies

Plasma cell malignancies consist of neoplastic monoclonal plasma cells, the highly differentiated B cells that have undergone antigenic stimulation, have passed through germinal centers, and have differentiated further to become antibody-secreting cells. This is the last, or terminal, stage in B-cell differentiation. It is not entirely clear at which stage in B-cell development and differentiation the seminal molecular lesions occur that are necessary for the development of neoplasia. It is possible that some of the initial lesions that lead to the development of plasma cell tumors occur in the germinal centers and result from the same DNA-modifying

Table 5.5 Case–control studies examining atopic conditions and risk of Hodgkin lymphoma

Author	Design	Sample size cases/controls	Response rate	Source of subjects/ criteria	Disease validation	Exposure validation	Hodgkin subtype	Exposure	Exposed cases/ exposed controls	Odds ratio (95% CI[a])
Becker et al. [19]	Frequency matched	Cases: 340 Controls: 2,458	Cases: 87.7% Controls: 68.5%	Cases: hospitals/ offices Controls: population-based, clinic-based and hospital-based	Pathology reports	Questionnaire	All	Respiratory allergy	49/375	0.8 (0.6, 1.1)
								Food allergy	15/171	0.6 (0.3, 1.0)
								Medicine allergy	51/322	1.2 (0.8, 1.7)
Chang et al. [47]	Frequency matched	Cases: 565 Controls: 679	Cases: 77% Eligible controls: 58%	Cases: cancer registries and hospitals Controls: RDD[b] and Boston "Town Books" resource	Pathology reports and slide review	Questionnaire	Young adult (15–54)	Childhood allergy	Not given	0.9 (0.7, 1.2)
								Childhood asthma	Not given	0.9 (0.6, 1.3)
							Older age (55–79)	Childhood allergy	Not given	0.6 (0.4, 1.2)
								Childhood asthma	Not given	0.5 (0.2, 1.3)
Cozen [51]	Individually matched twins	Cases: 188 Controls: 188	Cases: 70% Controls:70%	Volunteer Twin Registry	Pathology reports and slide review	Questionnaire	Young adult (13–50)	Eczema	14/5	**2.8 (1.01, 7.77)**
								Hay fever	21/18	1.2 (0.6, 2.2)
								Allergic reaction	22/19	1.2 (0.5, 2.1)
								Drug allergy	16/21	0.8 (0.4, 1.5)
								Animal or egg allergy	10/12	0.8 (0.4, 1.5)

Table 5.5 (continued)

Author	Design	Sample size cases/ controls	Response rate	Source of subjects/ criteria	Disease validation	Exposure validation	Hodgkin subtype	Exposure	Exposed cases/ exposed controls	Odds ratio (95% CI[a])
Pahwa et al. [49]	Frequency-matched male farm workers and residents	Cases: 119 Controls: 673	Not given	Cases: provincial cancer and hospital registries Controls: provincial health insurance records, voters and telephone lists	Cancer registry or hospital record	Questionnaire	All (males only)	Allergy shots	7/44	0.7 (0.3, 1.7)
Soderberg et al. [11]	Population-based database linkage	Cases 2,394 Controls: 149,344	NA	Swedish Cancer Registry, Population Registry and Hospital Discharge Database	Cancer registry	National Hospital Discharge Database	All	Asthma Asthma > 10 years prior to diagnosis	18/2,176 8/not given	**0.6 (0.4, 0.9)** 0.7 (0.4, 1.5)
Vineis et al. [16]	Population-based cases; randomly selected controls	Cases: 354 Controls: 1,718	Cases: 90% Controls: 81%	Cases: all hospitals in catchment area Controls: randomly selected from census data and National Health Service	Hospital record	Questionnaire	All	Eczema Allergies Hay fever	Not given Not given Not given	0.7 (0.4, 1.3) 0.9 (0.5, 1.4) **0.5 (0.3, 0.8)**

[a]95% confidence interval;[b]random digit dial.

processes that lead to the development of several forms of B-cell lymphoma. What is clear is that these tumors accrue additional molecular lesions during the course of their development. It is also clear that there is a necessary precursor condition consisting of a non-neoplastic clone of identical plasma cells, termed monoclonal gammopathy of undetermined significance (MGUS), which increases with age to a prevalence of about 5% overall in the United States by age 70 [51], with a 1% per risk of transformation by unknown mechanisms to multiple myeloma [52].

Malignant plasma cell tumors consist of solitary (plasmacytoma) or metastatic (multiple myeloma) malignant clones of plasma cells that produce aberrant antibodies or components of antibodies. Plasma cell leukemia is a rarely seen manifestation of plasma cell myeloma [18]. Of all of the isotypes, IgE-producing plasma cell tumors are the least common; only a handful have been reported [53]. Little is known about risk factors for plasma cell tumors other than older age, African-American race, male sex, and obesity [27, 54–57]. Multiple myeloma has a higher mortality rate than other broadly defined types of hematopoietic cancers affecting adults and it is less common; the result is smaller studies with poorer response rates.

Six cohort studies and 10 case–control studies meeting our criteria have had sufficient numbers to evaluate atopy and risk of plasma cell tumors (Table 5.2) [22, 31–33, 58, 59]; (Table 5.6) [11, 16, 17, 19, 49, 60–64]. Questionnaire-based studies have examined the effect of atopic conditions on multiple myeloma risk but definitions range from "respiratory allergy" [19] to "severe allergic reactions" [63], making cross-study comparison sometimes difficult.

None of six studies based on self-report [32, 59, 62–64] or medical record [22] found a link between asthma and multiple myeloma. However, two cohort studies based on separate Swedish national pharmacy–death index record-based linkages found that asthmatics had a decreased risk of multiple myeloma [31, 33], limited to women only in one study [33]. Hay fever has not been linked to multiple myeloma whether measured by self-report [16, 22, 32, 59, 63, 64] or medical record [17].

Results for other atopic conditions have also been inconsistent. A medical record-based study conducted in a large health maintenance organization (HMO) [17] found that multiple myeloma was positively linked to eczema, but four questionnaire-based studies failed to confirm this finding [22, 59, 62, 63]. When stratified by isotype, eczema was associated with an increased risk of IgG, but not IgA, multiple myeloma subtype [63].

An inverse association between allergies and multiple myeloma was reported in one study [62] and in another associated with the IgG subtype only [63]; however, three other studies found no association [16, 49, 60]. Becker et al. reported an inverse link to respiratory allergy but not food or medicine allergy [19]. No association with specific allergies was found in African-Americans [63] or Seventh-Day Adventists [59]. Inoculations with allergen for purposes of desensitization (allergy shots) were not associated with multiple myeloma risk [61, 63], unless over 100 allergy shots were received [61].

Table 5.6 Case–control studies examining atopic conditions and risk of multiple myeloma

Author	Design	Sample size cases/controls	Response rate	Source of subjects/criteria	Disease validation	Exposure assessment	Exposure	Exposed cases/ exposed controls	Odds ratio (95% CI[a])
Becker et al. [19]	Frequency matched	Cases: 278 Controls: 2,458	Cases: 87.7% Controls: 68.5%	Cases: hospitals/clinics Controls: population-based, clinic-based, and hospital-based frequency matched to all 2,480 NHL[b] cases	Pathology reports	Questionnaire	Respiratory allergy	28/375	**0.7 (0.4, 0.98)**
							Food allergy	9/171	0.5 (0.3, 1.0)
							Medicine allergy	35/322	1.0 (0.7, 1.4)
Boffetta et al. [64]	Individually matched (4 controls per case)	Cases: 282 Controls: 1,128	NA	American Cancer Society volunteer cohort	Death certificate	Questionnaire	Hay fever	14/38	1.6 (0.8, 2.9)
							Asthma	5/21	1.0 (0.3, 2.7)
Doody et al. [17]	Individually matched (2 controls per case)	Cases: 175 Controls: 787	NA	Kaiser Permanente (HMO)	Medical record	Medical record	Hay fever	18/18	1.3 (0.6, 2.7)
							Eczema	25/15	**2.0 (1.1, 4.0)**
Eriksson [60]	Individually matched	Cases: 239 Controls: 220	NA	Cases: Swedish Cancer Registry Controls: Swedish National Population Register	Cancer registry and medical records validation	Questionnaire	Allergy	20/16	1.1 (0.5, 2.3)

Table 5.6 (continued)

Author	Design	Sample size cases/controls	Response rate	Source of subjects/criteria	Disease validation	Exposure assessment	Exposure	Exposed cases/ exposed controls	Odds ratio (95% CI[a])
Koepsell et al. [61]	Unmatched	Cases: 698 Controls:1,683	89% in cases (32% by proxy); 83% of controls	Cases: SEER[c] Cancer registries in Utah, Washington and Atlanta Controls: mixture of RDD[d]; and neighborhood controls	Cancer registry	Questionnaire	Allergy shots (desensitization)	43/121	0.8 (0.5, 1.2)
							Number of allergy shots		
							1–99	5/24	0.4 (0.1, 1.1)
							100+	14/33	**0.9 (0.5, 0.9)**
Landgren et al. [62]	Frequency matched (females only)	Cases: 183 Controls: 717	57% in cases; 69% in RDD[d] controls; 47% in Medicare/ Medicaid controls	Cases: Connecticut Tumor Registry Controls: RDD[d] and Medicare/ Medicaid for 65+	Connecticut Tumor Registry	Questionnaire	Allergy	18/142	**0.4 (0.3, 0.7)**
							Asthma	15/58	1.1 (0.6, 2.0)
							Eczema	10/58	0.8 (0.4, 1.7)

Table 5.6 (continued)

Author	Design	Sample size cases/controls	Response rate	Source of subjects/criteria	Disease validation	Exposure assessment	Exposure	Exposed cases/ exposed controls	Odds ratio (95% CI[a])
Lewis et al. [63]	Frequency matched	Cases : 573 Controls : 2,131	63% white cases 67% African-American cases 67% all RDD[d] controls; 73% whites and 78% African-Americans for HCFA[e] controls	Cases: Cancer registries Controls: RDD[d] from 4 centers for 4 cancers	Population-based cancer registry; Ig isotype from medical record (SPEP[f])	Questionnaire	All cases ($n = 573$ cases; 2,131 controls)		
							Allergy shots	26/126	0.8 (0.5, 1.2)
							Asthma	38/116	1.2 (0.8, 1.8)
							Hay fever	94/411	1.0 (0.8, 1.3)
							Eczema	25/82	1.1 (0.7, 1.8)
							Severe allergic reactions	53/181	1.1 (0.8, 1.5)
							Allergies to :		
							Drugs	72/213	1.2 (0.9, 1.5)
							Dust	22/95	0.9 (0.5, 1.4)
							Household products	12/36	1.2 (0.6, 2.3)
							Whites ($n = 367$ cases; 1,164 controls)		
							Allergy shots	18/89	0.7 (0.4, 1.3)
							Asthma	22/63	1.3 (0.7, 2.1)
							Hay fever	54/240	0.9 (0.7, 1.3)
							Eczema	19/57	1.2 (0.7, 2.0)
							Severe allergic reactions	35/124	0.9 (0.6, 1.4)

Table 5.6 (continued)

Author	Design	Sample size cases/controls	Response rate	Source of subjects/criteria	Disease validation	Exposure assessment	Exposure	Exposed cases/ exposed controls	Odds ratio (95% CI[a])
							Allergies to:		
							Drugs	53/161	1.1 (0.8, 1.5)
							Dust	13/61	0.8 (0.4, 1.5)
							Household products	6/21	0.9 (0.3, 2.4)
							African-Americans ($n = 206$ cases; 967 controls)		
							Allergy shots	8/37	0.9 (0.4, 2.0)
							Asthma	16/53	1.2 (0.7, 2.3)
							Hay fever	40/171	1.1 (0.7, 1.6)
							Eczema	6/25	1.1 (0.4, 2.7)
							Severe allergic reactions	18/57	1.4 (0.9, 2.6)
							Allergies to:		
							Drugs	19/52	1.5 (0.9, 2.9)
							Dust	9/32	1.2 (0.5, 2.5)
							Household products	6/15	1.6 (0.4, 1.3)

Table 5.6 (continued)

Author	Design	Sample size cases/controls	Response rate	Source of subjects/criteria	Disease validation	Exposure assessment	Exposure	Exposed cases/ exposed controls	Odds ratio (95% CI[a])
Pahwa et al. [49]	Frequency-matched case–control study of male farm workers and residents	Cases: 178 Controls: 673	NA	Cases: provincial cancer and hospital registries Controls: provincial health insurance records, voters' lists, or telephone lists	Cancer registry or hospital record	Questionnaire	Allergies Skin prick allergy test	34/166 22/71	0.8 (0.5, 1.2) 1.5 (0.9, 2.7)
Soderberg et al. [11]	Swedish National Database Study; randomly selected controls	Cases: 7,189 Controls: 149,344	NA	Swedish Cancer Registry, Population Registry and Hospital Discharge Database	Cancer registry	National Hospital Discharge Database	Asthma	125/2,176	1.0 (0.9, 1.2)
Vineis et al. [16]	Population-based cases; randomly selected controls	Cases: 263 Controls:1,718	Cases: 90% Controls: 81%	Cases: all hospitals in catchment area Controls: Census and National Health Service	Hospital record	Questionnaire	Eczema Allergies Hay fever	Not given Not given Not given	0.6 (0.3, 1.3) 1.1 (0.6, 1.8) 0.8 (0.4, 1.5)

[a]95% confidence interval; [b]non-Hodgkin lymphoma; [c]surveillance epidemiology and end results;[d]random digit dial; [e]health care financing administration; [f]serum protein electrophoresis.

In summary, there is no consistent evidence for an etiological connection between atopic conditions and multiple myeloma. Studies with larger numbers using validated exposure history may help us to clarify this relationship.

5.7 Conclusion – Epidemiologic Findings

Epidemiologic studies of atopic conditions and risk of hematopoietic neoplasms are often limited by lack of power, since these cancers are much less common than solid tumors, and also by the relatively subjective measures of atopy and allergy, usually by self-report and not always reliable [65, 66]. In addition, the etiologic heterogeneity of the various subtypes of hematopoietic neoplasms is not fully understood; to the extent that etiologically distinct subtypes are presented as combined entities, subtype-specific relationships with atopy may be obscured.

In spite of these caveats, some patterns emerged. Atopic conditions have been most strongly and consistently inversely linked to childhood leukemia, especially ALL. The cumulative evidence for an inverse association between atopy and NHL is suggestive, but the inconsistency of the associations with specific types of atopy and allergy, the lack of any associations observed in most cohort studies, and the correlation between timing of diagnosis and decreasing IgE levels warrant further clarification. We found no consistent evidence to support an association between atopy and plasma cell neoplasms or Hodgkin lymphoma based on currently available data.

5.8 Potential Mechanistic Interactions between Allergy/Atopy Associated with the Development of Hematopoietic Cancers

There are several potential mechanisms by which atopy/allergy could contribute to the risk for the development of hematopoietic cancers. There may be trivial reasons for any atopy-lymphoid malignancy associations. For example, the presence of a lymphoid malignancy may dampen allergic responses, leading to an apparent protective association of allergy, while, in fact, this association would be a result of the disease process rather than an etiologic factor [20]. However, as indicated above, there is suggestive evidence for an etiologic effect, especially for childhood lymphocytic leukemia and possibly NHL.

Certainly, there are features of allergic responses (IgE, mast cell products) that have the potential to directly inhibit tumor cell growth, including the growth of hematopoietic cancers, by mediating enhanced antitumor immune responses. However, there is little evidence to directly support such a role for IgE and allergy-associated antitumor immune responses in humans, so such mechanisms remain speculative, with further studies needed to elucidate any contribution of antitumor cell IgE-mediated immune responses to protection from these cancers. There are other potential mechanisms that may provide an explanation for decreased risk of

lymphoid malignancies in atopic people, including a relative dampening of B-cell responses mediated by the interaction between IgE and CD23, and/or by a relative decrease in T-helper type 17 (Th17) cytokine responses in atopic individuals (see below). Decreased B-cell activation would be expected to result in a lower frequency of activation-associated oncogenic molecular lesions, which lead to the generation of neoplasms of mature lymphoid origin, such as NHL and multiple myeloma. Additionally, both soluble CD23 (sCD23) and Th17 cytokines have the potential to enhance the viability and growth of B-cell ALL, based on laboratory studies [67, 68].

5.8.1 IgE/Allergy-Mediated Enhancement of Antitumor Immunity

Several recent studies have pointed to a key role for IgE and other allergy-associated forms of immune function in the protection from cancer. In fact, the other chapters in this volume present many specific examples of the important role that IgE and allergy-associated immune responses can play in mediating protection from cancer. These allergy-associated and/or IgE-mediated antitumor immune responses may potentially play a role in protection from the growth of hematopoietic cancers. It is clear that IgE can mediate antitumor responses via the enhancement of various immune effector mechanisms, including antibody-dependent cellular cytotoxicity (ADCC), antibody-dependent cellular phagocytosis (ADCP), antigen presentation, and mast cell responses [69–73].

The especially high affinity of both the high- and low-affinity Fc receptors for IgE are thought to make antitumor antibodies of the IgE subclass more effective at mediating ADCC and additionally may allow enhanced antigen presentation of antigens bound by IgE, resulting in enhancement of the generation of antitumor cytotoxic T cells (CTLs) [69, 70, 74–77]. The two IgE Fc receptors, FcεRI (the so-called high-affinity IgE Fc receptor) and FcεRII (CD23, the "low-affinity" IgE Fc receptor) are actually both relatively high-affinity receptors ($K_d \sim 10^{-10}$ M and $K_d \sim 10^{-7}$M, respectively) [78, 79], binding affinities that are higher than those seen for most IgG or IgA Fc receptors. This feature of the IgE Fc receptors, combined with their widespread expression on immune system effector cells, including antigen-presenting cells, mast cells, basophiles, eosinophils, Langerhan's cells, macrophages, dendritic cells, and B cells [73, 80–83], and their signal-transducing properties [83–86], allows the potential for the effective IgE-mediated enhancement of ADCC and CTL directed to tumor cells. Additionally, IgE has been seen to bind to murine NK cells via FcRIII (CD16), the Fc receptor that is responsible for IgG-mediated cellular cytotoxicity, with IgE bound to NK cells in this manner being effective in ADCC and in the induction of cytokine production by NK cells [76].

Other antitumor mechanisms that may enhance in IgE-mediated responses are eosinophil and/or mast cell-mediated antitumor immune responses [82]. Eosinophils have been seen to mediate cellular cytotoxicity directly, providing a potential means

by which these cells, which are stimulated in allergic immune responses, could help control the growth of hematopoietic tumors [70, 87]. Similarly, activated mast cells, which are degranulated on exposure to IgE + antigen, produce a wide range of mediators that can exert direct cytotoxic and growth-inhibitory effects on tumor cells [70, 88].

Therefore, the most direct and obvious mechanisms that might link allergic/IgE-mediated responses to protection from hematopoietic cancers involve direct enhancement of antitumor cell effector mechanisms and, in this way, are not fundamentally different from how allergy/IgE may protect from other cancers. It was recently observed that treatment of allergic patients with an anti-IgE antibody (omalizumab, Xolair), which is used for the treatment of asthma [89], results in a doubling of cancer risk, with cancer seen in 20/4127 (0.5%) of omalizumab-treated patients (including one NHL) versus 5/2236 (0.2%) placebo recipients in unpublished studies sponsored by the manufacturer of this agent (Food and Drug Administration, Center for Biologics Evaluation and Research. BLA STN 103976/0, review of clinical safety data: original BLS submitted on June 2, 2000, and response to complete review letter submitted on December 18, 2002). [89]. Another study found that multiple myeloma patients with relatively higher IgE levels had a better survival than patients with lower levels of IgE [90]. These findings are consistent with the view that IgE, or allergic responses associated with the presence of IgE, may participate in anti-myeloma immune responses, even if a history of allergy is not associated with a decreased risk for the development of multiple myeloma (see Section 5.6).

5.8.2 Stabilization of CD23 Expression by IgE

Stabilization of cell-surface CD23 by IgE binding, preventing the release of sCD23, has the potential to dampen activities that may lead to the development of hematopoietic cancers. As noted earlier, errors in DNA-modifying activities that are associated with B-cell activation, including *IgH* CSR and SHM of Ig genes, can contribute to the development of mature B-cell malignancies, such as many subtypes of B-cell NHL. In fact, there is ample evidence that chronic stimulation of B cells, by infection (e.g., HIV, *H. pylori*, EBV, hepatitis C virus (HCV)) or forms of autoimmunity that involve autoantibody production (e.g., Sjogren's), is associated with an increased risk for the development of B-cell NHL [91]. Therefore, activities that generically promote B-cell activation should increase risk for the development of these mature B-cell cancers, while dampening of B-cell activation should, conversely, decrease risk for these cancers. Similarly, factors that promote the growth and viability of pre-B cells and immature B cells may be expected to support the emergence and growth of leukemic cells.

At first glance, it might be expected that IgE-mediated allergies would be associated with an overall enhancement of B-cell stimulation. However, IgE has the potential to dampen the stimulation of mature or immature B cells. One way by

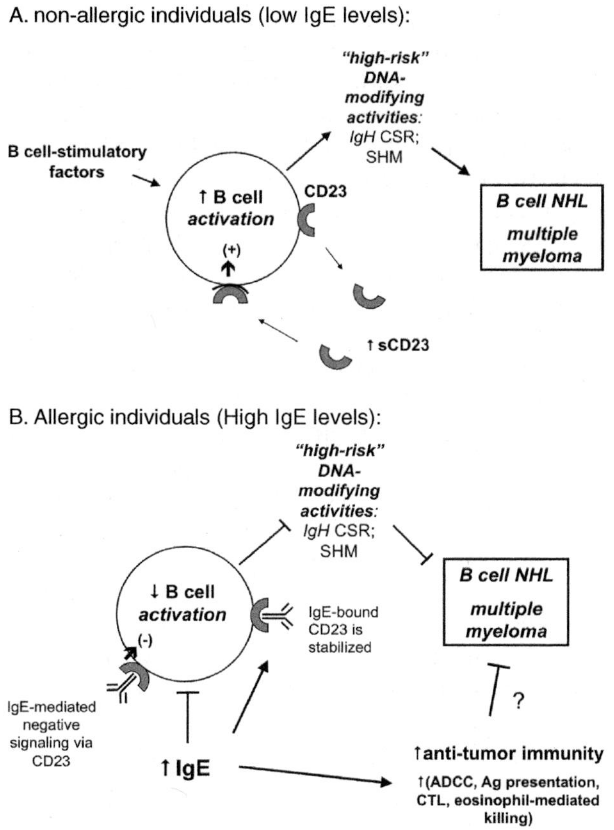

Fig. 5.1 Potential mechanisms by which IgE may prevent the development and/or growth of B-cell tumors. IgE has the potential to dampen B-cell stimulation, and thereby prevents the occurrence of DNA-modifying oncogenic events associated with the genesis of many B-cell cancers, by stabilizing cell-surface CD23, preventing the release of sCD23, which can act as a potent B-cell-stimulatory factor. In addition to this, IgE binding to CD23 also can result in negative signaling. Finally, IgE has the potential to function in antitumor immunity

which IgE could potentially inhibit the stimulation of B cells is by decreasing the release of sCD23 by stabilizing the cell-surface form of this molecule (Fig. 5.1). CD23 is a B-cell surface molecule that is induced on B-cell activation and which also is an Fc receptor for IgE (FcεRII) [78, 79]. Other types of hematopoietic cells also can express CD23. CD23 can be proteolytically cleaved to generate sCD23, a molecule that has cytokine-like B-cell-stimulatory activity, such as the enhancement of CSR [92]. In fact, elevated serum levels of sCD23 have been seen to precede the clinical diagnosis of NHL [93–96]. Additionally, sCD23 has been seen to prevent the apoptosis of ALL cells [67]. Therefore, sCD23 has B- and pre-B-cell-stimulatory properties that are consistent with a role in promoting lymphomagenesis and the viability of leukemic cells.

Binding of IgE to CD23, as would occur in atopic individuals who have elevated IgE levels, can result in the downregulation of sCD23-mediated B-cell activation in several ways: IgE binding to cell-surface FcεRII (CD23) can stabilize this molecule and prevent its cleavage and secretion, thereby preventing sCD23-mediated stimulation of B and pre-B cells [97, 98]. Additionally, IgE binding to FcεRII (CD23) on activated mature B cells may result in negative signaling, again resulting in the downregulation of B-cell activation [99, 100]. There is experimental and observational evidence that supports such a role for IgE: (1) people who have elevated serum levels of IgE have relatively decreased serum sCD23 levels and increased cellular expression of CD23 [101, 102], suggesting that IgE is able to stabilize cell-surface expressed CD23. Additionally, IgE can dampen switching to Ig isotypes other than IgE (inhibits *IgH* CSR), which would be consistent with a role for IgE in downregulating sCD23-mediated activities [101].

Therefore, IgE can interact with FcεRII (CD23) in ways that result in the inhibition of sCD23 release and activity, potentially dampening B-cell stimulation, and thereby decreasing the risk for oncogenic events that can result in the genesis of cancers of mature B cells and/or preventing the enhanced viability of pre-B cell cancer cells by sCD23. This is consistent with a protective role for IgE and atopy for the development of NHL and/or ALL. Interestingly, these interactions do not involve a role for IgE in mediating a direct antitumor cell immune response and would be expected to be unique to the pathogenesis hematopoietic cancers such as NHL or ALL. Future studies, including prospective cohort-based studies, should examine the association of sCD23 levels with the development of hematopoietic cancers of B-cell origin, including ALL and NHL, to more definitively define the association of allergy, sCD23 levels, and the development of these cancers.

5.8.3 The Immune Regulatory Milieu Associated with Allergy may be Less Supportive for the Stimulation of B-Cell Activation and/or Resistance to Apoptosis

People who have IgE-mediated allergies appear to be at decreased risk for the development of ALL and possibly some forms of NHL, while those who have autoimmune diseases that are mediated by aberrant B-cell anti-self responses have a marked increase in risk for the development of B-cell NHL [91, 103]. Both allergy and autoimmunity are characterized by changes in the host immunoregulatory environment, with IgE-mediated responses involving enhanced Th2 activity and autoimmune responses involving the enhanced activity of a recently recognized T-cell subset, Th17 cells [104–106] (Fig. 5.2). These epidemiologic observations suggest, then, that enhanced Th17 activity may be associated with the development of B-cell NHL, a hypothesis that can be addressed in future studies, especially in prospective cohort studies.

Are the properties of Th17 cells consistent with a role in the pathogenesis of these hematopoietic cancers? Th17 cells are a distinct, proinflammatory T-cell subset,

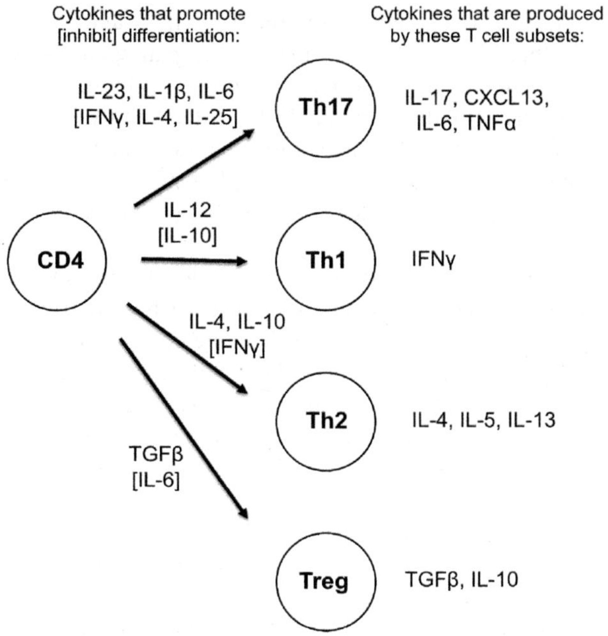

Fig. 5.2 T-cell subsets: distinct patterns of cytokine production. Several subsets of CD4-positive helper T cells have been defined, based on the pattern of cytokines produced by these different subsets, as well as by their unique biological activities

which is functionally characterized by mediating protection against extracellular bacteria and by its pathogenic role in autoimmune disorders [104, 107–110]. Th17 cells characteristically produce interleukin- (IL-) 17, CXCL13 (a B-cell stimulatory chemokine), IL-6, and tumor necrosis factor alpha (TNFα), in contrast to Th2 cells, which characteristically produce IL-4, IL-5, IL-9, and IL-13, or Th1 cells, which produce interferon gamma (IFNγ) [104, 111] (Fig. 5.2).

Extensive evidence links elevated IL-6 and TNFα production with B-cell NHL, including functional, observational, and genetic studies [112–136]. IL-6, another Th17 cytokine, has long been known to induce *IgH* CSR, with IL-6 transgenic mice developing lymphoma-like tumors (plasmacytomas) that are characterized by *myc:Ig* translocations [137]. In prior work, we also saw that elevated levels of serum IL-6 were seen to precede the development of AIDS-associated Burkitt lymphoma [114]. Therefore, Th17 cells produce several B-cell-stimulatory molecules, including several that are known to be associated with an increased risk for the development of B-cell NHL and/or which exert biological effects that can promote the development and/or growth of NHL. Additionally, CXCL13, a Th17 cytokine, has been seen to prevent apoptosis in B-cell lineage ALL [68], suggesting that this Th17 cytokine has the potential to promote the growth of these cancers.

The generation of Th17 cells from naïve Th precursor cells is stimulated by exposure of these cells to IL-23 (an IL-12-like cytokine), IL-1β, and IL-6 (in mice),

while the generation of Th17 cells is inhibited by IL-4 and IL-25 [104]. Given this, it is unlikely that Th17 cells contribute to the pathogenesis of allergic IgE-mediated disorders, because IL-4 and IL-25 (a powerful inducer of IL-4) are both potent inhibitors of Th17 cell development [104]. Interestingly, Th17 cells appear to be virtually missing in people who have autosomal dominant hyper-IgE syndrome (HIES, "Job's syndrome") and decreased in people who have severe allergies [138, 139], suggesting that lack of Th17 activity may be associated with enhanced IgE production.

Several animal studies have examined IL-17 levels in asthma, finding that IL-17 acts as a potent negative regulator of established allergic asthma [140]. Paradoxically, IL-17 also appears to play a role in the initiation of asthma-associated inflammation [141]. Therefore, IL-17 and TH17 cells appear to play complex roles in asthma and may contribute to inflammation associated with asthma but also downregulate the allergic response in sensitized animals [140]. However, little is known about the role of IL-17 or Th17 cells in allergic conditions not associated with asthma.

Although the known properties of Th17 cells are consistent with the activity of this Th subset being decreased in allergy and increased in autoimmunity, therefore, having a potential role in the pathogenesis of NHL and/or ALL, much additional work needs to be done to elucidate the role of Th17 cells and cytokines in allergy and in the etiology of hematopoietic cancers. Are levels of Th17 activity decreased in allergic individuals? Is Th17 activity (elevated levels of Th17-produced cytokines) associated with the subsequent development of NHL or ALL? These hypotheses can be tested, in both epidemiologic and functional studies, especially in prospective cohort studies that have access to precancer diagnosis materials and accurate clinical information on allergic and autoimmune diseases.

5.8.4 Conclusion – Potential Interactions between Allergy/Atopy Associated with the Development of Hematopoietic Cancers

There are several potential mechanisms by which atopy/allergy could contribute to the risk for the development of hematopoietic cancers, including but not limited to: (1) features of allergic responses (IgE, mast cell products) that may mediate enhanced antitumor immune responses and/or (2) a dampening of B-cell responses, mediated by the interaction between IgE and CD23 and/or by allergy-associated changes in the relative levels of B-cell-activating cytokines, resulting in less exposure to DNA mutating and potentially oncogenic activities associated with B-cell activation. Additionally, it remains a possibility that the presence of a lymphoid malignancy may dampen allergic responses, leading to an apparent etiological protective association of allergy. Studies to better define the associations between allergy and the development of hematopoietic cancers, including both laboratory-focused studies and epidemiologic studies, are needed.

Acknowledgments This work was supported, in part, by NIH grants R01-CA57152, R01-CA73475, P50-CA96888, P50-CA100707, P30-CA014089, and R01-CA121195, as well as by grants from the Department of Defense Peer-Reviewed Medical Research Program (PR054600) and the Leukemia and Lymphoma Society (6155-03 and 6137-07).

References

1. Eriksson N, Holmen A, Hogstedt B, Mikoczy Z, Hagmar L (1995) A prospective study of cancer incidence in a cohort examined for allergy. Allergy 50: 718–722
2. Lindelof B, Granath F, Tengvall-Linder M, Ekbom A (2005) Allergy and cancer. Allergy 60: 1116–1120
3. Lochmann O, Benes J, Vymola F, Pokorny J (1978) Observation of antibody activity against antibiotics in patients with atopic disease. J Hyg Epidemiol Microbiol Immunol 22: 344–353
4. Ellison-Loschmann L, Benavente Y, Douwes J, Buendia E, Font R, Alvaro T, Kogevinas M, de Sanjose S (2007) Immunoglobulin E levels and risk of lymphoma in a case-control study in Spain. Cancer Epidemiol Biomarkers Prev 16: 1492–1498
5. Holly E, Chitra L (1997) Non-Hodgkin's lymphoma in HIV-positive and HIV-negative homosexual men in the San Francisco Bay area: Allergies, prior medication use, and sexual practices. J AIDS 15: 211–222
6. Groves FD, Linet MS, Devesa SS (1995) Patterns of occurrence of the leukaemias. Eur J Cancer 31A: 941–949
7. Jourdan-Da Silva N, Perel Y, Mechinaud F, Plouvier E, Gandemer V, Lutz P, Vannier J, Lamagnere J, Margueritte G, Boutard P, Robert A, Armari C, Munzer M, Millot F, de Lumley L, Berthou C, Rialland X, Pautard B, Hemon D, Clavel J (2004) Infections diseases in the first year of life, perinatal characteristics and childhood acute leukemia. Br J Cancer 90: 139–145
8. Rosenbaum P, Buck G, Brecher M (2005) Allergy and infectious disease histories and the risk of childhood acute lymphoblastic leukaemia. Paediatric Perinatal Epidemiol 19: 152–164
9. Schuz J, Morgan G, Bohler E, Kaatsch P, Michaelis J (2003) Atopic disease and childhood acute lymphoblastic leukemia. Int J Cancer 105: 255–260
10. Wen W, Shu X, Linet M, Neglia J, Potter J, Trigg M, Robison L (2000) Allergic disorders and the risk of childhood acute lymphoblastic leukemia (United States). Cancer Causes Contr 11: 303–307
11. Soderberg K, Jonsson F, Winqvist O, Hagmar L, Feychting M (2006) Autoimmune diseases, asthma and risk of haematological malignancies: a nationwide case-control study in Sweden. Eur J Cancer 42: 3028–3033.
12. Hughes A, Lightfoot T, Simpson J, Ansell P, McKinney P, Kinsey S, Mitchell C, Eden T, Greaves M, Roman E, United Kingdom Childhood Cancer Study Investigators (2007) Allergy and risk of childhood leukemia: Results from the UKCCS. Int J Cancer 121: 819–824
13. Spector L, Groves F, DeStefano F, Liff J, Klein M, Mullooly J, Black S, Shinefield H, Ward J, Marcy M, Vaccine Safety Datalink Project (2004) Medically recorded allergies and the risk of childhood acute lymphoblastic leukemia. Eur J Cancer 40: 579–584
14. Cooper G, Kamel F, Sandler D, Davey F, Bloomfield C (1996) Risk of adult acute leukemia in relation to prior immune-related conditions. Cancer Epidemiol Biomarkers Prev 5: 867–872
15. Severson R, Davis S, Thomas D, Stevens E, Heuser L, Sever L (1989) Acute myelocytic leukemia and prior allergies. J Clin Epidemiol 42: 995–1001
16. Vineis P, Crosignani P, Sacerdote C, Fontana A, Masala G, Miligi L, Nanni O, Ramazzotti V, Rodella S, Stagnaro E, Tumino R, Viganò C, Vindigni C, Costantini AS (2000) Haematopoietic cancer and medical history: A multicentre case control study. J Epidemiol Community Health 54: 4331–4436

17. Doody M, Linet M, Glass A, Friedman GD, Pottern LM, Boice JD Jr, Fraumeni JF Jr. (1992) Leukemia, lymphoma and multiple myeloma following selected medical conditions. Cancer Causes Contr 3: 449–456
18. Jaffe E, Harris N, Stein H, Vardiman J (2001) Pathology & genetics of tumours of haematopoietic and lymphoid tissues. In: Kleihues P, Sobin L (eds) World Health Organization Classification of Tumours. International Agency for Research on Cancer (IARC) Press, Lyon, France.
19. Becker N, De Sanjose S, Nieters A, Maynadie M, Foretova L, Cocco P, Staines A, Alvaro T, Vornanen M, Brennan P, Boffetta P (2007) Birth order, allergies and lymphoma risk: Results of the European collaborative reserach project Epilymph. Leuk Res 31: 1365–1372
20. Melbye M, Smedby K, Lehtinen T, Rostgaard K, Glimelius B, Munksgaard L, Schöllkopf C, Sundström C, Chang ET, Koskela P, Adami H-O, Hjalgrim H (2007) Atopy and risk of non-Hodgkin lymphoma. JNCI 99: 158–166
21. Zhang Y, Holdford T, Leaderer B, Zahm SH, Boyle P, Morton LM, Zhang B, Zou K, Flynn S, Tallini G, Owens PH, Zheng T (2004) Prior medical conditions and medication use and risk of non-Hodgkin lymphoma in Connecticut, United States women. Cancer Causes Contr 15: 419–428
22. Soderberg K, Hagmar K, Schwartzbaum J, Feychting M (2004) Allergic conditions and risk of hematopoietic malignancies in adults: A cohort study. BMC Public Health 4: 51–57
23. Morton L, Wang S, Cozen W, Linet M, Chatterjee N, Davis S, Severson R, Colt J, Vasef M, Rothman N, BLair A, Bernstein L, Cross A, De Roos A, Engels E, Hein D, Hill D, Keleman L, Lim U, Lynch C, Schenk M, Wacholder S, Ward M, Hoar Zahm S, Chanoock S, Cerhan J, Hartge P (2008) Etiologic heterogeneity among non-Hodgkin lymphoma subtypes. Blood 112: 5150–5160
24. Morton L, Wang S, SS D, Hartge P, Weisenburger D, Linet M (2006) Lymphoma incidence patterns by WHO subtype in the United States, 1992–2001. Blood 107: 265–276
25. Bernstein L, Ross R (1992) Prior medication use and health history as risk factors for non-Hodgkin's lymphoma: Preliminary results from a case-control study in Los Angeles County. Cancer Res 52: 5510s–5515s
26. Briggs N, Levine R, Brann E (2002) Allergies and risk of non-Hodgkin's lymphoma by subtype. Cancer Epidemiol Biomarkers Prev 11: 401–407
27. Cozen W, Cerhan J, Martinez-Maza O, Ward M, Linet M, Colt J, Davis S, Severson R, Hartge P, Bernstein L (2007) The effect of atopy, childhood crowding and other immune-related factors on non-Hodgkin lymphoma risk. Cancer Causes Contr 18: 821–831
28. Fabbro-Peray P, Daures J-P, Rossi J-F (2001) Environmental risk factors for non-Hodgkin's lymphoma: A population-based case-control study in Languedoc-Rousillon, France. Cancer Causes Contr 12: 201–212
29. Grulich A, Vajdic C, Kaldor J, Hughes AM, Kricker A, Fritschi L, Turner JJ, Milliken S, Benke G, Armstrong BK (2005) Birth order, atopy, and risk of non-Hodgkin lymphoma. JNCI 97: 587–594
30. Holly E, Lele C, Bracci P, McGrath MS (1999) Case-control study of non-Hodgkin's lymphoma among women and heterosexual men in the San Francisco Bay area, California. Am J Epidemiol 150: 375–389
31. Kallen B, Gunnarskog J, Conradson T (1993) Cancer risk in asthmatic subjects selected from hospital discharge registry. Eur Resp J 6: 694–697
32. Turner M, Chen Y, Krewski D, Ghadirian P, Thun M, Calle E (2005) Cancer mortality among US men and women and asthma and hay fever. Am J Epidemiol 162: 212–221
33. Vesterinen E, Pukkala E, Timonen T, Aromaa A (1993) Cancer incidence among 78,000 asthmatic patients. Int J Cancer 22: 976–982
34. Bracci P, Dalvi T, Holly E (2006) Residential history, family characteristics and non-Hodgkin's lymphoma, a population-based case-control study in the San Francisco Bay are. . Cancer Epidemiol Biomarkers Prev 15: 1287–1294

35. Holly E, Bracci P (2003) Population-based study of non-Hodgkin lymphoma, histology and medical history among human immunodeficiency virus-negative participants in San Francisco. Am J Epidemiol 158: 316–327
36. Whittemore A, Holly E, Lee I-M, Abel E, Adams R, Nickoloff B, Bley L, Peters J, Gibney C (1989) Mycosis fungoides in relation to environmental exposures and immune response: A case-control study. J Natl Cancer Inst 81: 1560–1567
37. Vajdic CM, Falster MO, de Sanjose S, Martínez-Maza O, Becker N, Bracci PM, Melbye M, Smedby KE, Engels EA, Turner J, Vineis P, Costantini AS, Holly EA, Kane E, Spinelli JJ, La Vecchia C, Zheng T, Chiu BC, Maso LD, Cocco P, Maynadié M, Foretova L, Staines A, Brennan P, Davis S, Severson R, Cerhan JR, Breen EC, Birmann B, Cozen W, Grulich AE (2009) Atopic Disease and Risk of Non-Hodgkin Lymphoma: An InterLymph Pooled Analysis. Cancer Res 69: 6482–6489
38. Jarrett R (2006) Viruses and lymphoma/leukemia. J Pathol 208: 176–186
39. Cozen W, Katz J, Mack T (1992) Hodgkin's disease varies by cell type in Los Angeles. Cancer Epidemiol Biomarkers Preven 1: 261–268
40. Glaser S, Gulley M, Clarke C, Keegan T, Chang E, Shema S, Craig F, Diguiseppe J, Dorfman R, Mann R, Anton-Culver H, Ambinder R (2008) Racial/ethnic variation in EBV-positive classical Hodgkin lymphoma in California. Int J Cancer 123: 1499–1507
41. Skinnider B, Mak T (2002) The role of cytokines in classical Hodgkin lymphoma. Blood 99: 4283–4297
42. Romagnani S, Biagiotti R, Amadori A, Maggi E, Biti G, Bellesi G, Ricci M (1980) Hyperproduction of IgE and T-cell dysfunction in Hodgkin's disease. Int Arch Allergy Appl Immunol 63: 64–72
43. Amlot P, Green L (1978) Atopy and immunoglobulin E concentrations in Hodgkin's disease and other lymphomas. BMJ 1: 327–329
44. Samoszuk M, Ramzi E (1992) IgE, Reed-Sternberg cells, and eosinophilia in Hodgkin's Disease. Leuk Lymphoma 9: 315–319
45. Amlot P, Slaney J, Brown R (1983) Atopy—a favourable prognostic factor for survival in Hodgkin's disease. Br J Cancer 48: 209–215
46. Slivnik D, Ellis T, Nawrocki J, Risher R (1990) The impact of Hodgkin's disease on the immune system. Semin Oncol 17: 673–682
47. Chang E, Tongzhang Z, Weir E, Borowitz M, Mann R, Spiegelman D, Mueller N (2004a) Childhood social environment and Hodgkin's lymphoma: New findings from a population-based case-control study. Cancer Epidemiol Biomarkers Prev 13: 1361–1370
48. Chang E, Zhang T, Lennette E, Weir E, Borowitz M, Mann R, Spiegelman D, Mueller N (2004b) Heterogeneity of risk factors and antibody profiles in Epstein-Barr virus genome-positive and -negative Hodgkin lymphoma. J Infect Dis 189: 2271–2281
49. Pahwa P, McDuffie H, Dosman J, Robson D, McLaughlin J, Spinelli J, Fincham S (2003) Exposure to animals and selected risk factors among Canadian farm residents with Hodgkin's Disease, multiple myeloma, or soft tissue sarcoma. J Occup Environ Med 45: 857–868
50. Kyle R, Thermeau T, Rajkumar S, Larson D, Plevak M, Offord J, Dispenzieri A, Katzmann J, Melton L, III (2006) Prevalence of monoclonal gammopathy of undetermined sigficance. N Eng J Med 354: 1362–1369
51. Cozen W, Hamilton AS, Zhao P, Salam MT, Deapen DK, Nathwani BN, Weiss LM, Mack TM (2009) A protective role for early childhood exposures and young adult Hodgkin lymphoma. Blood, epub doi: 10.1182/blood-2009-03-209601
52. Kyle R, Therneau T, Rajkumar S, Offord J, Larson D, Plevak M, Melton L, III (2002) A long-term study of prognosis in monoclonal gammopathy of undetermined significance. N Eng J Med 346: 564–569
53. Kairemo K, Lindberg M, Pyrtz M (1999) IgE myeloma: A case presentation and a review of the literature. Scan J Clin Lab Invest 59: 451–456
54. Gebregziabher M, Bernstein L, Wang Y, Cozen W (2006) Risk patterns of multiple myeloma in Los Angeles County, 1972–1999. Cancer Causes Control 17: 931–938

55. Cozen W, Gebregziabher M, Conti D, Van Den Berg D, Coetzee G, Wang S, Rothman N, Bernstein L, Hartge P, Morhbacher A, Coetzee S, Salam M, Wang W, Zadnick J, Ingles S (2006) Interleukin-6 related genotypes, body mass index and risk of multiple myeloma and plasmacytoma. . Cancer Epidemiol Biomarkers Preven 15: 2285–2291
56. Larsson S, Wolk A (2007) Body mass index and multiple myeloma: A meta-analysis. Int J Cancer 121: 2512–2516
57. Alexander DD, Mink PJ, Adami HO, Cole P, Mandel JS, Oken MM, Trichopoulos D (2007) Multiple myeloma: A review of the epidemiologic literature. Int J Cancer 120(Suppl 12): 40–61, doi: 10.1002/ijc.22718
58. Bourguet C, Logue E (1993) Antigenic stimulation and multiple myeloma: A prospective study. Cancer 72: 2148–2154
59. Mills P, Beeson W, Fraser G, Phillips RL (1992) Allergy and cancer: Organ-site specific results from the Adventist Health Study. Am J Epidemiol 136: 287–295
60. Eriksson M (1993) Rheumatoid arthritis as a risk factor for multiple myeloma: A case-control study. Eur J Cancer 29A: 259–263
61. Koepsell T, Daling J, Weiss N, Taylor J, Olshan A, Lyon J, Swanson G, Child M (1987) Antigenic stimulation and the occurrence of multiple myeloma. Am J Epidemiol 126: 1051–1062
62. Landgren O, Zhang Y, Zham S, Inskip P, Zheng T, Baris D (2006) Risk of multiple myeloma following medication use and medical conditions: A case-control study in Connecticut women. Cancer Epidemiol Biomarkers Prev 15: 2342–2347
63. Lewis D, Pottern L, Brown L, Silverman D, Hayes R, Schoenberg J, Greenberg R, Swanson G, Schwartz A, Liff J, Hoover R (1994) Multiple myeloma among Blacks and Whites in the United States: The role of chronic antigenic stimulation Cancer Causes Contr 5: 529–539
64. Boffetta P, Stellman S, Garfinkel L (1989) A case-control study of multiple myeloma nested in the American Cancer Society prospective study. Int J Cancer 43: 554–559
65. Linet M, Harlow S, McLaughlin J, McCaffrey L (1989) A comparison of interview data and medical records for previous medical conditions and surgery. J Clin Epidemiol 42: 1207–1213
66. Burgess J, Walteres E, Byrnes G, Wharton C, Jenkins M, Abramson M, Hopper J, Dharmage S (2006) Who remembers whether they had asthma as children? J Asthma 43: 727–730
67. White LJ, Ozanne BW, Graber P, Aubry JP, Bonnefoy JY, Cushley W (1997) Inhibition of apoptosis in a human pre-B-cell line by CD23 is mediated via a novel receptor. Blood 90: 234–243
68. Chunsong H, Yuling H, Li W, Jie X, Gang Z, Qiuping Z, Qingping G, Kejian Z, Li Q, Chang AE, Youxin J, Jinquan T (2006) CXC chemokine ligand 13 and CC chemokine ligand 19 cooperatively render resistance to apoptosis in B cell lineage acute and chronic lymphocytic leukemia CD23+CD5+ B cells. J Immunol 177: 6713–6767.
69. Fu SL, Pierre J, Smith-Norowitz TA, Hagler M, Bowne W, Pincus MR, Mueller CM, Zenilman ME, Bluth MH (2008) Immunoglobulin E antibodies from pancreatic cancer patients mediate antibody-dependent cell-mediated cytotoxicity against pancreatic cancer cells. Clin Exp Immunol 153: 401–409
70. Jensen-Jarolim E, Achatz G, Turner MC, Karagiannis S, Legrand F, Capron M, Penichet ML, Rodriguez JA, Siccardi AG, Vangelista L, Riemer AB, Gould H (2008) AllergoOncology: The role of IgE-mediated allergy in cancer. Allergy 63: 1255–1266
71. Hartman ML, Lin SY, Jouvin MH, Kinet JP (2008) Role of the extracellular domain of Fc epsilon RI alpha in intracellular processing and surface expression of the high affinity receptor for IgE Fc epsilon RI. Mol Immunol 45: 2307–2311
72. Ozdemir O (2005) Immunosurveillance function of human mast cell? World J Gastroenterol 11: 7054–7056

73. Stingl G, Maurer D (1997) IgE-mediated allergen presentation via Fc epsilon RI on antigen-presenting cells. Int Arch Allergy Immunol 113: 24–29
74. Karagiannis SN, Bracher MG, Beavil RL, Beavil AJ, Hunt J, McCloskey N, Thompson RG, East N, Burke F, Sutton BJ, Dombrowicz D, Balkwill FR, Gould HJ (2008) Role of IgE receptors in IgE antibody-dependent cytotoxicity and phagocytosis of ovarian tumor cells by human monocytic cells. Cancer Immunol Immunother 57: 247–263
75. Karagiannis SN, Bracher MG, Hunt J, McCloskey N, Beavil RL, Beavil AJ, Fear DJ, Thompson RG, East N, Burke F, Moore RJ, Dombrowicz DD, Balkwill FR, Gould HJ (2007) IgE-antibody-dependent immunotherapy of solid tumors: Cytotoxic and phagocytic mechanisms of eradication of ovarian cancer cells. J Immunol 179: 2832–2843
76. Arase N, Arase H, Hirano S, Yokosuka T, Sakurai D, Saito T (2003) IgE-mediated activation of NK cells through Fc gamma RIII. J Immunol 170: 3054–3058
77. Gould HJ, Mackay GA, Karagiannis SN, O'Toole CM, Marsh PJ, Daniel BE, Coney LR, Zurawski VR, Jr., Joseph M, Capron M, Gilbert M, Murphy GF, Korngold R (1999) Comparison of IgE and IgG antibody-dependent cytotoxicity in vitro and in a SCID mouse xenograft model of ovarian carcinoma. Eur J Immunol 29: 3527–3537
78. Sarfati M, Fournier S, Wu CY, Delespesse G (1992) Expression, regulation and function of human Fc epsilon RII (CD23) antigen. Immunol Res 11: 260–272
79. Bonnefoy JY, Lecoanet-Henchoz S, Gauchat JF, Graber P, Aubry JP, Jeannin P, Plater-Zyberk C (1997) Structure and functions of CD23. Int Rev Immunol 16: 113–128
80. Ochiai K, Wang B, Rieger A, Kilgus O, Maurer D, Fodinger D, Kinet JP, Stingl G, Tomioka H (1994) A review on Fc epsilon RI on human epidermal Langerhans cells. Int Arch Allergy Immunol 104(Suppl 1): 63–64
81. Wang B, Rieger A, Kilgus O, Ochiai K, Maurer D, Fodinger D, Kinet JP, Stingl G (1992) Epidermal Langerhans cells from normal human skin bind monomeric IgE via Fc epsilon RI. J Exp Med 175: 1353–1365
82. Prussin C, Metcalfe DD (2006) 5. IgE, mast cells, basophils, and eosinophils. J Allergy Clin Immunol 117: S450–S456
83. Kikutani H, Yokota A, Uchibayashi N, Yukawa K, Tanaka T, Sugiyama K, Barsumian EL, Suemura M, Kishimoto T (1989) Structure and function of Fc epsilon receptor II (Fc epsilon RII/CD23): A point of contact between the effector phase of allergy and B cell differentiation. Ciba Found Symp 147: 23–31; discussion 31–25
84. Rivera J, Olivera A (2008) A current understanding of Fc epsilon RI-dependent mast cell activation. Curr Allergy Asthma Rep 8: 14–20
85. Kolb JP, Abadie A, Paul-Eugene N, Capron M, Sarfati M, Dugas B, Delespesse G (1993) Ligation of CD23 triggers cyclic AMP generation in human B lymphocytes. J Immunol 150: 4798–4809
86. Paul-Eugene N, Kolb JP, Abadie A, Gordon J, Delespesse G, Sarfati M, Mencia-Huerta JM, Braquet P, Dugas B (1992) Ligation of CD23 triggers cAMP generation and release of inflammatory mediators in human monocytes. J Immunol 149: 3066–3071
87. Costain DJ, Guha AK, Liwski RS, Lee TD (2001) Murine hypodense eosinophils induce tumour cell apoptosis by a granzyme B-dependent mechanism. Cancer Immunol Immunother 50: 293–299
88. Strik MC, de Koning PJ, Kleijmeer MJ, Bladergroen BA, Wolbink AM, Griffith JM, Wouters D, Fukuoka Y, Schwartz LB, Hack CE, van Ham SM, Kummer JA (2007) Human mast cells produce and release the cytotoxic lymphocyte associated protease granzyme B upon activation. Mol Immunol 44: 3462–3472
89. Strunk RC, Bloomberg GR (2006) Omalizumab for asthma. N Engl J Med 354: 2689–2695
90. Matta GM, Battaglio S, Dibello C, Napoli P, Baldi C, Ciccone G, Coscia M, Boccadoro M, Massaia M (2007) Polyclonal immunoglobulin E levels are correlated with hemoglobin values and overall survival in patients with multiple myeloma. Clin Cancer Res 13: 5348–5354

91. Ekstrom Smedby K, Vajdic CM, Falster M, Engels EA, Martinez-Maza O, Turner J, Hjalgrim H, Vineis P, Seniori Costantini A, Bracci PM, Holly EA, Willett E, Spinelli JJ, La Vecchia C, Zheng T, Becker N, De Sanjose S, Chiu BC, Dal Maso L, Cocco P, Maynadie M, Foretova L, Staines A, Brennan P, Davis S, Severson R, Cerhan JR, Breen EC, Birmann B, Grulich AE, Cozen W (2008) Autoimmune disorders and risk of non-Hodgkin lymphoma subtypes: A pooled analysis within the InterLymph Consortium. Blood 111: 4029–4038
92. Gordon J (1992) CD23 and B cell activation. Clin Exp Allergy 22: 199–204
93. Yawetz S, Cumberland WG, van der Meyden M, Martinez-Maza O (1995) Elevated serum levels of soluble CD23 (sCD23) precede the appearance of acquired immunodeficiency syndrome–associated non-Hodgkin's lymphoma. Blood 85: 1843–1849
94. Schroeder JR, Saah AJ, Ambinder RF, Martinez-Maza O, Crabb Breen E, Variakojis D, Margolick JB, Jacobson LP, Rowe DT, Hoover DR (1999) Serum sCD23 level in patients with AIDS-related non-Hodgkin's lymphoma is associated with absence of Epstein-Barr virus in tumor tissue. Clin Immunol 93: 239–244
95. Schroeder JR, Saah AJ, Hoover DR, Margolick JB, Ambinder RF, Martinez-Maza O, Breen EC, Jacobson LP, Variakojis D, Rowe DT, Armenian HK (1999) Serum soluble CD23 level correlates with subsequent development of AIDS-related non-Hodgkin's lymphoma. Cancer Epidemiol Biomarkers Prev 8: 979–984
96. Hannig H, Buske C, Matz-Rensing K, Hunsmann G, Hiddemann W, Bodemer W (1998) Elevated serum level of soluble CD23 precedes development of B-non-Hodgkin's lymphoma in SIV-infected Rhesus monkeys. Int J Cancer 77: 734–740
97. Kawabe T, Takami M, Hosoda M, Maeda Y, Sato S, Mayumi M, Mikawa H, Arai K, Yodoi J (1988) Regulation of Fc epsilon R2/CD23 gene expression by cytokines and specific ligands (IgE and anti-Fc epsilon R2 monoclonal antibody). Variable regulation depending on the cell types. J Immunol 141: 1376–1382
98. Ford JW, Kilmon MA, Haas KM, Shelburne AE, Chan-Li Y, Conrad DH (2006) In vivo murine CD23 destabilization enhances CD23 shedding and IgE synthesis. Cell Immunol 243: 107–117
99. Fournier S, Delespesse G, Rubio M, Biron G, Sarfati M (1992) CD23 antigen regulation and signaling in chronic lymphocytic leukemia. J Clin Invest 89: 1312–1321
100. Conrad DH, Ford JW, Sturgill JL, Gibb DR (2007) CD23: An overlooked regulator of allergic disease. Curr Allergy Asthma Rep 7: 331–337
101. Yamada T, Zhu D, Zhang K, Saxon A (2003) Inhibition of interleukin-4-induced class switch recombination by a human immunoglobulin Fc gamma-Fc epsilon chimeric protein. J Biol Chem 278: 32818–32824
102. Oettgen HC, Geha RS (2001) IgE regulation and roles in asthma pathogenesis. J Allergy Clin Immunol 107: 429–440
103. Smedby KE, Hjalgrim H, Askling J, Chang ET, Gregersen H, Porwit-MacDonald A, Sundstrom C, Akerman M, Melbye M, Glimelius B, Adami HO (2006) Autoimmune and chronic inflammatory disorders and risk of non-Hodgkin lymphoma by subtype. J Natl Cancer Inst 98: 51–60
104. Romagnani S (2008) Human Th17 cells. Arthritis Res Ther 10: 206
105. Annunziato F, Cosmi L, Santarlasci V, Maggi L, Liotta F, Mazzinghi B, Parente E, Fili L, Ferri S, Frosali F, Giudici F, Romagnani P, Parronchi P, Tonelli F, Maggi E, Romagnani S (2007) Phenotypic and functional features of human Th17 cells. J Exp Med 204: 1849–1861
106. Annunziato F, Cosmi L, Liotta F, Maggi E, Romagnani S (2008) The phenotype of human Th17 cells and their precursors, the cytokines that mediate their differentiation and the role of Th17 cells in inflammation. Int Immunol 20: 1361–1368
107. Korn T, Oukka M, Kuchroo V, Bettelli E (2007) Th17 cells: Effector T cells with inflammatory properties. Semin Immunol 19: 362–371
108. Katsifis GE, Moutsopoulos NM, Wahl SM (2007) T lymphocytes in Sjogren's syndrome: Contributors to and regulators of pathophysiology. Clin Rev Allergy Immunol 32: 252–264

109. Stockinger B, Veldhoen M (2007) Differentiation and function of Th17 T cells. Curr Opin Immunol 19: 281–286
110. Weaver CT, Harrington LE, Mangan PR, Gavrieli M, Murphy KM (2006) Th17: An effector CD4 T cell lineage with regulatory T cell ties. Immunity 24: 677–688
111. Ouyang W, Kolls JK, Zheng Y (2008) The biological functions of T helper 17 cell effector cytokines in inflammation. Immunity 28: 454–467
112. Legouffe E, Rodriguez C, Picot MC, Richard B, Klein B, Rossi JF, Commes T (1998) C-reactive protein serum level is a valuable and simple prognostic marker in non Hodgkin's lymphoma. Leuk Lymphoma 31: 351–357
113. Pluda JM, Venzon DJ, Tosato G, Lietzau J, Wyvill K, Nelson DL, Jaffe ES, Karp JE, Broder S, Yarchoan R (1993) Parameters affecting the development of non-Hodgkin's lymphoma in patients with severe human immunodeficiency virus infection receiving antiretroviral therapy. J Clin Oncol 11: 1099–1107
114. Breen EC, van der Meijden M, Cumberland W, Kishimoto T, Detels R, Martinez-Maza O (1999) The development of AIDS-associated Burkitt's/small noncleaved cell lymphoma is preceded by elevated serum levels of interleukin-6. Clin Immunol 92: 293–299
115. el-Far M, Fouda M, Yahya R, el-Baz H (2004) Serum IL-10 and IL-6 levels at diagnosis as independent predictors of outcome in non-Hodgkin's lymphoma. J Physiol Biochem 60: 253–258
116. Pedersen LM, Klausen TW, Davidsen UH, Johnsen HE (2005) Early changes in serum IL-6 and VEGF levels predict clinical outcome following first-line therapy in aggressive non-Hodgkin's lymphoma. Ann Hematol 84: 510–516
117. Niitsu N, Okamato M, Nakamine H, Yoshino T, Tamaru J, Nakamura S, Higashihara M, Hirano M (2002) Simultaneous elevation of the serum concentrations of vascular endothelial growth factor and interleukin-6 as independent predictors of prognosis in aggressive non-Hodgkin's lymphoma. Eur J Haematol 68: 91–100
118. Fayad L, Cabanillas F, Talpaz M, McLaughlin P, Kurzrock R (1998) High serum interleukin-6 levels correlate with a shorter failure-free survival in indolent lymphoma. Leuk Lymphoma 30: 563–571
119. Kato H, Kinoshita T, Suzuki S, Nagasaka T, Hatano S, Murate T, Saito H, Hotta T (1998) Production and effects of interleukin-6 and other cytokines in patients with non-Hodgkin's lymphoma. Leuk Lymphoma 29: 71–79
120. Voorzanger N, Touitou R, Garcia E, Delecluse HJ, Rousset F, Joab I, Favrot MC, Blay JY (1996) Interleukin (IL)-10 and IL-6 are produced in vivo by non-Hodgkin's lymphoma cells and act as cooperative growth factors. Cancer Res 56: 5499–5505
121. Kato H, Kinoshita T, Suzuki S, Nagasaka T, Murate T, Saito H, Hotta T (1996) Elevated serum interleukin-6 (IL-6) is derived from neoplastic lymphoid cells in patients with B-cell non-Hodgkin's lymphoma: Correlation with extent of IL-6 expression and serum concentration. Br J Haematol 92: 1014–1021
122. Suematsu S, Matsuda T, Aozasa K, Akira S, Nakano N, Ohno S, Miyazaki J, Yamamura K, Hirano T, Kishimoto T (1989) IgG1 plasmacytosis in interleukin-6 transgenic mice. Proc Natl Acad Sci USA 86: 7547–7551
123. Wang SS, Cozen W, Cerhan JR, Colt JS, Morton LM, Engels EA, Davis S, Severson RK, Rothman N, Chanock SJ, Hartge P (2007) Immune mechanisms in non-Hodgkin lymphoma: Joint effects of the TNF G308A and IL10 T3575A polymorphisms with non-Hodgkin lymphoma risk factors. Cancer Res 67: 5042–5054
124. Purdue MP, Lan Q, Kricker A, Grulich AE, Vajdic CM, Turner J, Whitby D, Chanock S, Rothman N, Armstrong BK (2007) Polymorphisms in immune function genes and risk of non-Hodgkin lymphoma: Findings from the New South Wales non-Hodgkin Lymphoma Study. Carcinogenesis 28: 704–712
125. Wang SS, Cerhan JR, Hartge P, Davis S, Cozen W, Severson RK, Chatterjee N, Yeager M, Chanock SJ, Rothman N (2006) Common genetic variants in proinflammatory and other immunoregulatory genes and risk for non-Hodgkin lymphoma. Cancer Res 66: 9771–9780

126. Rothman N, Skibola CF, Wang SS, Morgan G, Lan Q, Smith MT, Spinelli JJ, Willett E, De Sanjose S, Cocco P, Berndt SI, Brennan P, Brooks-Wilson A, Wacholder S, Becker N, Hartge P, Zheng T, Roman E, Holly EA, Boffetta P, Armstrong B, Cozen W, Linet M, Bosch FX, Ennas MG, Holford TR, Gallagher RP, Rollinson S, Bracci PM, Cerhan JR, Whitby D, Moore PS, Leaderer B, Lai A, Spink C, Davis S, Bosch R, Scarpa A, Zhang Y, Severson RK, Yeager M, Chanock S, Nieters A (2006) Genetic variation in TNF and IL10 and risk of non-Hodgkin lymphoma: A report from the InterLymph Consortium. Lancet Oncol 7: 27–38
127. Sappino AP, Seelentag W, Pelte MF, Alberto P, Vassalli P (1990) Tumor necrosis factor/cachectin and lymphotoxin gene expression in lymph nodes from lymphoma patients. Blood 75: 958–962
128. Macia J, Gomez X, Esquerda A, Perez B, Callao V, Marzo C (1996) Value of the determination of TNF-alpha in the plasma of patients with non-Hodgkins lymphoma. Leuk Lymphoma 20: 481–486
129. Warzocha K, Salles G, Bienvenu J, Bastion Y, Dumontet C, Renard N, Neidhardt-Berard EM, Coiffier B (1997) Tumor necrosis factor ligand-receptor system can predict treatment outcome in lymphoma patients. J Clin Oncol 15: 499–508
130. Warzocha K, Ribeiro P, Bienvenu J, Roy P, Charlot C, Rigal D, Coiffier B, Salles G (1998) Genetic polymorphisms in the tumor necrosis factor locus influence non-Hodgkin's lymphoma outcome. Blood 91: 3574–3581
131. Lissoni P, Bolis S, Mandala M, Viviani S, Pogliani E, Barni S (1999) Blood concentrations of tumor necrosis factor-alpha in malignant lymphomas and their decrease as a predictor of disease control in response to low-dose subcutaneous immunotherapy with interleukin-2. Int J Biol Markers 14: 167–171
132. Seidemann K, Zimmermann M, Book M, Meyer U, Burkhardt B, Welte K, Reiter A, Stanulla M (2005) Tumor necrosis factor and lymphotoxin alfa genetic polymorphisms and outcome in pediatric patients with non-Hodgkin's lymphoma: Results from Berlin-Frankfurt-Munster Trial NHL-BFM 95. J Clin Oncol 23: 8414–8421
133. Spink CF, Keen LJ, Mensah FK, Law GR, Bidwell JL, Morgan GJ (2006) Association between non-Hodgkin lymphoma and haplotypes in the TNF region. Br J Haematol 133: 293–300
134. Bel Hadj Jrad B, Chatti A, Laatiri A, Ahmed SB, Romdhane A, Ajimi S, Chouchane L (2007) Tumor necrosis factor promoter gene polymorphism associated with increased susceptibility to non-Hodgkin's lymphomas. Eur J Haematol 78: 117–122
135. Nowak J, Kalinka-Warzocha E, Juszczynski P, Bilinski P, Mika-Witkowska R, Zajko M, Bienvenu J, Coiffier B, Salles G, Warzocha K (2007) Association of human leukocyte antigen ancestral haplotype 8.1 with adverse outcome of non-Hodgkin's lymphoma. Genes, Chromosomes & Cancer 46: 500–507
136. Skibola CF, Curry JD, Nieters A (2007) Genetic susceptibility to lymphoma. Haematologica 92: 960–969
137. Suematsu S, Hibi M, Sugita T, Saito M, Murakami M, Matsusaka T, Matsuda T, Hirano T, Taga T, Kishimoto T (1990) Interleukin 6 (IL-6) and its receptor (IL-6R) in myeloma/plasmacytoma. Curr Top Microbiol Immunol 166: 13–22
138. Ma CS, Chew GY, Simpson N, Priyadarshi A, Wong M, Grimbacher B, Fulcher DA, Tangye SG, Cook MC (2008) Deficiency of Th17 cells in hyper IgE syndrome due to mutations in STAT3. J Exp Med 205: 1551–1557
139. Milner JD, Brenchley JM, Laurence A, Freeman AF, Hill BJ, Elias KM, Kanno Y, Spalding C, Elloumi HZ, Paulson ML, Davis J, Hsu A, Asher AI, O'Shea J, Holland SM, Paul WE, Douek DC (2008) Impaired T(H)17 cell differentiation in subjects with autosomal dominant hyper-IgE syndrome. Nature 452: 773–776
140. Schnyder-Candrian S, Togbe D, Couillin I, Mercier I, Brombacher F, Quesniaux V, Fossiez F, Ryffel B, Schnyder B (2006) Interleukin-17 is a negative regulator of established allergic asthma. J Exp Med 203: 2715–2725
141. Wang YH, Liu YJ (2008) The IL-17 cytokine family and their role in allergic inflammation. Curr Opin Immunol 20: 697–702

Chapter 6
Mast Cells in Allergy and Tumor Disease

Anna Wasiuk, Victor C. de Vries, Elizabeth C. Nowak, and Randolph J. Noelle

Abstract In allergy, mast cells (MCs) are known for the notoriously detrimental role they play. MC mediators like histamine, prostaglandins, leukotrienes and thromboxane are released during the early phase of an allergic reaction and produce inflammation and local tissue responses. One pervasive roadblock in the effective development of therapeutic immunity to cancer is the fact that tumors create immune privileged sites that are resistant to the development of effective inflammation and effective anti-tumor responses. In this chapter we will present the current knowledge of the inflammatory responses elicited in allergies by IgE and MCs as well as the current knowledge on how the responses of MCs may regulate tumor growth and the immune response to tumors.

6.1 Introduction

There are a few, if any, inflammatory responses that are more rapid or intense than those mediated by IgE. IgE exerts its massive and sometimes deadly pro-inflammatory effects by triggering the release of a vast array of pro-inflammatory mediators from mast cells. MCs, first termed by Paul Ehrlich in his graduate thesis, are best known for their protective role in helminth infections and allergy [1]. During helminth infections, MCs accumulate in numbers (mastocytosis) at the site of infection (skin, intestines and lung), eosinophils are recruited, there is an induction of goblet cell hyperplasia, high levels of IgE are elicited and a Th2 inflammatory environment is created, leading to the development of protective immunity. In allergy, MCs are known for the notoriously detrimental role they play. MC mediators like histamine, prostaglandins, leukotrienes and thromboxane during the early phase of an allergic reaction are released and produce local tissue responses. In the respiratory tract, the classic symptoms of sneezing, edema and mucus secretion

R.J. Noelle (✉)
Department of Microbiology and Immunology, Dartmouth Medical School, Lebanon, NH, USA
e-mail: Randolph.J.Noelle@Dartmouth.edu

Anna Wasiuk and Victor C. de Vries contributed equally to this manuscript.

M.L. Penichet, E. Jensen-Jarolim (eds.), *Cancer and IgE*,
DOI 10.1007/978-1-60761-451-7_6,

are evident, with vasodilatation in the nose and bronchoconstriction in the lung. As allergies proceed in the lung, there is accumulating cellular infiltration, fibrin deposition and tissue destruction as a result of a sustained allergic response leading to edema and further inflammatory cell recruitment. Immunologically, helminth infections and allergies show striking similarities such as induction of Th2 responses, eosinophilia, goblet cell hyperplasia, mastocytosis and high levels of IgE [2]. However, helminth infection and allergy seem to be mutually exclusive as has been shown by several epidemiological studies [3–5].

One pervasive roadblock in the effective development of therapeutic immunity to cancer is the fact that tumors create immune privileged sites that are resistant to the development of effective inflammation. Given this fact and the extraordinary capacity of IgE to mediate intense inflammatory responses a series of studies starting in the 1950s were undertaken to induce allergic reactions against tumors [6]. This novel approach in the context of the newly emerging field of AllergoOncology, the use of "allergy" as anti-tumor therapy, was later strengthened by epidemiological studies that show a protective effect of the presence of IgE on the development of malignancies [7–10]. Given the state of advanced antibody engineering, the widespread use of therapeutic antibodies and the ease with which one can produce fully human tumor-specific antibodies, IgE monoclonal antibodies directed at tumor antigens can be vigorously tested for their therapeutic value. In this chapter we will present the current knowledge of the inflammatory responses elicited in allergies by IgE and MCs as well as the current knowledge on how the responses of MCs may regulate tumor growth and the immune response to tumors.

6.2 Mast Cells in Allergy

6.2.1 Allergies and Mast Cell Subsets

In non-atopic individuals, B cells are skewed toward the production of allergen-specific IgG4 or IgA and to lesser extent IgG1, whereas in atopic patients B cells are driven to switch to IgE production [11]. However, IgE production is not a prerequisite for the development of disease, as allergy can be either IgE or cell (non-IgE) mediated or a combination of both. Although allergies are multifaceted, the involvement of MCs is considered one of the hallmarks in both mouse models and humans, and depending on the model, MCs have been proven to be the critical effector cells in allergy [11, 12]. MCs are divided into two subsets based on location and content: mucosal (MMC) and connective tissue (CTMC) MCs. These subsets can be distinguished based upon the presence of proteolytic enzymes in the granules. MMCs contain both chymases, chymotryptic peptidases, and tryptases, serine-class peptidases, whereas CTMCs only contain chymases [12]. Activation of MCs after allergen encounter leads to the release of chymases among many other mediators and does not seem to be dependent on subset. Chymases are mainly involved in

tissue remodeling [13], and thus MCs degranulation could exert a profound impact on the tumor microenvironment.

MMCs and CTMCs may be involved in Th2 versus Th1 responses, respectively. MMCs and CTMCs differ in the expression of STAT4, in that the latter express STAT4 and may play a role in driving Th1 responses. These findings suggest that CTMCs might not be prominently involved in Th2-driven allergies [14]. STAT4 seems to be dispensable for Th1 skewing in T cells, but the presence of STAT4 in CTMCs leads to the production of interferon gamma (INF-γ) and nitric oxide (NO) and is involved in the response to interleukin-18 (IL-18), IL-4, and IL-13. Additionally, Th1 skewing by CTMCs shows increased tumor cell lytic activity [14, 15]. The contrast of CTMCs with MMCs is even more striking when both subsets get triggered by IL-18, a cytokine that synergizes with IL-12 to induce cell-mediated immunity. CTMCs produce INF-γ when stimulated with IL-12 and IL-18, the same treatment elicits the production of IL-4 and IL-13 in MMCs, hallmark cytokines of IgE-mediated allergy [14, 16]. However, a strict demarcation of MC subsets into mediating Th1 versus Th2 responses cannot be delineated based on the current definitions of CTMCs versus MMCs. Allergens can enter the body through ingestion (food allergies are mainly MMCs mediated), inhalation (allergic rhinitis and asthma are mediated by both CTMCs and MMCs) or via the skin (atopic dermatitis is mainly CTMCs mediated) suggesting that both subsets play a role in allergy. It is likely that there are additional phenotypic distinctions among MC subsets that would further delineate them into MCs that play a role in Th1 versus Th2 responses. No doubt, it is critical to develop a more comprehensive understanding of the functional and transcriptional profile of subsets of MCs if they are going to be exploited to mediate anti-tumor immunity.

6.2.2 Mast Cells and Dendritic Cells

There is little doubt that the presentation and cross-presentation of tumor antigens by dendritic cells (DCs) is essential for the development of tumor-specific $CD4^+$ and $CD8^+$ T cells and protective anti-tumor immunity. Emerging data illustrate that MCs play an early role in DC migration and function, and it is in this context that MCs may contribute to the development of tumor immunity. Contact hypersensitivity (CHS) was regarded a Th1 cell-mediated allergy and has been studied extensively [17]. However, Th2-dependent CHS has been reported and seems to be dependent on allergen [18, 19]. One of the important early events in the development of CHS is the degranulation of MCs leading to the release of vasoactive and inflammatory mediators, like IL-α/β, histamine, tumor necrosis factor (TNF)-α, leukotrienes and granulocyte–macrophage colony-stimulating factor (GM-CSF) [20–22]. It has been shown that these mediators can dramatically modulate DC maturation and induce DC migration. Especially in Th2-driven CHS, TNF-α plays a crucial role in controlling DC migration [23]. Late phase disease is characterized by the infiltration of the skin by MCs, local swelling and recruitment of antigen-specific T cells, and

other leukocytes, to the site where the hapten is applied [24–26]. Additionally, the role of MCs in CHS has been refined very recently and even though the disease still develops in the absence of MCs, this study showed that MCs are regulators of the magnitude and the cytokine microenvironment [27]. Many insights on the interplay between MCs and DCs/Langerhans cells (LCs) come from CHS studies.

As mentioned earlier, TNF-α plays an important role in the development of CHS and can be produced by MCs in soluble and membrane-bound "cell-associated" form [28–30]. TNF-α is necessary for optimal response at the site where the hapten is applied during challenge [28]. Additionally, MC-deficient mice show impaired migration of LCs to the draining lymph nodes (dLN), a delay of approximately 18 h was observed while activation of MCs by IgE and allergen showed enhanced migration of LCs from the epidermis [31, 32]. The two observations were elegantly fused to show that cell-membrane-associated TNF-α produced by MCs regulating DCs/LCs migration, both in the skin and in the lung [33]. This implies that under atopic conditions, MCs modulate the adaptive immune responses by triggering increased antigen presentation in the dLN through enhanced DC migration.

There are TNF-α-independent ways MCs promote DC/LC migration. Patients with atopic dermatitis (AD) and CHS show a diminished defense against pathogens by reduced amounts of antimicrobial peptides (AMPs) and increased permeability of the skin by delayed repair [34–36]. Therefore, the lesions formed during encounter with the allergen are confronted with a wide array of Toll-like receptor (TLR) activation signals. It is known from studies with TLR2 agonist *Staphylococcus aureus* peptidoglycan (PGN) that MCs can induce LC migration equally well in wild type (WT) or $TNF^{-/-}$ mice [22]. The authors concluded that this was TLR2/MyD88 independent but complement dependent, which is plausible since PGN can activate complement efficiently. This observation could implicate that PGN leads to IgE-independent complement-dependent degranulation since IgE/antigen-mediated degranulation yielded the same results although the latter is dependent on TNF-α [22, 37]. Another study shows that MC cells up-regulate IL-1β when activated with imiquimod, a TLR7 agonist. Even though there was a trend suggesting involvement of TNF-α, there was a significant reduction in LC migration in IL-1α/$\beta^{-/-}$ mice [38]. MCs also express a functional TLR4 receptor [39, 40]. Upon infection of gram-negative bacteria MCs respond by the release of TNF-α as the main pro-inflammatory cytokine, thereby promoting DC maturation and migration [39]. Additionally IL-1β, IL-6 and IL-13 are produced and in the presence of IgE-mediated degranulation as seen in allergies IL-5 and IL-10 are released as well, thereby creating a Th2 cytokine environment [41]. These studies clearly show that multiple different responses to infection during CHS or AD can lead to aggravation of disease that is independent of the allergen but dependent on MCs which are abundantly present.

Another mechanism by which MCs influence DC function is through indirectly modulating the allergic microenvironment. It has been shown that MCs regulate thymic stromal lymphopoietin (TSLP) expressed by epithelial cells. TSLP activates DCs and lead to the induction of Th2 cells from naive $CD4^+$ T cells [42, 43]. It has been shown in a murine allergic rhinitis model that allergen challenge leads to

upregulation of TSLP in a MC- and IgE-dependent manner, thereby contributing to the Th2 environment and enhanced DC migration and maturation [44].

These modulatory properties imprinted by MCs on DCs are reflected in the development of the subsequent T-cell responses. In allergy models, it has been shown that MCs induce a Th2 profile by the production of PGE2 and histamine. These mediators induce DCs to produce CCL17/22, which are Th2-cell recruitment factors and also suppress the frequency of Th1 allergen-specific cells both in vivo and in vitro [45–47]. This further emphasizes the important role of MCs during allergic responses. Altogether, the current understanding is that there is an intimate and complex network of communication between MCs and DCs, which can exert profound effects on the development of acquired immunity.

6.2.3 Mast Cells and T-Cells

Although MCs indirectly influence T-cell responses via DCs, there is a body of information that shows MCs may also directly impact the T-cell compartment. During allergen encounter, IgE-sensitized MCs degranulate and release a wide array of mediators in the environment. Many of these factors affect the migration, development, proliferation and phenotype of T cells as has been reviewed extensively. As such, this represents another way in which MCs can orchestrate the development of the adaptive immune response [48–52]. The observation that MCs and T cells can be found in close proximity to each other suggests that cell-to-cell contact and/or regional cytokine production play key roles in this interaction [53]. Although MCs are not present in high numbers in secondary lymphoid organs, under inflammatory conditions, like during allergic reactions, MCs migrate from the periphery to the regional node [54, 55]. This suggests that MCs can interact with T cells both in tissue and in lymphoid organs. Additionally, since MCs express MHC-I and MHC-II, a role as antigen-presenting cells has been suggested and in fact demonstrated in vitro [56–58].

The idea of MCs acting as antigen-presenting cells (APCs) is not a novel concept. In 1993, Frandji et al. observed that MCs can activate T cell in vitro in an antigen-dependent manner leading to T-cell proliferation [56]. Yet even 10 years earlier, it was reported that MC progenitors could up-regulate MHC-II in the presence of IFN-γ [59]. Paradoxically, IFN-γ leads to the down-regulation of co-stimulatory molecules CD80 and CD86 on MCs [60]. More recently, MCs have been shown to express other co-stimulatory molecules of both the TNF-super family (OX40L, CD30L, Fas and GITR) as well as the B7 family CD80, CD86, programmed death ligand (PD-L)1 and PD-L2 [61]. IL-4 up-regulates MHC-II, albeit less than with IFN-γ but in combination with the up-regulation of co-stimulatory molecules [62]. Additionally, IL-4-cultured MCs but not IFN-γ-cultured MCs induce T-cell proliferation in vitro [52, 60]. These results suggest that MCs can enhance Th2 responses by positive feedback of IL-4 but dampen Th1 by negative regulation of IFN-γ.

Engagement of TLR4 on MCs induces MHC-II expression, and MCs can phagocytose, process and present bacterial antigens in the context of MHC-I [58]. All

these studies clearly show that MCs can be functional APCs; however, whether the same occurs in vivo is not yet clear. Since it appears that MCs undergo a cytokine-dependent up-regulation of MHC molecules it is feasible that the antigen-presenting function of MCs is to activate T cells locally in the peripheral tissues, where pro-inflammatory cytokines are released.

Although the role of MCs as *bone fide* APCs in vivo is debatable, antigen-independent regulation of T-cell response has been widely studied and recognized. The release of a wide array of immune-modulatory mediators induces recruitment, activation, skewing and proliferation of T cells. When activated, MCs release their granular content with the first effects being thought to involve recruitment of T cells and other leukocytes from the blood. The release of soluble TNF-α leads to up-regulation of several adhesion molecules, such as ICAM1, VCAM1 and VAP1, on endothelial cells needed for extravasation of T cells from the blood to the site of inflammation [63, 64]. Although seemingly contradictory, TNF-α also induces T-cell migration to the dLN during infection [65]. In this context, we speculate that TNF-α may function as a gatekeeper leading the T cells through the site of inflammation by recruiting them from the blood and directing them toward the dLN. Another factor known to promote extravasation is histamine. During allergies, the release of histamine increases the permeability of the vasculature, thereby increasing the efflux of T-effectors among other leukocytes [66].

A long list of chemokines can be released to fine tune the inflammatory response locally [51, 67, 68]. Once the T cells reach the location of allergen challenge, the release of IL-4, IL-13 and IL-10 by MCs sets the stage for a Th2 response [68]. Although not always the case, it seems that MCs preferentially skew toward a Th2 response. For instance histamine can both promote Th1 responses or suppress Th2 and Th1 T-cell activation depending on the receptor engaged [69].

In addition to the role of MCs during allergic inflammation by their influence on the adaptive immune response MCs have a well-established innate immune function and play an important role in wound healing and in the eradication of nematodes. These innate functions are also revealed during adaptive immune responses as tissue remodeling and destruction.

6.2.4 Mast Cells and Airway Tissue Remodeling

MCs products can directly affect airway epithelium and airway smooth muscle (ASM) function to enhance airway inflammation and hyperresponsiveness. Persistent MC activation during asthma can also lead to airway remodeling. This process is associated with damage and aberrant repair to lung tissue, including epithelial damage both at the surface of the lung and in the underlying basal lamina, increased development of myofibroblasts from fibroblasts, increased size and number of smooth muscle cells, and increased numbers of goblet cells (which produce mucus) [70]. One of the principle MC mediators of this process is β-tryptase, which enhances the proliferation of fibroblasts, airway epithelial and endothelial cells,

and smooth muscle cells, leading to global airway thickening [71–73]. Other products that contribute to airway remodeling are transforming growth factor (TGF)-β, which drives the differentiation of fibroblasts and ASM cells, and amphiregulin, which causes the proliferation of lung fibroblasts as well up-regulates mucin gene expression [74–76]. In addition, the MC products histamine, prostaglandin D_2 and leukotriene C_4 can cause ASM contraction [77, 78].

There is increasing evidence that angiogenesis plays an important role during tissue remodeling to provide oxygen and nutrients to the inflamed tissue as well as to allow the influx of inflammatory cells to the site. The most compelling evidence for this is that increased vascularity of the airways is observed in patients with both severe and mild asthma in comparison to healthy controls [79–82]. MCs derived IL-4, IL-5, IL-13 and TGF-β that can induce the production of vascular endothelial growth factor (VEGF) by fibroblasts and ASM cells contributing strongly to neovascularization [83, 84]. In addition, VEGF can to some extent regulate immune responses by inhibiting DC maturation and serve as a chemoattractant for other lymphocytes [85, 86].

6.3 Mast Cells in Cancer

6.3.1 Introduction

It has been proposed that the infiltration of MCs at the tumor site can greatly enhance tumorigenesis; MC accumulation has been confirmed in both experimental models in rodents and in primary human tumor biopsies; and MC accumulation in tumors is often associated with a poor prognosis [87, 88]. It has been suggested that MCs contribute to enhanced tumor growth by enhancing tumor-associated angiogenesis and by facilitating tissue remodeling. As noted above, MC production and induction of pro-angiogenic factors, as observed in asthma, may support the creation of a supportive environment for the growth of tumor cells. Likewise, the same mediators responsible for tissue remodeling in asthma may help to degrade the extracellular matrix and facilitate tumor growth and metastasis. Furthermore, MCs may enhance tumor growth through the release of tumor growth factors and by means of suppressing the development of protective anti-tumor immunity.

6.3.2 Mast Cells and Angiogenesis

Several factors underscore the importance of vasculature and angiogenesis for neoplastic growth and spread [89]. The original observations that tumor-associated vasculature plays an important role in the growth of neoplasms were made by Goldmann in 1907 [90]. Half a decade later (1970), a positive correlation of tumor growth and induced vasculature became evident. During the early stages of tumor development, tumors need oxygen and nutrients for continued growth and differentiation. Excessive tumor growth creates a hypoxic environment which in turn

promotes new blood vasculature through the up-regulation of angiogenic mediators released by tumor as well as non-tumor cells.

The impact of MCs on tumor angiogenesis was initially described in 1988 when it was shown that the angiogenic response was impaired in mast cell-deficient (W/Wv) mice in comparison to WT mice. In these studies, fewer W/Wv mice than WT mice developed spontaneous lung metastases and W/Wv mice exhibited fewer lung metastases per mouse. Bone-marrow reconstitution of W/Wv mice restored the angiogenic responses and also the incidence of hematogenous metastases to that of WT mice [91]. These studies implicated a role of MCs in vivo for tumor angiogenesis. Later Coussens and co-workers demonstrated that early angiogenic activity was greatly reduced in W/Wv mice using the HPV16 transgenic mouse model of squamous cell carcinoma, showing that up-regulated expression of the matrix metalloproteinase (MMP)-9 coincided with the angiogenic switch in early tumor lesions [92].

Recent studies confirmed these earlier observations establishing that MCs are an essential hematopoietic component for pre-neoplastic polyp development. It was seen that from the onset, adenomatous polyps are infiltrated with MCs and their precursors. Depletion of MCs either pharmacologically or by using MC-deficient animals resulted in a profound remission of existing polyps [93]. In addition, MCs have been shown to be necessary for the angiogenesis and macroscopic expansion of c-Myc-induced pancreatic β-cell tumors [94].

MCs have been shown to be selectively recruited to the site of tumor growth by means of tumor-derived peptides, RANTES and MCP-1 [95, 96], and several important angiogenic factors are expressed and secreted by MCs, such as IL-8, IL-1, VEGF, fibroblast growth factor-2 (FGF-2), TGF-β, TGF-α, MMP-2, MMP-9, nerve growth factor (NGF), platelet-derived growth factor (PDGF), leptin, tryptase, chymase, histamine and heparin [97].

IL-8 acts both as an angiogenic factor as well as a tumor cell chemotactic factor and tumor mitogen [97]. Inhibition of IL-8 by neutralizing antibodies reduces human non-small cell lung carcinoma progression in mice [98].

IL-1 secreted by MCs contributes to neovascularization by stimulating the secretion of VEGF from stroma surrounding tumor as well as directly acting on tumor growth [99]. In addition, IL-1 can induce selective secretion of IL-6 without overt degranulation in cultures of human MCs. High levels of circulating IL-6 are observed in almost every type of tumor studied and predict a poor patient outcome [100].

MC MMPs contribute to tumor metastases and invasiveness due to their proteolytic activity [101]. MC MMP products, for instance, have been seen to contribute to brain tumor metastases by regulating the permeability of the blood–brain barrier [102].

Currently MC involvement in tumor growth by means of neovascularization is relatively well accepted due to studies in murine tumor models. Below we will review observations linking MCs and tumor growth from human studies and will further elaborate on potential roles of MCs on tumor growth.

6.3.3 Mast Cells in Human Tumors

Some of the most aggressive human tumors, including breast carcinoma, malignant melanoma and colorectal adenocarcinoma, are notably populated with MCs at their periphery [87, 88, 103]. MCs have been found in the connective tissue surrounding tumor and in the environment of lymphatic and blood vessels. In mammary tumors, MCs are found on the invading, growing front of the tumor, and they contain elevated tryptase expression as compared to MCs in benign lesions.

Similar observations have been made about MCs in renal tumor tissue, and increased MC density correlates with poor prognosis in non-small lung carcinoma and increased VEGF expression [104]. Increased VEGF expression found in clinical samples may be the basis for the studies reported by Norrby and Wooley in 1993 [105], demonstrating a positive correlation of MCs with increased tumor angiogenesis. In the 1990s, a closer correlation was seen between angiogenesis and MCs in several different tumor models, such as angioma, lymphoma and multiple myeloma [106]. In Table 6.1we summarize several important mouse and human studies investigating the connection between MCs and tumor and list the major outcomes of the studies.

MCs are represented throughout the literature as contributing to tumorigenesis and poor prognosis. In tumor specimens from Hodgkin's lymphoma (HL), where sections were stained with MC-specific antibody that detects tryptase, MCs were seen in virtually every case. Furthermore, higher MC infiltration correlated with increased tumor aggressiveness [107]. If there is a case to be made for MCs contributing to enhanced tumor growth and metastasis, then lessening the infiltration or function of MCs in tumors might be an attractive therapeutic approach. In a study of advanced human breast carcinoma it was seen that recombinant human stem cell factor (SCF) (c-kit ligand) promoted human MC activation in vivo. As such, neutralization of c-kit ligand on MCs may represent a potential therapeutic target [108].

6.3.4 Mast Cells Mediators of Tumor Growth or Rejection

The link between inflammation and cancer has long been recognized and has been recently reviewed by Coussens et al. [109]. The inflammatory nature of the MCs may allow them to act as both beneficiaries of tumor growth and contributors of tumor rejection.

With the wealth of correlative clinical data, the early infiltration of MCs into human tumors appears to correlate with a poor prognosis. Given this evidence, animal cancer models have been used to try to understand whether MCs contribute to tumor growth and demise of the host, or in fact protect the host from cancer. Contrary to many human clinical observations, studies in one murine model have shown that MCs can exert a protective role for the host in a genetic model of intestinal tumorigenesis. This model of spontaneous intestinal adenomas in the

Table 6.1 Mast cell infiltration and role in tumor progression in human and murine tumor models

Tumor	Mouse model	Outcome of study	References
Murine, pro-tumor			
Mouse plasmacytoma	BALB/c nu/nu mice	Primary mast cells accelerate tumor growth through Ang-1 and VEGF-A	Nakayama et al. [127]
K14-HPV16 spontaneous murine model (models human cervical cancer)	(KitW/KitWWv) HPV16 transgenic mice	Mast cell infiltration and activation of MMP-9 coincides with the angiogenic switch in premalignant lesions. Premalignant angiogenesis is diminished in MC-deficient HPV16 transgenic mice	Coussens et al. [128]
b-cell carcinoma	pIns-mycERTAM;RIP7-bcl-xL;KitW-sh;KitW-sh	Mast cells are necessary for angiogenesis and macroscopic expansion of Myc-induced pancreatic islet tumors	Soucek et al. [93]
Murine, anti-tumor			
Murine mammary adenocarcinoma cell line (4T1)	BALB/c mice	Imatinib mesylate (Gleevec) accelerated the growth and peri-tumoral blood clotting of mammary adenocarcinoma in mice by inhibiting the survival and function of MCs	Samoszuk et al. [129]
Human, pro-tumor			
MM	–	Angiogenesis parallels progression of MM and MC participate in the induction by release of angiogenic factors. Poor prognosis in MM correlates directly with increased MC number	Ribatti et al. [130]
Rectal cancer	–	In a study of 331 rectal cancer samples a correlation was found of worsened overall survival rate with increase in MC present around tumor	Fisher et al. [131]
Melanoma	–	A high correlation was demonstrated between microvessel counts and total metachromatic and tryptase-reactive MCs. Suggesting that tryptase secreted by MCs cooperate in angiogenesis induction in human melanoma and as such increasing tumor progression	Ribatti et al. [132]
Oral SCC	–	MCs in all lesions and normal mucosa express tryptase. Density of MCs and microvessels increase with disease progression	Iamaroon et al. [133]
Lung adenocarcinoma	–	MCs correlate with angiogenesis and poor outcome in stage I lung adenocarcinoma	Imada et al. [134]
HL	–	MCs were detected in all tumor samples and increased number of MCs correlated with nodular sclerosis histology and a worse relapse-free survival	Molin et al. [106]

Table 6.1 (continued)

Tumor	Mouse model	Outcome of study	References
Pterygium	–	Angiogenesis was highly correlated with MC tryptase-positive cell count in pterygium tissues. Neovascularization in pterygium may be sustained by MC angiogenic mediators	Ribatti et al. [135]
Human, anti-tumor			
Breast, head and neck, lung, ovarian, NHL, HD	–	MCs are present in fibrotic regions of cancer and MC heparin is a inhibitor of tumor growth	Samoszuk et al. [136]
Breast carcinoma	–	A high number of MCs in tumor stroma were related to low S phase fraction, DNA diploidy, high proportion of intraductal growth and a high degree of tubule formation. A high MC count was related to a favorable prognosis	Aaltomaa et al. [137]
Breast carcinoma	–	Tissue microarrays of invasive breast carcinoma demonstrated the presence of MCs in the stroma correlating with a good prognosis. The presence of MCs showed an inverse correlation with CD68 positive macrophages and no correlation with the presence of B cells or T cells	Dabiri et al. [138]
Ovarian cancer	–	There was no significant association between angiogenesis and mast cell density. Peri-tumoral MC infiltration in tumors with high MVD predicts for improved survival in women with advanced epithelial ovarian cancer	Chan et al. [139]
Human, neutral			
RCC	–	The correlation between microvessels and MC counts was established and compared with tumor stage, grade and additional clinicopathologic parameters. No correlation was found between MC number and tumor size, stage, grade or patient survival	Tuna et al. [140]
Breast cancer	–	No difference in 10-year disease-free survival was established in patients with and without MC infiltration suggesting no correlation between MC numbers and prognosis	Fisher et al. [141]
NSCLC	–	Macrophage and MC infiltration of tumor cell islets confers a marked survival advantage in NSCLC	Welsh et al. [142]

Abbreviations: MM, multiple myeloma; SCC, small cell carcinoma; HL, Hodgkin's lymphoma; NHL, non-Hodgkin's lymphoma; HD, Hodgkin's disease; RCC, renal cell carcinoma; NSCLC, non-small cell lung carcinoma; VEGF, vascular endothelial growth factor; MVD, mean vessel density

multiple intestinal neoplasia (Min, $APC^{Min/+}$) mouse was seen to have an increased number of MCs and increased abundance of MC-associated proteinases. The MC-deficient Min (Min-Sash) mice developed 50% more adenomas than littermate controls, and the tumors were 33% larger in Min-Sash mice. These results suggest a protective, anti-tumor role for MCs in a genetic model of early-stage intestinal tumorigenesis [110]. Indeed, many of the cytokines produced by MCs can conceivably lead to impaired tumor growth. For example, the IL-4 receptor (IL-4R) is expressed on human breast carcinoma and signaling through the IL-4R can lead to tumor cell apoptosis, allowing for the possibility that MCs may act in a protective role to the host by directly killing tumor cells via IL-4 or other apoptosis-producing cytokines like TNF-α. Additionally, TNF-α contributes to leukocyte infiltration into the tumor which may also be protective [29, 111].

However, the overwhelming evidence in animal models suggests that MCs facilitate tumor growth and progression. In mammary tumor development MCs allow for tumor angiogenesis, contribute to tissue remodeling and metastasis through the release of MMPs and the release of growth factors such as SCF and NGF [112].

Using the mouse model of MC deficiency of the Kit^{W}/Kit^{Wv} mice Galli et al. conclusively demonstrated that these mice have decreased susceptibility to the development of 1,2-dimethylhydrazine-induced intestinal tumors [113]. These results were later supported, as described above, by studies in spontaneous human colorectal cancers where MCs are essential for polyp development and play a protective role to the tumor in intestinal tumorigenesis [93, 110]. Furthermore, the same studies show that TNF-α is required for the growth of adenomatous polyps, and it is proposed that MC-derived TNF-α is acting in an autocrine loop as a MC recruiting factor to increase the concentration of MCs at the site. Figure 6.1 summarizes the multiple ways by which MCs may either promote tumor growth or contribute to tumor rejection.

6.3.5 Mast Cells Regulate Adaptive Immune Responses to Tumors

In addition to the generally accepted role of MCs influencing tumor growth by means of angiogenesis and tissue remodeling, MCs may exert an immunomodulatory role in the generation of anti-tumor immune responses. Tumors utilize several mechanisms by which they evade the immune response including the induction of T-cell ignorance and anergy and by means of active suppression of effector cells [114–118]. The idea that MCs are beneficial for tumor formation together with the fact that MCs can selectively release cytokines and other mediators without degranulation raises the question weather MCs contribute in the development of an immune privilege within the tumor microenvironment. Such selective release of MC mediators is called piece meal degranulation and is a critical factor in MC versatility and their ability to release certain products without others and without degranulation [119].

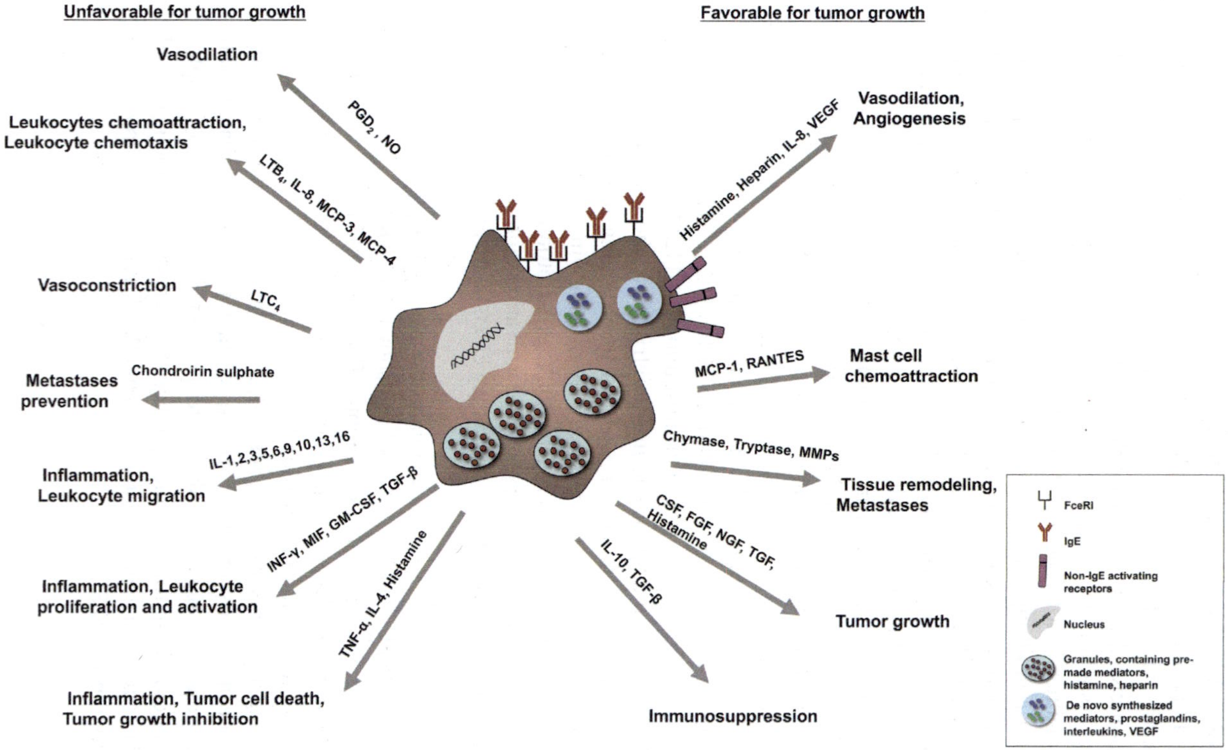

Fig. 6.1 Mast cell mediators and their effect on tumor growth. MCs carry and release multiple mediators that can both favorably and unfavorably affect tumor growth. Among the MC mediators thought to be unfavorable to tumor growth are those which cause leukocyte infiltration to the tumor site, vasoconstriction, prevent metastases, cause inflammation, cause leukocyte proliferation and activation and have direct anti-tumor effect by means of tumor cell death and tumor growth inhibition. Conversely, other factors, such as the pro-angiogenic mediators IL-8 and VEGF, are thought to contribute favorably to tumor growth by inducing angiogenesis; chymases and tryptases are known for their role in tissue remodeling and tumor metastasis and other factors such as FGF and NGF act directly on tumor growth. Factors such as IL-10 act in an immunosuppressive manner and yet others in the increased chemoattraction of additional MCs. What role MCs play during tumor progression likely varies depending on their immediate environment and the stimuli they encounter

Some of the immunoregulatory components of MC function are believed to be mediated by the release of histamine. Histamine released from MCs has been shown to play a dual role in that it can stimulate the proliferation of tumor cells through the H1 receptors (H1R) and act as a negative modulator of immune cells through H2 receptors (H2R) [112]. Results suggest that histamine in tumor tissue suppresses local tumor immunity via HR2 activation that results in tumor growth promotion. In addition, and somewhat conflicting with the immune stimulatory role of signaling through H1R, histamine has been seen to enhance growth of melanoma in a H1R-dependent manner [120]. The effect of histamine directly on tumor growth is currently quiet a conflicting topic as studies report differing results depending on dosage of histamine used as well as type of tumor studied. While it is likely that tumor-infiltrating MCs provide enough histamine to act as a tumor growth factor, exogenous administration of high-dose histamine seems to instead result in an anti-tumor effect of histamine in both a direct and an indirect manner [121].

MCs may contribute to tumor growth via immune modulation in the same way described above due to their interactions and influence on DC migration and functionality as well as by directly modulating T-cell responses. MCs produce IL-10, a common immunomodulatory cytokine produced by a variety of T-cells including T-regulatory cells (T_{reg}). Interestingly, MC-derived IL-10 has been shown to play a significant role in the suppression of UV-B-induced CHS [122]. MC-derived IL-10 is also seen to reduce immune responses after mosquito bites [123]. Hence, the production of IL-10 by MCs at the tumor site may contribute to the generation of an immunosuppressive microenvironment. In addition to providing immunosuppressive factors, MCs may also act in a suppressive way by removing proinflammatory mediators from the tumor microenvironment such as serotonin. Serotonin was recently shown to promote T-cell proliferation and activation, and MCs express the serotonin-specific transporter (SERT) by which they can take up and store serotonin [124–126].

As reviewed earlier, MCs can up-regulate the expression of several co-stimulatory molecules, and in addition it has been shown that MCs express PD-L1 and PD-L2, the ligands for the inhibitory receptor PD1 expressed on T cells [61]. These inhibitory ligands are expressed on tumors and tumor-infiltrating DCs and in doing so contribute to tumor immune evasion [127].

Further supporting a suppressive immunoregulatory role of MCs, it was recently shown that MCs are necessary intermediaries in regulatory T-cell-mediated graft tolerance. In this context, MCs were shown to prevent the rejection of haplo-mismatched skin allografts in tolerant mice. Hence, further investigation is needed to establish whether MCs and their mediators can alter the development of protective T-cell immunity to tumors [128].

6.4 Conclusion

Altogether, the role of MCs during allergic inflammation is very complex, and it is clear that MCs can influence the adaptive immune response by influencing antigen

presentation, as well as T-cell recruitment, activation, skewing and proliferation. It is perhaps easy to see then how these MC-mediated effects in the immune system may as well play an important role in tumor disease. Many studies show that MCs mediate processes that modify the tumor microenvironment in terms of angiogenesis and tissue remodeling that can help tumor grow and metastasize. Furthermore, MCs may also play an influential role in the development of adaptive immunity within the tumor microenvironment. It seems feasible to hypothesize that MCs may act in a tumor-friendly manner through a controlled release of certain mediators while having an anti-tumor effect upon a robust and immediate release of their granular content. As such MCs may play a dual role in propagating the development of cancer. Whether MCs truly regulate the development of anti-tumor immunity, how they do it and the identity of the molecular mediators are currently being studied.

References

1. Krishnaswamy G. (2005) Mast Cells: Methods and Protocols. Humana Press, New York.
2. Yazdanbakhsh, M., A. van den Biggelaar, and R. M. Maizels. (2001) Th2 responses without atopy: immunoregulation in chronic helminth infections and reduced allergic disease. Trends Immunol 22:372–377.
3. Lynch, N. R., R. I. Lopez, M. C. Di Prisco-Fuenmayor, I. Hagel, L. Medouze, G. Viana, C. Ortega, and G. Prato. (1987) Allergic reactivity and socio-economic level in a tropical environment. Clin Allergy 17:199–207.
4. Masters, S., and E. Barrett-Connor. (1985) Parasites and asthma – predictive or protective? Epidemiol Rev 7:49–58.
5. Scrivener, S., H. Yemaneberhan, M. Zebenigus, D. Tilahun, S. Girma, S. Ali, P. McElroy, A. Custovic, A. Woodcock, D. Pritchard, A. Venn, and J. Britton. (2001) Independent effects of intestinal parasite infection and domestic allergen exposure on risk of wheeze in Ethiopia: a nested case-control study. Lancet 358:1493–1499.
6. Molomut, N., D. M. Spain, L. Kreisler, and L. J. Warshaw. (1955) The effect of an allergic inflammatory response in the tumor bed on the fate of transplanted tumors in mice. Cancer Res 15:181–183.
7. Augustin, R., S. O'Sullivan, and I. Davies. (1971) Isolation of grass pollen antigens failing to induce IgE reagin formation although capable of inducing IgG antibody formation. Int Arch Allergy Appl Immunol 41:144–147.
8. Jacobs, D., J. Landon, M. Houri, and T. G. Merrett. (1972) Circulating levels of immunoglobulin E in patients with cancer. Lancet 2:1059–1061.
9. McCormick, D. P., A. J. Ammann, K. Ishizaka, D. G. Miller, and R. Hong. (1971) A study of allergy in patients with malignant lymphoma and chronic lymphocytic leukemia. Cancer 27:93–99.
10. Ure, D. M. (1969) Negative association between allergy and cancer. Scott Med J 14:51–54.
11. Pereira, E. A., D. A. Silva, J. P. Cunha-Junior, K. C. Almeida, R. Alves, S. J. Sung, and E. A. Taketomi. (2005) IgE, IgG1, and IgG4 antibody responses to Blomia tropicalis in atopic patients. Allergy 60:401–406.
12. Maurer, M., T. Theoharides, R. D. Granstein, S. C. Bischoff, J. Bienenstock, B. Henz, P. Kovanen, A. M. Piliponsky, N. Kambe, H. Vliagoftis, F. Levi-Schaffer, M. Metz, Y. Miyachi, D. Befus, P. Forsythe, Y. Kitamura, and S. Galli. (2003) What is the physiological function of mast cells? Exp Dermatol 12:886–910.
13. Algermissen, B., B. Hermes, I. Feldmann-Boeddeker, F. Bauer, and B. M. Henz. (1999) Mast cell chymase and tryptase during tissue turnover: analysis on in vitro mitogenesis

of fibroblasts and keratinocytes and alterations in cutaneous scars. Exp Dermatol 8: 193–198.
14. Kataoka, T. R., N. Komazawa, E. Morii, K. Oboki, and T. Nakano. (2005) Involvement of connective tissue-type mast cells in Th1 immune responses via Stat4 expression. Blood 105:1016–1020.
15. Kaplan, M. H., A. L. Wurster, and M. J. Grusby. (1998) A signal transducer and activator of transcription (Stat)4-independent pathway for the development of T helper type 1 cells. J Exp Med. 188:1191–1196.
16. Yoshimoto, T., H. Tsutsui, K. Tominaga, K. Hoshino, H. Okamura, S. Akira, W. E. Paul, and K. Nakanishi. (1999) IL-18, although antiallergic when administered with IL-12, stimulates IL-4 and histamine release by basophils. Proc Natl Acad Sci USA 96:13962–13966.
17. Grabbe, S., and T. Schwarz. (1998) Immunoregulatory mechanisms involved in elicitation of allergic contact hypersensitivity. Immunol Today 19:37–44.
18. Takeshita, K., T. Yamasaki, S. Akira, F. Gantner, and K. B. Bacon. (2004) Essential role of MHC II-independent CD4+ T cells, IL-4 and STAT6 in contact hypersensitivity induced by fluorescein isothiocyanate in the mouse. Int Immunol 16:685–695.
19. Yokozeki, H., M. Ghoreishi, S. Takagawa, K. Takayama, T. Satoh, I. Katayama, K. Takeda, S. Akira, and K. Nishioka. (2000) Signal transducer and activator of transcription 6 is essential in the induction of contact hypersensitivity. J Exp Med 191:995–1004.
20. Askenase, P. W., M. Szczepanik, A. Itakura, C. Kiener, and R. A. Campos. (2004) Extravascular T-cell recruitment requires initiation begun by Valpha14+ NKT cells and B-1 B cells. Trends Immunol 25:441–449.
21. Galli, S. J., J. Kalesnikoff, M. A. Grimbaldeston, A. M. Piliponsky, C. M. Williams, and M. Tsai. (2005) Mast cells as "tunable" effector and immunoregulatory cells: recent advances. Annu Rev Immunol 23:749–786.
22. Jawdat, D. M., G. Rowden, and J. S. Marshall. (2006) Mast cells have a pivotal role in TNF-independent lymph node hypertrophy and the mobilization of Langerhans cells in response to bacterial peptidoglycan. J Immunol 177:1755–1762.
23. Pasparakis, M., L. Alexopoulou, V. Episkopou, and G. Kollias. (1996) Immune and inflammatory responses in TNF alpha-deficient mice: a critical requirement for TNF alpha in the formation of primary B cell follicles, follicular dendritic cell networks and germinal centers, and in the maturation of the humoral immune response. J Exp Med 184:1397–1411.
24. Hwang, J. M., J. Yamanouchi, P. Santamaria, and P. Kubes. (2004) A critical temporal window for selectin-dependent CD4+ lymphocyte homing and initiation of late-phase inflammation in contact sensitivity. J Exp Med 199:1223–1234.
25. Van Loveren, H., K. Kato, R. Meade, D. R. Green, M. Horowitz, W. Ptak, and P. W. Askenase. (1984) Characterization of two different Ly-1+ T cell populations that mediate delayed-type hypersensitivity. J Immunol 133:2402–2411.
26. van Loveren, H., R. Meade, and P. W. Askenase. (1983) An early component of delayed-type hypersensitivity mediated by T cells and mast cells. J Exp Med 157:1604–1617.
27. Norman, M. U., J. Hwang, S. Hulliger, C. S. Bonder, J. Yamanouchi, P. Santamaria, and P. Kubes. (2008) Mast cells regulate the magnitude and the cytokine microenvironment of the contact hypersensitivity response. Am J Pathol 172:1638–1649.
28. Biedermann, T., M. Kneilling, R. Mailhammer, K. Maier, C. A. Sander, G. Kollias, S. L. Kunkel, L. Hultner, and M. Rocken. (2000) Mast cells control neutrophil recruitment during T cell-mediated delayed-type hypersensitivity reactions through tumor necrosis factor and macrophage inflammatory protein 2. J Exp Med 192:1441–1452.
29. Gordon, J. R., and S. J. Galli. (1990) Mast cells as a source of both preformed and immunologically inducible TNF-alpha/cachectin. Nature 346:274–276.
30. Gordon, J. R., and S. J. Galli. (1991) Release of both preformed and newly synthesized tumor necrosis factor alpha (TNF-alpha)/cachectin by mouse mast cells stimulated via the Fc epsilon RI. A mechanism for the sustained action of mast cell-derived TNF-alpha during IgE-dependent biological responses. J Exp Med 174:103–107.

31. Bryce, P. J., M. L. Miller, I. Miyajima, M. Tsai, S. J. Galli, and H. C. Oettgen. (2004) Immune sensitization in the skin is enhanced by antigen-independent effects of IgE. Immunity 20:381–392.
32. Jawdat, D. M., E. J. Albert, G. Rowden, I. D. Haidl, and J. S. Marshall. (2004) IgE-mediated mast cell activation induces Langerhans cell migration in vivo. J Immunol 173: 5275–5282.
33. Suto, H., S. Nakae, M. Kakurai, J. D. Sedgwick, M. Tsai, and S. J. Galli. (2006) Mast cell-associated TNF promotes dendritic cell migration. J Immunol 176:4102–4112.
34. Roelandt, T., C. Heughebaert, and J. P. Hachem. (2008) Proteolytically active allergens cause barrier breakdown. J Invest Dermatol 128:1878–1880.
35. Schittek, B., M. Paulmann, I. Senyurek, and H. Steffen. (2008) The role of antimicrobial peptides in human skin and in skin infectious diseases. Infect Disord Drug Targets 8: 135–143.
36. Schmid-Wendtner, M. H., and H. C. Korting. (2006) The pH of the skin surface and its impact on the barrier function. Skin Pharmacol Physiol 19:296–302.
37. Nilsson, G., M. Johnell, C. H. Hammer, H. L. Tiffany, K. Nilsson, D. D. Metcalfe, A. Siegbahn, and P. M. Murphy. (1996) C3a and C5a are chemotaxins for human mast cells and act through distinct receptors via a pertussis toxin-sensitive signal transduction pathway. J Immunol 157:1693–1698.
38. Heib, V., M. Becker, T. Warger, G. Rechtsteiner, C. Tertilt, M. Klein, T. Bopp, C. Taube, H. Schild, E. Schmitt, and M. Stassen. (2007) Mast cells are crucial for early inflammation, migration of Langerhans cells, and CTL responses following topical application of TLR7 ligand in mice. Blood 110:946–953.
39. McCurdy, J. D., T. J. Lin, and J. S. Marshall. (2001) Toll-like receptor 4-mediated activation of murine mast cells. J Leukoc Biol 70:977–984.
40. Supajatura, V., H. Ushio, A. Nakao, K. Okumura, C. Ra, and H. Ogawa. (2001) Protective roles of mast cells against enterobacterial infection are mediated by Toll-like receptor 4. J Immunol 167:2250–2256.
41. Varadaradjalou, S., F. Feger, N. Thieblemont, N. B. Hamouda, J. M. Pleau, M. Dy, and M. Arock. (2003) Toll-like receptor 2 (TLR2) and TLR4 differentially activate human mast cells. Eur J Immunol 33:899–906.
42. Liu, Y. J. (2006) Thymic stromal lymphopoietin: master switch for allergic inflammation. J Exp Med 203:269–273.
43. Ziegler, S. F., and Y. J. Liu. (2006) Thymic stromal lymphopoietin in normal and pathogenic T cell development and function. Nat Immunol 7:709–714.
44. Miyata, M., K. Hatsushika, T. Ando, N. Shimokawa, Y. Ohnuma, R. Katoh, H. Suto, H. Ogawa, K. Masuyama, and A. Nakao. (2008) Mast cell regulation of epithelial TSLP expression plays an important role in the development of allergic rhinitis. Eur J Immunol 38:1487–1492.
45. Mazzoni, A., R. P. Siraganian, C. A. Leifer, and D. M. Segal. (2006) Dendritic cell modulation by mast cells controls the Th1/Th2 balance in responding T cells. J Immunol 177: 3577–3581.
46. McIlroy, A., G. Caron, S. Blanchard, I. Fremaux, D. Duluc, Y. Delneste, A. Chevailler, and P. Jeannin. (2006) Histamine and prostaglandin E up-regulate the production of Th2-attracting chemokines (CCL17 and CCL22) and down-regulate IFN-gamma-induced CXCL10 production by immature human dendritic cells. Immunology 117:507–516.
47. Theiner, G., A. Gessner, and M. B. Lutz. (2006) The mast cell mediator PGD2 suppresses IL-12 release by dendritic cells leading to Th2 polarized immune responses in vivo. Immunobiology 211:463–472.
48. Galli, S. J., S. Nakae, and M. Tsai. (2005) Mast cells in the development of adaptive immune responses. Nat Immunol 6:135–142.
49. Galli, S. J., M. Grimbaldeston, and M. Tsai. (2008) Immunomodulatory mast cells: negative, as well as positive, regulators of immunity. Nat Rev Immunol 8:478–486.

50. Metz, M., M. A. Grimbaldeston, S. Nakae, A. M. Piliponsky, M. Tsai, and S. J. Galli. (2007) Mast cells in the promotion and limitation of chronic inflammation. Immunol Rev 217: 304–328.
51. Sayed, B. A., and M. A. Brown. (2007) Mast cells as modulators of T-cell responses. Immunol Rev 217:53–64.
52. Stelekati, E., Z. Orinska, and S. Bulfone-Paus. (2007) Mast cells in allergy: innate instructors of adaptive responses. Immunobiology 212:505–519.
53. Mekori, Y. A. (2004) The mastocyte: the "other" inflammatory cell in immunopathogenesis. J Allergy Clin Immunol 114:52–57.
54. Tanzola, M. B., M. Robbie-Ryan, C. A. Gutekunst, and M. A. Brown. (2003) Mast cells exert effects outside the central nervous system to influence experimental allergic encephalomyelitis disease course. J Immunol 171:4385–4391.
55. Wang, H. W., N. Tedla, A. R. Lloyd, D. Wakefield, and P. H. McNeil. (1998) Mast cell activation and migration to lymph nodes during induction of an immune response in mice. J Clin Invest 102:1617–1626.
56. Frandji, P., C. Oskeritzian, F. Cacaraci, J. Lapeyre, R. Peronet, B. David, J. G. Guillet, and S. Mecheri. (1993) Antigen-dependent stimulation by bone marrow-derived mast cells of MHC class II-restricted T cell hybridoma. J Immunol 151:6318–6328.
57. Koch, N., and A. W. Harris. (1984) Differential expression of the invariant chain in mouse tumor cells: relationship to B lymphoid development. J Immunol 132:12–15.
58. Malaviya, R., N. J. Twesten, E. A. Ross, S. N. Abraham, and J. D. Pfeifer. (1996) Mast cells process bacterial Ags through a phagocytic route for class I MHC presentation to T cells. J Immunol 156:1490–1496.
59. Wong, G. H., I. Clark-Lewis, J. L. McKimm-Breschkin, and J. W. Schrader. (1982) Interferon-gamma-like molecule induces Ia antigens on cultured mast cell progenitors. Proc Natl Acad Sci USA 79:6989–6993.
60. Frandji, P., C. Tkaczyk, C. Oskeritzian, B. David, C. Desaymard, and S. Mecheri. (1996) Exogenous and endogenous antigens are differentially presented by mast cells to CD4+ T lymphocytes. Eur J Immunol 26:2517–2528.
61. Nakae, S., H. Suto, M. Iikura, M. Kakurai, J. D. Sedgwick, M. Tsai, and S. J. Galli. (2006) Mast cells enhance T cell activation: importance of mast cell costimulatory molecules and secreted TNF. J Immunol 176:2238–2248.
62. Frandji, P., C. Tkaczyk, C. Oskeritzian, J. Lapeyre, R. Peronet, B. David, J. G. Guillet, and S. Mecheri. (1995) Presentation of soluble antigens by mast cells: upregulation by interleukin-4 and granulocyte/macrophage colony-stimulating factor and downregulation by interferon-gamma. Cell Immunol 163:37–46.
63. Walsh, L. J. (1995) Ultraviolet B irradiation of skin induces mast cell degranulation and release of tumor necrosis factor-alpha. Immunol Cell Biol 73:226–233.
64. Meng, H., M. J. Marchese, J. A. Garlick, A. Jelaska, J. H. Korn, J. Gailit, R. A. Clark, and B. L. Gruber. (1995) Mast cells induce T-cell adhesion to human fibroblasts by regulating intercellular adhesion molecule-1 and vascular cell adhesion molecule-1 expression. J Invest Dermatol 105:789–796.
65. McLachlan, J. B., J. P. Hart, S. V. Pizzo, C. P. Shelburne, H. F. Staats, M. D. Gunn, and S. N. Abraham. (2003) Mast cell-derived tumor necrosis factor induces hypertrophy of draining lymph nodes during infection. Nat Immunol 4:1199–1205.
66. Zhuang, X., A. J. Silverman, and R. Silver. (1996) Brain mast cell degranulation regulates blood-brain barrier. J Neurobiol 31:393–403.
67. Marshall, J. S., C. A. King, and J. D. McCurdy. (2003) Mast cell cytokine and chemokine responses to bacterial and viral infection. Curr Pharm Des 9:11–24.
68. Mekori, Y. A., and D. D. Metcalfe. (1999) Mast cell-T cell interactions. J Allergy Clin Immunol 104:517–523.
69. Jutel, M., T. Watanabe, S. Klunker, M. Akdis, O. A. Thomet, J. Malolepszy, T. Zak-Nejmark, R. Koga, T. Kobayashi, K. Blaser, and C. A. Akdis. (2001) Histamine regulates T-cell and antibody responses by differential expression of H1 and H2 receptors. Nature 413:420–425.

70. Holgate, S. T. (2008) Pathogenesis of asthma. Clin Exp Allergy 38:872–897.
71. Cairns, J. A., and A. F. Walls. (1996) Mast cell tryptase is a mitogen for epithelial cells. Stimulation of IL-8 production and intercellular adhesion molecule-1 expression. J Immunol 156:275–283.
72. Compton, S. J., J. A. Cairns, S. T. Holgate, and A. F. Walls. (1998) The role of mast cell tryptase in regulating endothelial cell proliferation, cytokine release, and adhesion molecule expression: tryptase induces expression of mRNA for IL-1 beta and IL-8 and stimulates the selective release of IL-8 from human umbilical vein endothelial cells. J Immunol 161: 1939–1946.
73. Berger, P., D. W. Perng, H. Thabrew, S. J. Compton, J. A. Cairns, A. R. McEuen, R. Marthan, J. M. Tunon De Lara, and A. F. Walls. (2001) Tryptase and agonists of PAR-2 induce the proliferation of human airway smooth muscle cells. J Appl Physiol 91:1372–1379.
74. Okumura, S., H. Sagara, T. Fukuda, H. Saito, and Y. Okayama. (2005) FcepsilonRI-mediated amphiregulin production by human mast cells increases mucin gene expression in epithelial cells. J Allergy Clin Immunol 115:272–279.
75. Wang, S. W., C. K. Oh, S. H. Cho, G. Hu, R. Martin, S. Demissie-Sanders, K. Li, M. Moyle, and Z. Yao. (2005) Amphiregulin expression in human mast cells and its effect on the primary human lung fibroblasts. J Allergy Clin Immunol 115:287–294.
76. Woodman, L., S. Siddiqui, G. Cruse, A. Sutcliffe, R. Saunders, D. Kaur, P. Bradding, and C. Brightling. (2008) Mast cells promote airway smooth muscle cell differentiation via autocrine up-regulation of TGF-beta 1. J Immunol 181:5001–5007.
77. Black, P. N., R. W. Fuller, G. W. Taylor, P. J. Barnes, and C. T. Dollery. (1989) Effect of inhaled leukotriene B4 alone and in combination with prostaglandin D2 on bronchial responsiveness to histamine in normal subjects. Thorax 44:491–495.
78. Rajah, R., S. E. Nunn, D. J. Herrick, M. M. Grunstein, and P. Cohen. (1996) Leukotriene D4 induces MMP-1, which functions as an IGFBP protease in human airway smooth muscle cells. Am J Physiol 271:L1014–1022.
79. Dunnill, M. S. (1960) The pathology of asthma, with special reference to changes in the bronchial mucosa. J Clin Pathol 13:27–33.
80. Li, X., and J. W. Wilson. (1997) Increased vascularity of the bronchial mucosa in mild asthma. Am J Respir Crit Care Med 156:229–233.
81. Orsida, B. E., X. Li, B. Hickey, F. Thien, J. W. Wilson, and E. H. Walters. (1999) Vascularity in asthmatic airways: relation to inhaled steroid dose. Thorax 54:289–295.
82. Redington, A. E., W. R. Roche, J. Madden, A. J. Frew, R. Djukanovic, S. T. Holgate, and P. H. Howarth. (2001) Basic fibroblast growth factor in asthma: measurement in bronchoalveolar lavage fluid basally and following allergen challenge. J Allergy Clin Immunol 107:384–387.
83. Horiuchi, T., and P. F. Weller. (1997) Expression of vascular endothelial growth factor by human eosinophils: upregulation by granulocyte macrophage colony-stimulating factor and interleukin-5. Am J Respir Cell Mol Biol 17:70–77.
84. Richter, A., S. M. Puddicombe, J. L. Lordan, F. Bucchieri, S. J. Wilson, R. Djukanovic, G. Dent, S. T. Holgate, and D. E. Davies. (2001) The contribution of interleukin (IL)-4 and IL-13 to the epithelial-mesenchymal trophic unit in asthma. Am J Respir Cell Mol Biol 25:385–391.
85. Lee, C. G., H. Link, P. Baluk, R. J. Homer, S. Chapoval, V. Bhandari, M. J. Kang, L. Cohn, Y. K. Kim, D. M. McDonald, and J. A. Elias. (2004) Vascular endothelial growth factor (VEGF) induces remodeling and enhances TH2-mediated sensitization and inflammation in the lung. Nat Med 10:1095–1103.
86. Puxeddu, I., D. Ribatti, E. Crivellato, and F. Levi-Schaffer. (2005) Mast cells and eosinophils: a novel link between inflammation and angiogenesis in allergic diseases. J Allergy Clin Immunol 116:531–536.
87. Amini, R. M., K. Aaltonen, H. Nevanlinna, R. Carvalho, L. Salonen, P. Heikkila, and C. Blomqvist. (2007) Mast cells and eosinophils in invasive breast carcinoma. BMC Cancer 7:165.

88. Lachter, J., M. Stein, C. Lichtig, S. Eidelman, and M. Munichor. (1995) Mast cells in colorectal neoplasias and premalignant disorders. Dis Colon Rectum 38:290–293.
89. Sivridis, E., A. Giatromanolaki, and M. I. Koukourakis. (2003) The vascular network of tumours – what is it not for? J Pathol 201:173–180.
90. Goldmann, E. (1908) The growth of malignant disease in man and the lower animals, with special reference to the Vascular system. Proc R Soc Med 1:1–13.
91. Starkey, J. R., P. K. Crowle, and S. Taubenberger. (1988) Mast-cell-deficient W/Wv mice exhibit a decreased rate of tumor angiogenesis. Int J Cancer 42:48–52.
92. Coussens, L. M., W. W. Raymond, G. Bergers, M. Laig-Webster, O. Behrendtsen, Z. Werb, G. H. Caughey, and D. Hanahan. (1999) Inflammatory mast cells up-regulate angiogenesis during squamous epithelial carcinogenesis. Genes Dev 13:1382–1397.
93. Gounaris, E., S. E. Erdman, C. Restaino, M. F. Gurish, D. S. Friend, F. Gounari, D. M. Lee, G. Zhang, J. N. Glickman, K. Shin, V. P. Rao, T. Poutahidis, R. Weissleder, K. M. McNagny, and K. Khazaie. (2007) Mast cells are an essential hematopoietic component for polyp development. Proc Natl Acad Sci USA 104:19977–19982.
94. Soucek, L., E. R. Lawlor, D. Soto, K. Shchors, L. B. Swigart, and G. I. Evan. (2007) Mast cells are required for angiogenesis and macroscopic expansion of Myc-induced pancreatic islet tumors. Nat Med 13:1211–1218.
95. Conti, P., X. Pang, W. Boucher, R. Letourneau, M. Reale, R. C. Barbacane, J. Thibault, and T. C. Theoharides. (1997) Impact of Rantes and MCP-1 chemokines on in vivo basophilic cell recruitment in rat skin injection model and their role in modifying the protein and mRNA levels for histidine decarboxylase. Blood 89:4120–4127.
96. Conti, P., M. Reale, R. C. Barbacane, R. Letourneau, and T. C. Theoharides. (1998) Intramuscular injection of hrRANTES causes mast cell recruitment and increased transcription of histidine decarboxylase in mice: lack of effects in genetically mast cell-deficient W/WV mice. FASEB J 12:1693–1700.
97. Crivellato, E., B. Nico, and D. Ribatti. (2008) Mast cells and tumour angiogenesis: new insight from experimental carcinogenesis. Cancer Lett 269:1–6.
98. Brew, R., J. S. Erikson, D. C. West, A. R. Kinsella, J. Slavin, and S. E. Christmas. (2000) Interleukin-8 as an autocrine growth factor for human colon carcinoma cells in vitro. Cytokine 12:78–85.
99. Salven, P., K. Hattori, B. Heissig, and S. Rafii. (2002) Interleukin-1alpha promotes angiogenesis in vivo via VEGFR-2 pathway by inducing inflammatory cell VEGF synthesis and secretion. FASEB J 16:1471–1473.
100. Hong, D. S., L. S. Angelo, and R. Kurzrock. (2007) Interleukin-6 and its receptor in cancer: implications for translational therapeutics. Cancer 110:1911–1928.
101. Almholt, K., and M. Johnsen. (2003) Stromal cell involvement in cancer. Recent Results Cancer Res 162:31–42.
102. Esposito, P., N. Chandler, K. Kandere, S. Basu, S. Jacobson, R. Connolly, D. Tutor, and T. C. Theoharides. (2002) Corticotropin-releasing hormone and brain mast cells regulate blood-brain-barrier permeability induced by acute stress. J Pharmacol Exp Ther 303: 1061–1066.
103. Ch'ng, S., R. A.Wallis, L. Yuan, F. P. Davis, and S. T. Tan. (2006) Mast cells and cutaneous malignancies. Mod Pathol 19:149–159.
104. Beil, W. J., W. Fureder, H. Wiener, K. Grossschmidt, U. Maier, A. Schedle, H. C. Bankl, K. Lechner, and P. Valent. (1998) Phenotypic and functional characterization of mast cells derived from renal tumor tissues. Exp Hematol 26:158–169.
105. Wooley, D., and Norrby K. (1993) Role of mast cells in mitogenesis and angiogenesis in normal tissue and tumor tissue. Adv Biosci 89:71–115.
106. Ribatti, D., E. Crivellato, A. M. Roccaro, R. Ria, and A. Vacca. (2004) Mast cell contribution to angiogenesis related to tumour progression. Clin Exp Allergy 34:1660–1664.
107. Molin, D., A. Edstrom, I. Glimelius, B. Glimelius, G. Nilsson, C. Sundstrom, and G. Enblad. (2002) Mast cell infiltration correlates with poor prognosis in Hodgkin's lymphoma. Br J Haematol 119:122–124.

108. Costa, J. J., G. D. Demetri, T. J. Harrist, A. M. Dvorak, D. F. Hayes, E. A. Merica, D. M. Menchaca, A. J. Gringeri, L. B. Schwartz, and S. J. Galli. (1996) Recombinant human stem cell factor (kit ligand) promotes human mast cell and melanocyte hyperplasia and functional activation in vivo. J Exp Med 183:2681–2686.
109. Coussens, L. M., and Z. Werb. (2002) Inflammation and cancer. Nature 420:860–867.
110. Sinnamon, M. J., K. J. Carter, L. P. Sims, B. Lafleur, B. Fingleton, and L. M. Matrisian. (2008) A protective role of mast cells in intestinal tumorigenesis. Carcinogenesis 29: 880–886.
111. Gooch, J. L., A. V. Lee, and D. Yee. (1998) Interleukin 4 inhibits growth and induces apoptosis in human breast cancer cells. Cancer Res 58:4199–4205.
112. Theoharides, T. C., and P. Conti. (2004) Mast cells: the Jekyll and Hyde of tumor growth. Trends Immunol 25:235–241.
113. Wedemeyer, J., and S. J. Galli. (2005) Decreased susceptibility of mast cell-deficient Kit(W)/Kit(W-v) mice to the development of 1, 2-dimethylhydrazine-induced intestinal tumors. Lab Invest 85:388–396.
114. Cuenca, A., F. Cheng, and H. Wang. (2003) Extra-lymphatic solid tumor growth is not immunologically ignored and results in early induction of antigen-specific T-cell anergy: dominant role of cross-tolerance to tumor antigens. Cancer Res 63:9007–9015.
115. Gajewski, T. F., Y. Meng, C. Blank, I. Brown, A. Kacha, J. Kline, and H. Harlin. (2006) Immune resistance orchestrated by the tumor microenvironment. Immunol Rev 213: 131–145.
116. Ochsenbein, A. F., P. Klenerman, U. Karrer, B. Ludewig, M. Pericin, H. Hengartner, and R. M. Zinkernagel. (1999) Immune surveillance against a solid tumor fails because of immunological ignorance. Proc Natl Acad Sci USA 96:2233–2238.
117. Sotomayor, E. M., I. Borrello, D. M. Rattis, A. G. Cuena, J. Abrams, K. Staveley-O'Carroll, and H. I. Levitsky. (2001) Cross-presentation of tumor antigens by bone marrow-derived antigen-presenting cells is the dominant mechanism in the induction of T-cell tolerance during B-cell lymphoma progression. Blood 98:1070–1077.
118. Zou, W. (2006) Regulatory T cells, tumour immunity and immunotherapy. Nat Rev Immunol. 6:295–307.
119. Theoharides, T. C., D. Kempuraj, M. Tagen, P. Conti, and D. Kalogeromitros. (2007) Differential release of mast cell mediators and the pathogenesis of inflammation. Immunol Rev 217:65–78.
120. Pos, Z., Z. Wiener, P. Pocza, M. Racz, S. Toth, Z. Darvas, V. Molnar, H. Hegyesi, and A. Falus. (2008) Histamine suppresses fibulin-5 and insulin-like growth factor-II receptor expression in melanoma. Cancer Res 68:1997–2005.
121. Cianchi, F., M. C. Vinci, and E. Masini. (2008) Histamine in cancer: the dual faces of the coin. Cancer Biol Ther 7:36–37.
122. Hart, P. H., M. A. Grimbaldeston, G. J. Swift, A. Jaksic, F. P. Noonan, and J. J. Finlay-Jones. (1998) Dermal mast cells determine susceptibility to ultraviolet B-induced systemic suppression of contact hypersensitivity responses in mice. J Exp Med 187: 2045–2053.
123. Depinay, N., F. Hacini, W. Beghdadi, R. Peronet, and S. Mecheri. (2006) Mast cell-dependent down-regulation of antigen-specific immune responses by mosquito bites. J Immunol 176:4141–4146.
124. Aune, T. M., H. W. Golden, K. M. McGrath. (1994) Inhibitors of serotonin synthesis and antagonists of serotonin 1A receptors inhibit T lymphocyte function in vitro and cell-mediated immunity in vivo. J Immunol 153:489–498.
125. Laberge, S., W. W. Cruikshank, D. J. Beer, and D. M. Center. (1996) Secretion of IL-16 (lymphocyte chemoattractant factor) from serotonin-stimulated CD8+ T cells in vitro. J Immunol 156:310–315.
126. León-Ponte, M., G. P. Ahern, and P. J. O'Connell. (2007) Serotonin provides an accessory signal to enhance T-cell activation by signaling through the 5-HT7 receptor. Blood 109:3139–3146.

127. Keir, M. E., M. J. Butte, G. J. Freeman, and A. H. Sharpe. (2008) PD-1 and its ligands in tolerance and immunity. Annu Rev Immunol 26:677–704.
128. Lu, L. F., E. F. Lind, D. C. Gondek, K. A. Bennett, M. W. Gleeson, K. Pino-Lagos, Z. A. Scott, A. J. Coyle, J. L. Reed, J. Van Snick, T. B. Strom, X. X. Zheng, and R. J. Noelle. (2006) Mast cells are essential intermediaries in regulatory T-cell tolerance. Nature 442: 997–1002.
129. Samoszuk, M., and M. A. Corwin. (2003) Acceleration of tumor growth and peri-tumoral blood clotting by imatinib mesylate (Gleevec). Int J Cancer 106:647–652.
130. Ribatti, D., A. Vacca, B. Nico, F. Quondamatteo, R. Ria, M. Minischetti, A. Marzullo, R. Herken, L. Roncali, and F. Dammacco. (1999) Bone marrow angiogenesis and mast cell density increase simultaneously with progression of human multiple myeloma. Br J Cancer 79:451–455.
131. Fisher, E. R., S. M. Paik, H. Rockette, J. Jones, R. Caplan, and B. Fisher. (1989) Prognostic significance of eosinophils and mast cells in rectal cancer: findings from the National Surgical Adjuvant Breast and Bowel Project (protocol R-01). Hum Pathol 20:159–163.
132. Ribatti, D., M. G. Ennas, A. Vacca, F. Ferreli, B. Nico, S. Orru, and P. Sirigu. (2003) Tumor vascularity and tryptase-positive mast cells correlate with a poor prognosis in melanoma. Eur J Clin Invest 33:420–425.
133. Iamaroon, A., S. Pongsiriwet, S. Jittidecharaks, K. Pattanaporn, S. Prapayasatok, and S. Wanachantararak. (2003) Increase of mast cells and tumor angiogenesis in oral squamous cell carcinoma. J Oral Pathol Med 32:195–199.
134. Imada, A., N. Shijubo, H. Kojima, and S. Abe. (2000) Mast cells correlate with angiogenesis and poor outcome in stage I lung adenocarcinoma. Eur Respir J 15:1087–1093.
135. Ribatti, D., B. Nico, C. Maxia, V. Longo, D. Murtas, D. Mangieri, M. T. Perra, M. De Giorgis, F. Piras, E. Crivellato, and P. Sirigu. (2007) Neovascularization and mast cells with tryptase activity increase simultaneously in human pterygium. J Cell Mol Med 11:585–589.
136. Samoszuk, M., E. Kanakubo, and J. K. Chan. (2005) Degranulating mast cells in fibrotic regions of human tumors and evidence that mast cell heparin interferes with the growth of tumor cells through a mechanism involving fibroblasts. BMC Cancer 15:121.
137. Aaltomaa, S., P. Lipponen, S. Papinaho, and V. M. Kosma. (1993) Mast cells in breast cancer. Anticancer Res 13:785–788.
138. Dabiri, S., D. Huntsman, N. Makretsov, M. Cheang, B. Gilks, C. Bajdik, K. Gelmon, S. Chia, and M. Hayes. (2004) The presence of stromal mast cells identifies a subset of invasive breast cancers with a favorable prognosis. Mod Pathol 17:690–695.
139. Chan, J. K., A. Magistris, V. Loizzi, F. Lin, J. Rutgers, K. Osann, P. J. DiSaia, and M. Samoszuk. (2005) Mast cell density, angiogenesis, blood clotting, and prognosis in women with advanced ovarian cancer. Gynecol Oncol 99:20–25.
140. Tuna, B., K. Yorukoglu, M. Unlu, M. U. Mungan, and Z. Kirkali. (2006) Association of mast cells with microvessel density in renal cell carcinomas. Eur Urol 50:530–534.
141. Fisher, E. R., R. Sass, G. Watkins, J. Johal, and B. Fisher. (1985) Tissue mast cells in breast cancer. Breast Cancer Res Treat 5:285–291.
142. Welsh, T. J., R. H. Green, D. Richardson, D. A. Waller, K. J. O'Byrne, and P. Bradding. (2005) Macrophage and mast-cell invasion of tumor cell islets confers a marked survival advantage in non-small-cell lung cancer. J Clin Oncol 23:8959–8967.

Chapter 7
The IgE Antibody and Its Use in Cancer Immunotherapy

Tracy R. Daniels, José A. Rodríguez, Elizabeth Ortiz-Sánchez, Gustavo Helguera, and Manuel L. Penichet

Abstract The immunoglobulin E (IgE) is a class of antibody that is capable of mounting a robust immune response resulting in anaphylaxis, which plays a central role in allergic reactions against environmental agents and immunity against parasites. Multiple studies also suggest that IgE plays a role in cancer immunosurveillance, which implies that this class of antibody can be exploited for the treatment of cancer. While most therapeutic antibodies developed for cancer therapy are of the IgG class, IgE has several advantages including the exceptionally high affinity for its Fc receptors (FcεRs) and its low serum concentration that provides less competition for Fc receptor occupancy. In addition, FcεRs are expressed on relevant effector cells involved in antibody-dependent cell-mediated cytotoxicity (ADCC) and/or antibody-dependent cell-mediated phagocytosis (ADCP) including antigen-presenting cells (APC). In fact, multiple IgEs targeting different tumor-associated antigens (TAA) have been developed and shown to be effective against cancer cells in vitro and in animal models. Further advances of current technologies and experimental models, coupled with a better understanding of IgE-mediated immune effector mechanisms against targeted tumors, are expected to help elucidate the full potential of tumor-specific IgE antibodies for cancer immunotherapy.

7.1 IgE and Its Relevance in Cancer Therapy

7.1.1 Immunoglobulins

Immunoglobulins (Ig, also known as antibodies) are glycoproteins and are central effector molecules of the humoral immune response [1–3]. They are highly selective for a broad spectrum of antigens including pathogens as well as tumor-associated

---

M.L. Penichet (✉)
Division of Surgical Oncology, Department of Surgery and Department of Microbiology, Immunology, and Molecular Genetics, Molecular Biology Institute, Jonsson Comprehensive Cancer Center, David Geffen School of Medicine, University of California, Los Angeles (UCLA), Los Angeles, CA, USA
e-mail: penichet@mednet.ucla.edu

M.L. Penichet, E. Jensen-Jarolim (eds.), *Cancer and IgE*,
DOI 10.1007/978-1-60761-451-7_7,

antigens (TAA) and potentiate the immune response by activating host effector systems against the targeted antigen. Antibodies are composed of heavy (H) and light (L) chains and exhibit a H_2L_2 heterotetramer configuration. In humans there are five classes of antibodies that are distinguished by their heavy chain structure designated by lower-case Greek letters: α (IgA), δ (IgD), ε (IgE), γ (IgG), and μ (IgM) [1–3]. There are two subclasses of IgA (IgA1 and IgA2) and four subclasses of IgG (IgG1, IgG2, IgG3, and IgG4). The light chains are designated κ and λ and are shared by all heavy chain classes. IgD, IgE and IgG are monomeric, while IgA can also be dimeric and IgM is usually pentameric (Fig. 7.1). Multimeric antibodies contain a joining (J) chain, which is a 15-kilodalton (kDa) polypeptide that promotes polymerization [1]. The IgM molecule exists as a pentamer with the J chain or occasionally as a hexamer without the J chain. In addition, polymeric antibodies contain an 18-amino acid extension, known as the "tailpiece," in the carboxy-terminus that contains a cysteine residue that is also required for polymerization. The approximate molecular weights (m.w.) of the different classes are as follows: 180 kDa for IgD; 190 kDa for IgE; 150 kDa for IgG1, IgG2 and IgG4; 170 kDa for IgG3 due to an extended hinge region; 160 kDa for both subclasses of monomeric IgA in serum and 300–360 kDa for secretory dimeric IgA and 900–970 kDa for IgM [1]. Similar to humans, mice also have five classes of antibodies (IgA, IgD, IgE, IgG and IgM) [4]. However, there is only one murine subclass of IgA that is approximately 160 kDa as a monomer and 350–400 kDa as a secretory dimer. The murine IgG subclasses are also different when compared to the human IgG subclasses. The murine IgG subclasses are IgG1, IgG2a, IgG2b and IgG3 (which are all approximately 160 kDa). Murine IgM is about 900 kDa, while the IgD and the IgE are comparable in size to their human counterparts (180 and 190 kDa, respectively) [4].

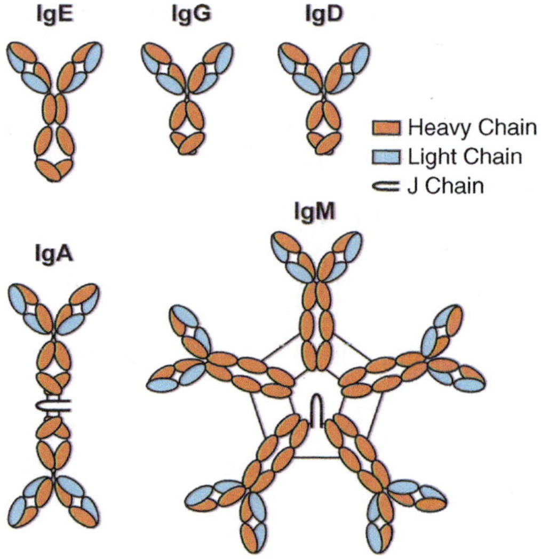

Fig. 7.1 Comparative structure of the human antibody classes. All five classes of antibodies share the basic H_2L_2 heterotetrameric structure that is organized into discrete domains. Antibodies of the IgE, IgG and IgD class are monomeric, while IgA (dimer) and IgM (pentamer) are polymeric. The polymeric antibodies contain a J chain, a polypeptide that promotes polymerization

7.1.2 The Structure of the IgE Antibody and Its Binding Properties

The heavy chains of IgE are composed of five domains: four constant domains (Cε1, Cε2, Cε3, and Cε4) and one variable domain (V_H) (Fig. 7.2) [5]. The light chains are composed of two domains: one variable (V_L) and one constant domain each (C_L) (Fig. 7.2). Like the other classes of antibodies, the variable regions are responsible for antigen binding while the constant region is responsible for effector functions. IgG, the most abundant Ig in human serum and the most widely used in clinical applications [5–7], has a structure similar to that of IgE but lacks the fourth constant domain of the heavy chain (Fig. 7.2). Thus, the IgG heavy chain contains only three constant domains (Cγ1, Cγ2, and Cγ3). Moreover, IgE has six N-linked glycosylation sites compared to only one for IgG. The additional domain of the IgE (Cε4) increases the overall size of the molecule compared to that of IgG; however, the crystallographic structure of the molecule has revealed a bent conformation in solution, and when bound to its high-affinity receptor Fc epsilon receptor (FcεRI), implying that the constant heavy region of the molecule may fold on itself to reduce its overall hydrodynamic radius [8, 9]. It has been suggested that the Cε2 domain of the IgE takes the place of the hinge region in IgG [8]. The effect of this domain on the structure and function of the molecule remains to be clearly established.

The binding affinity of human IgE for FcεRI ($K_a = 10^{10}\ M^{-1}$) is two orders of magnitude higher than that of IgG for its high-affinity receptor FcγRI (CD64;

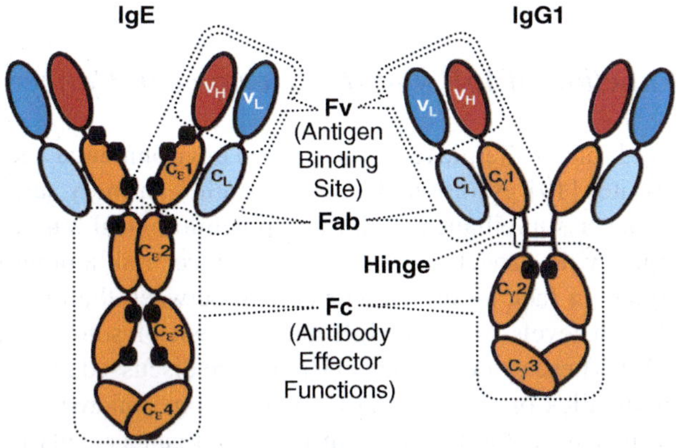

Fig. 7.2 Schematic diagram comparing the domain structures of human IgE and IgG1. Antibodies are composed of two pairs of identical heavy (H) and light (L) chain proteins linked by disulfide bonds forming H_2L_2 heterotetramers. The Fab region consists of one constant and one variable domain from each heavy and light chain. The variable region (Fv), composed of both the heavy and light chain variable domains, is responsible for antigen binding and is located at the amino-terminus of the antibody. The remaining constant region includes the Fc portion of the antibody and is responsible for its effector functions. Black circles denote N-linked glycosylation sites. Note the hinge region in the IgG1 joining the Cγ1 and Cγ2 domains. This region, which provides flexibility, is absent in the IgE

$K_a = 10^8\ M^{-1}$) [10–12]. This high-affinity interaction is attributed in part to a conformational change observed upon binding to its receptor [9, 13, 14]. In fact, K_{on} and K_{off} rates of IgE binding to its high-affinity receptor suggest that the main difference between IgE and IgG binding is in the K_{off} rate of their interactions, where the IgE FcεRI K_{off} rate is four orders of magnitude lower than that of IgG for FcγRIII (CD16) [15–17]. The region of the IgE associated with FcεRI binding resides within the Cε2 and Cε3 domains and involves two distinct sites [18]. The human IgE Cε3 domain is also responsible for binding to the low-affinity IgE receptor, FcεRII (CD23). Membrane-bound CD23 has three lectin domain "heads" that are connected to the membrane via a triple α-helical coiled-coil "stalk" [19]. CD23 is known as the "low-affinity" FcεR since the affinity of human IgE for a single lectin domain "head" is about 10^6–$10^7\ M^{-1}$ [19–22]. However, the avidity of human IgE for the naturally occurring CD23 molecule with its three "heads" is about 10^8–$10^9\ M^{-1}$, which approaches the affinity of human IgE for FcεRI [19, 21, 22]. Each Cε3 region contains a glycosylated asparagine residue (N394), which allows two branched glycosylated chains to reside at the center of the IgE. The structure of the branching sugars consists of two *N*-acetyl-glucosamine and five mannose units per chain [8]. These branching chain glycosylations are not essential for the binding of IgE to its low-affinity receptor CD23. Instead a lysine residue (K352) also present in the Cε3 domain facilitates the interaction to a large extent [23]. In addition to binding FcεRI and CD23, IgE antibodies can bind CD21 (a CD23 co-receptor) and galectin-3 (a carbohydrate-rich lectin also known as epsilon-binding protein) [19]. The effects of IgE interactions with these molecules are yet to be fully understood.

7.1.3 The Function of IgE and Its Relevance in Cancer Therapy

IgE plays a central role in allergic reactions against environmental agents and immunity against parasites [19]. Additionally, several studies strongly suggest a potential role of IgE in cancer surveillance. Relevant epidemiological studies on the association of allergies with cancer support a lower cancer risk among people with a history of allergies. In fact, an inverse correlation between the incidence of atopic conditions and high levels of serum IgE and the risk of some cancers has been demonstrated [24]. These epidemiological studies are discussed in Chapters 4 and 5. Furthermore, antibodies of the IgE class isolated from pancreatic cancer patients were shown to mediate cytotoxicity against targeted cancer cells [25]. Moreover, levels of polyclonal IgE are directly correlated with the overall survival in patients with multiple myeloma [26]. Taken together, these studies suggest a natural role of IgE in the immunosurveillance of cancer. Interestingly, treatment of patients affected with moderate to severe asthma with omalizumab (Xolair®), a recombinant humanized IgG1 specific for the constant region of human IgE, has raised some concerns regarding the safety of anti-IgE therapy. Omalizumab interacts with the IgE molecule in the region where it binds to the FcεRI and thus binds to all circulating IgE regardless of antibody specificity, leading to the downregulation of IgE

levels and FcεRI expression [27–29]. However, in patients treated with omalizumab, 0.5% (20 out of 4,127) developed cancer compared to 0.2% (5 out of 2,236) treated with placebo [29]. These results are supported by an earlier study that revealed 1 in 200 patients treated with the antibody developed breast, prostate, melanoma, non-melanoma skin, or parotid gland malignancies during the median observation period of 1 year [30]. Due to a possible increase in cancer risk, it has been suggested that omalizumab should not be used in asthma patients with a personal or family history of cancer [29]. It is tempting to speculate that the general interference of the interaction between IgE and FcεRI caused by omalizumab may be blocking the cancer immunosurveillance activity of endogenous IgE leading to an increased risk of cancer development.

The potential role of IgE in cancer immunosurveillance strongly suggests that this class of antibody should be exploited as a therapeutic for the treatment of cancer. However, regardless of whether IgE plays a role in cancer surveillance, this antibody has several intrinsic advantages that increase its therapeutic potential compared to the commonly used IgG in cancer therapy. One of the major advantages of IgE over IgG that can be exploited for the treatment of human cancers is the low serum levels of IgE. The average serum concentration of IgE is less than 0.0003 mg/ml in non-atopic adults [31]. The level of IgE in circulation is lowest of all the antibody classes, consisting of only 0.02% of total circulating Igs, whereas IgG is the most abundant at 85% [31]. The low serum levels of IgE compared to IgG provides less competition for FcR occupancy. In fact, the loss of specific IgG from effector cells due to the high levels of competing serum IgG for host FcγR-expressing cells is a limitation of IgG antibody-dependent cell-mediated cytotoxicity (ADCC) [32], a critical mechanism of anti-tumor protection. The extremely low levels of IgE in the serum have been attributed both to its low synthesis rate and to its short serum half-life (2.5 days, when not bound to FcεRs) [31]. Chapter 2 describes the tight regulatory mechanisms involved in maintaining the low serum concentrations of IgE.

Another advantage of IgE-mediated cancer therapeutics is that IgE binds its FcεRs with exceptionally high affinity. As mentioned above, FcεRI binds IgE with an affinity (K_a) of 10^{10} M^{-1}, which is two orders of magnitude higher than that of IgG for the FcγRI (CD64) [10–12]. Human FcεRI is expressed on human monocytes, macrophages, eosinophils, basophils, mast cells, Langerhans cells, dendritic cells (DC), and platelets [33]. In contrast to the human receptor, murine FcεRI is expressed only on mast cells and basophils [33]. Even though FcεRII (CD23) is the low-affinity FcεR, its affinity for IgE is as high as that of IgG for its high-affinity receptor FcγRI (CD64) [24, 33]. CD23 is expressed on eosinophils, monocytes, lymphocytes, follicular DC, Langerhans cells, and platelets [34, 35]. Additionally, there is no known inhibitory FcεR for IgE, while IgG binds to the inhibitory FcγRIIB (CD32b) that decreases ADCC and antibody-mediated antigen presentation for IgG molecules [36, 37]. The fact that IgE does not elicit complement-dependent cytotoxicity (CDC) like IgG does should not dampen its therapeutic efficacy since CDC does not seem to be a major player in the anti-tumor activity of many therapeutic antibodies targeting cancer cells, such as rituximab [38]

and trastuzumab [39, 40], and it has been reported that complement activation may interfere with ADCC activity [41].

Through the interaction with FcεRI, IgE mediates many downstream events that lead to the induction of a potent immune response characterized by immediate hypersensitivity, an acute inflammatory response followed by a late phase reaction 6–8 hours thereafter [42]. The uniqueness of the IgE-mediated allergic (anaphylactic) response is due to the presence of mast cells in the tissue that are sensitized by IgE bound to FcεRI. When these FcεRs are crosslinked due to the binding of antigens (allergens) to multiple IgE on the surface of the mast cell, these cells are rapidly, or "explosively," degranulated releasing a variety of factors. These factors include enzymes such as tryptase that lead to the breakdown of tissue matrix proteins, chemical mediators such as histamine that increase blood vessel permeability and blood flow to the area, and lipid mediators such as leukotrienes that stimulate smooth muscle contraction and the infiltration of eosinophils, basophils, and other lymphocytes to the tissue [42]. All of these factors together trigger tissue damage and the acute inflammatory response. If this response occurs in the tumor microenvironment due to the presence of a tumor-specific IgE, it is expected to lead to massive tumor cell death and phagocytosis of these dying cells by professional antigen-presenting cells (APC) such as DC. These activated APC will then migrate to the local lymph nodes and stimulate cognate T cells that will initiate adaptive (cellular and humoral) immune responses against the tumor. Importantly, this immune response will not only be against the IgE-targeted TAA but will expand to a broad spectrum of antigens expressed by the cancer cells, a process known as epitope spreading. In addition, tumor-specific IgE can enhance this antigen uptake and presentation of TAA via the interaction with FcεR expressed on APC such as DC, Langerhans cells, and monocytes/macrophages, which are efficient stimulators of both primary and secondary T-cell responses [33, 43–46]. Therefore, IgE is able to prime naïve T cells to IgE-reactive antigens as well as amplify established T-cell responses.

It is well known that IgE can mediate ADCC of targeted cancer cells through the interaction of its Fc region with FcεRI on the surface of effector cells [47] (Fig. 7.3). IgE can also mediate antibody-dependent cell-mediated phagocytosis (ADCP) of cancer cells through the interaction with CD23 on the surface of effector cells [47] (Fig. 7.3). Effector cells such as DC and macrophages can potentially phagocytose live cancer cells as well as apoptotic cancer cells, entirely or as apoptotic bodies. This phagocytosis can occur in the absence of IgE, but the presence of the antibody is expected to enhance the uptake of targeted cells resulting in better antigen presentation. This suggests that the IgE antibody can be used as an adjuvant of cancer vaccines, a possibility that is discussed in detail in Chapter 9. It is important to note that depending on the effector cell type, certain effectors can preferentially act through ADCC (such as basophils and mast cells), while other effectors can act preferentially through ADCP (such as DC and Langerhans cells). Moreover, other cells such as monocytes/macrophages are capable of eliciting targeted cell cytotoxicity through both mechanisms: ADCC and ADCP [47–49]. It is also expected that antibodies of the IgE class would be able to target secreted or shed TAA in the

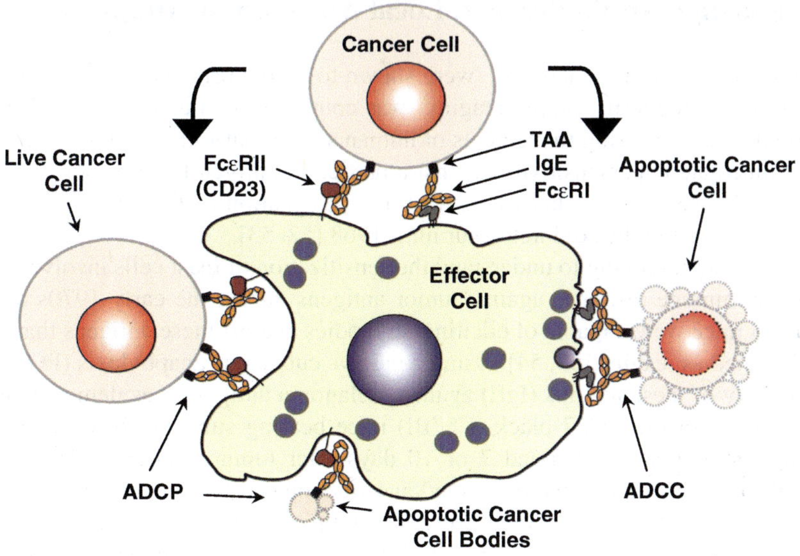

Fig. 7.3 Scheme of the possible interactions between immune effector cells and targeted tumor cells, mediated by an IgE specific for a tumor-associated antigen. The IgE specific for a TAA interacts with the FcεRI or the FcεRII expressed on the surface of the effector cell and may trigger cell killing through ADCC or ADCP. Antibodies bound to apoptotic cells or apoptotic bodies are also expected to trigger phagocytosis

circulation that will make complexes with the IgE leading to internalization of these antigens through endocytosis by professional APC expressing the FcεRs [33]. In fact, IgE-mediated soluble antigen uptake and presentation has been demonstrated [45, 46]. However, it is important to stress that the targeted soluble antigen should be preferentially monoepitope, resulting in the binding of one or two antigens to only one IgE. This is particularly relevant when the IgE is administered systemically to avoid the general crosslinking of FcεRIs on the surface of basophils and mast cells that may lead to systemic anaphylaxis. This enhanced antigen uptake and presentation is expected to activate an adaptive immune response without even targeting the tumor microenvironment. Finally, in the specific case of murine IgE, the activation of natural killer (NK) cells can be mediated through the binding of IgE to FcγRIII (CD16), the Fc receptor that is responsible for IgG-mediated cellular cytotoxicity [50]. This interaction between murine IgE and NK cells implicates IgE in ADCC and in the induction of cytokine production by NK cells [50].

In summary, there are several potential advantages of IgE over IgG that make this class of antibody an attractive anti-cancer agent. Antibodies of the IgE class, even if they are administered in a passive immunotherapy setting, are expected to be capable of a two-pronged attack against malignant cells. They are expected to directly target and eliminate cancer cells as well orchestrate a potent secondary and broad-spectrum anti-tumor immune response, thus linking passive and active immunotherapy.

7.2 Reaginic Antibodies and Local Anti-Tumor Anaphylaxis

Reaginic antibodies, namely IgE, were shown to be the primary mediators of anaphylaxis, and the term "atopic reagins" was coined by Arthur F. Coca and Ella F. Grove in 1925, referring to elements of human serum that were capable of transferring immediate hypersensitivity against a particular antigen from person to person [51, 52]. However, the acknowledgment and designation of the term "IgE" as the fifth class of antibodies did not occur until 1968 [52, 53].

Investigators seeking to understand the sensitization of mast cells involved in the adaptive immune response against tumor antigens during the early 1970s discovered that mice were capable of eliciting antibodies against these antigens that could be classified as reagins [52, 54]. Using a passive cutaneous anaphylaxis (PCA) test, the activity of these reagins (IgE) against melanoma antigens was demonstrated in vivo [54]. Sera from C57 black (C57Bl) mice bearing subcutaneous B16 murine melanoma cells were obtained 7 or 10 days after tumor challenge. In addition, the subcutaneous tumors were resected and fractionated to prepare extracts of presumed TAA. Splenocyte extracts were also prepared for use as negative controls [54]. BALB/c mice were intradermally injected with the serum samples from the B16-bearing C57Bl mice. Seventy-two hours later the tumor extracts combined with the Evans blue dye were injected intravenously. A positive PCA reaction against B16 extracts was observed as evidenced by the leakage of the dye from the blood vessels while no reaction was observed with splenocyte extracts. The existence of anti-tumor reaginic antibodies in both C57Bl and BALB/c mice used in this PCA experiment was demonstrated and served as initial proof-of-principle of the potential role of reaginic (IgE) antibodies as key effectors in local anaphylaxis against cancer [54]. These results indicate that IgE are produced in mice in response to tumor formation, leading the authors to suggest that basophils and mast cells sensitized with IgE may play a role in the host immune response against cancer cells.

It was not until half a decade later that a more detailed study established a potential connection between reaginic IgE antibodies inducing passive local anaphylaxis (PLA), also known as PCA, and a possible mechanism of anti-tumor activity in mice [55]. These studies found that if radioactively labeled splenocytes or an extracellular dye (Lissamine green) were administered intravenously, only small amounts would penetrate an established tumor. Conversely, if the labeled splenocytes or the dye were administered intratumorally, they remained trapped within the tumor for several days. These investigators concluded that C3H mice bearing syngeneic McC3 fibrosarcoma had reduced vascular permeability within established tumors. This phenomenon could be reversed by the intratumoral induction of PLA achieved by sequential injection of ovalbumin (as the antigen) and sera containing high titers of anti-ovalbumin reaginic antibodies [55]. Importantly, this PLA resulted in anti-fibrosarcoma activity. The active agent inducing these effects following the PLA event was found to be histamine-related given that administration of the histamine antagonist, cyproheptadine, into mice prior to inducing intratumoral PLA cancelled the beneficial effects of the procedure. The increased vascular permeability in the tumors that resulted from PLA induction facilitated the entry

of lymphoid cells and soluble molecules into the tumor microenvironment, a process cited as a possible "gatekeeper" mechanism of anti-tumor activity of the PLA reaction [55]. It is important to note that although these studies found no evidence of tumor-reactive IgE in the serum of the protected mice, the induction of PLA was mediated by ovalbumin antiserum with significantly high titers of IgE antibody. This study served to highlight the beneficial role of LPA within solid tumors and suggested that tumor-specific IgE may be effective for anti-cancer therapy.

7.3 Generating Tumor-Specific Monoclonal IgE

7.3.1 Development of Monoclonal and Recombinant IgE

Advances in the field of passive immunotherapy mediated by antibodies of the IgE class, as with other antibody classes such as IgG, have been propelled by parallel advances in the understanding of the responses elicited by these molecules and by advances in the molecular and cellular biology techniques that have facilitated the manipulation of these proteins. The production of monoclonal antibodies from rodent hybridomas in 1975 by Hans Köhler and César Milstein [56] was a significant breakthrough in the field of antibody therapy. The adaptation of these advances to the production and purification of recombinant antibodies of desired specificity [57] facilitated not only the development of novel IgE antibodies but also the manipulation of these proteins under controlled conditions to evaluate the mechanisms that underlie their physiological activity.

The first recombinant IgE was a mouse/human chimeric antibody composed of murine variable chains fused to human λ light and ε constant heavy chains specific for the hapten 4-hydroxy-3-nitro-phenacetyl (NP) [58]. The aim of this study was to produce large quantities of NP-specific IgE as a protective agent against severe allergies but would additionally serve as the foundation for further work describing tumor-specific recombinant IgE with human effector functions. The initial characterization of this recombinant IgE demonstrated its capacity to induce degranulation of basophils when crosslinked by the hapten (5-iodo-4-hydroxy-3-nitrophenacetyl caproate, NIP) coupled to bovine serum albumin [58]. This degranulation included histamine release and the passive sensitization of effector cells in vitro. Moreover, pre-incubation of this anti-NP IgE with basophils prevented their degranulation induced by a common house dust mite antigen combined with sera from allergic individuals with high levels of IgE specific for this antigen. This is most likely due to its effect as a competitor for FcεR occupancy. By generating the first recombinant IgE, this study proved to be an important milestone in understanding the physiological activity of IgE in the context of acute allergic reactions.

The technology for generating recombinant antibodies of different classes and subclasses with desired specificity also facilitated the first comparisons of the effector functions of human antibodies. A matched set of mouse/human chimeric antibodies specific for the hapten NP was expressed in murine myeloma cells [59].

The panel of chimeric Igs consisted of IgM, IgE, IgA2, and four IgGs (IgG1, IgG2, IgG3, and IgG4). As a measure of their activity, the panel of antibodies was tested for the capacity to bind the C1q complement protein, mediate the lysis of red blood cells derivatized with the hapten through CDC, or facilitate the cytotoxic killing (ADCC) of the hapten-derivatized human acute lymphoblastic leukemia cell line HPB-ALL using human peripheral blood mononuclear cells (PBMC) as effector cells [59]. The results indicated that the IgG subclasses IgG1 and IgG3 were far superior at eliciting both CDC and ADCC under the conditions used for this study. As expected, the recombinant chimeric IgE did not activate complement. It is important to note that the target cells used in the ADCC assay (HPB-ALL) were artificially labeled with the antigen. In addition, the studies were conducted in vitro and the repertoire of effector cells was limited to PBMC. The inability of IgE to induce complement activation along with the poor induction of ADCC compared to IgG1 and IgG3 together with the expected concern of induction of systemic anaphylaxis has discouraged the use of antibodies of the IgE class as a possible treatment for human cancer.

7.3.2 Use of Tumor-Specific IgE for the Passive Immunotherapy of Cancer

Although most antibodies in clinical use are of the IgG class, the use of IgE for the passive immunotherapy of cancer would offer some advantages over their IgG counterparts (as discussed in Section 7.1.3). These advantages include the higher affinity of IgE for its FcεRs, the low serum levels of IgE (which means less competition for binding to FcRs), the expression of the FcεRs on a broad spectrum of effector cells, and its capacity to trigger antigen processing and presentation leading to a secondary immune response. Moreover, as discussed below, several studies suggest that antibodies of the IgE class can be potent anti-cancer agents. Importantly, the use of antibodies of the IgE or IgG is not necessarily mutually exclusive since they can potentially be used in combination (simultaneously or sequentially), resulting in an additive or synergistic effect through the recruitment and engagement of different FcRs and effector cells.

7.3.2.1 Murine IgE Specific for the Glycoprotein 36 of the Mouse Mammary Tumor Virus

The use of monoclonal antibodies of the IgE class for the passive treatment of cancer was explored for the first time in the 1990s. Two murine monoclonal IgEs specific for the major envelope glycoprotein 36 (gp36) of the mouse mammary tumor virus (MMTV) were developed using the hybridoma technology [56] in which the spleens of immunized BALB/c mice producing the anti-gp36 IgE were fused with P3 $\times$ 20 myeloma cells [60]. These hybridoma cells were then injected intraperitoneally into BALB/c mice. Ten days following injection, ascites containing the anti-gp36 IgE were collected. In order to evaluate the anti-cancer potential of these IgE, syngeneic C3H/HeJ mice were subcutaneously challenged with H2712 murine mammary carcinoma ($MMTV^+$) cells in combination with 20% ascites fluid containing 12.5 μg

of the anti-gp36 IgE. These mice were subsequently treated with 25 μg of the anti-gp36 IgE via intraperitoneal injection every fourth day for 8 weeks. This treatment demonstrated a 50% protection rate from cancer development compared to control animals that received 20% normal mouse serum instead of the IgE-containing ascites fluid. Interestingly, all control mice ($n = 6$) died within 44 days, while 66% (4/6) treated with the anti-gp36 IgE survived during this time frame. One of these four mice died on day 72, but the three remaining mice were tumor-free 175 days after tumor challenge. A similar level of protection was observed when the H2712 tumor cells were injected intraperitoneally and mice were treated for 6 weeks at 4-day intervals with 25 μg of the anti-gp36 IgE. All mice treated with normal mouse serum died within 34 days while two of six mice treated with the IgE were still alive after 139 days after tumor challenge. Importantly, the anti-gp36 IgE was unable to protect mice from tumor development in mice challenged with murine MA16/C mammary carcinoma ($MMTV^-$) cells. These results demonstrate that the tumor specificity of the antibody is required for the anti-tumor effect of the anti-gp36 IgE.

7.3.2.2 Rat/Human Chimeric IgE Specific for Murine CD8

A rat/human chimeric IgE specific for the Ly-2 antigen was constructed for the initial purpose of evaluating antibody-mediated elimination of CD8-expressing target cells in vivo [61]. Murine CD8 is a cell surface glycoprotein that serves as a marker of cytotoxic T lymphocytes (CTL). It is a heterodimer consisting of the Ly-2 (α chain) and Ly-3 (β chain) [62]. The anti-tumor effects of this IgE were later explored [63]. One obstacle facing those evaluating the in vivo anti-cancer activity of recombinant IgE is the fact that human IgE does not interact with the mouse FcεRI [33, 64, 65]. In order to overcome this problem and to direct CTL to recognize TAA in a non-major histocompatibility (non-MHC)-dependent manner, a unique strategy utilizing a chimeric FcεRI was used [63]. This chimeric receptor was composed of three components: (1) the extracellular domain of human FcεRI, (2) the membrane proximal and transmembrane domains of human FcγRIIA, and (3) the cytoplasmic domain of human CD3ζ. The chimeric receptor was stably expressed in the CTLL-R8 murine T-cell line under the control of the mouse CTL-specific perforin promoter. In vitro assays demonstrated that the binding of human IgE to this chimeric receptor resulted in target cell cytotoxicity. In this IgE-mediated ADCC assay, murine E3 thymoma cells ($Ly\text{-}2^+$) pre-incubated with the chimeric rat/human anti-Ly-2 IgE were used as malignant target cells. Targeted cytotoxicity of the thymoma cells was observed when combined with CTLL-R8 cells expressing the chimeric FcεRI receptor on the cell surface (3H2 cells). The ability of 3H2 cells to lyse E3 thymoma cells in vivo was also explored using a Winn assay [63]. For this assay, 3H2 effector cells plus E3 target cells at an effector-to-target ratio of 10:1 in the presence or absence of the chimeric rat/human anti-Ly-2 IgE were incubated for 4 hours. E3 cells incubated in media alone (without 3H2 cells or antibody) were used as a control. The cells were then harvested, washed, and injected subcutaneously into C57BL/6 mice. E3 thymoma cells grew rapidly and caused mouse death within 5–7 days. The addition of 3H2 cells significantly prolonged survival; however, the anti-tumor effect was more prominent in mice treated with E3 and 3H2 cells pre-incubated with the chimeric

rat/human anti-Ly2 IgE. Only one of five of these mice developed a subcutaneous tumor (compared to four of five with 3H2 cells alone). In addition, the only tumor that developed in this group developed 1 week later than the tumors of the 3H2-alone treated mice. In a second experiment where the effector-to-target ratio was reduced to 3:1, all mice treated with only E3 tumor cells died in the first 15 days. Two of five mice treated with the mixture of E3 target tumor cells plus 3H2 effector cells, and a non-targeting IgE survived without the development of the tumor. Moreover, all five mice treated with the mixture of E3 target tumor cells, 3H2 effector cells plus the targeted anti-Ly2 IgE survived tumor-free. These results demonstrate that cancer-specific IgE can be used to redirect CTL that express a chimeric IgE receptor to lyse cancer cells providing further evidence for the potential use of IgE for cancer immunotherapy in humans.

The chimeric rat/human anti-Ly2 IgE used in the above studies has also been used in a similar approach using primary human T cells, genetically engineered to express a recombinant human FcεRI [66]. For this study, the chimeric receptor consisted of the extracellular domain of human FcεRI, the human FcγRII hinge and transmembrane regions, the cytoplasmic signaling domain of human CD28, and the cytoplasmic signaling domain of the human T cell receptor ζ chain. The anti-Ly2 IgE in combination with primary T-cells expressing the chimeric FcεRI (T-CL9) were shown to induce IgE-mediated murine E3 thymoma ($Ly\text{-}2^{+}$) cell lysis in vitro [66]. Lysis was not observed in 3LL ($Ly\text{-}2^{-}$) murine Lewis lung carcinoma cells. Importantly, anti-Ly2 IgE in combination with T-CL9 and E3 thymoma cells also resulted in the production of immune-stimulatory cytokine production (IFN-γ and GM-CSF) that was only observed with the combination of these three components. In addition, transfer of chimeric FcεRI-expressing T cells demonstrated in vivo anti-tumor activity [66]. E3 thymoma tumors were established via intraperitoneal injection in non-obese diabetic severe combined immunodeficient (SCID) mice. Mice were treated with T cells expressing the recombinant receptor (T-CL9) or mock transduced T cells that had been previously incubated with the anti-Ly2 IgE by intraperitoneal injection. Mice received treatment on days 0, 1, 2 and 4. T-CL9 cells significantly enhanced mouse survival from 18 to 27 days [66]. Pre-incubation of T-CL9 cells with a non-specific IgE did not enhance survival compared to control animals. Similarly enhanced survival was observed in mice with established tumors. Thus, the tumor-specific IgE is required for the in vivo ability of the anti-Ly2 IgE to redirect the cytotoxic effects of the recombinant T cells toward the targeted cancer cells.

7.3.2.3 Murine and Mouse/Human Chimeric IgE Specific for an Antigenic Determinant on the Surface of Colorectal Carcinoma Cells

In order to evaluate the cytotoxic effects of a cancer-specific IgE, a murine IgE (mIgE 30.6) was tested in parallel with a chimeric mouse/human IgE (chIgE 30.6) [67]. Both antibodies contain the variable region of the murine IgG2b antibody 30.6 and bind an antigen expressed on the surface of human colorectal carcinoma cells, such as COLO 205 cells. Neither of these antibodies demonstrated any direct in

vitro cytotoxicity against COLO 205 cells [67]. To evaluate the in vivo anti-tumor effects of the two IgE antibodies, BALB/c SCID mice subcutaneously xenografted with COLO 205 cells were treated intravenously with a single injection of 1 μg of mIgE 30.6, chIgE 30.6 or buffer (PBS) 5 days after tumor challenge. Only mice treated with mIgE 30.6 significantly inhibited tumor growth; however, the effect was transient and tumor growth returned to the same rate as control mice starting 48 hours after mIgE injection. Three consecutive treatments with 1 μg mIgE 30.6 every 2 days starting 5 days after tumor challenge did not enhance this anti-tumor effect [67]. A previous study by this group demonstrated that milligram quantities of a mouse/human chimeric IgG1 with the same variable regions (chIgG 30.6) are required to inhibit COLO 205 growth in SCID mice [68]. The superior in vivo activity of mIgE compared to that of the previously reported chIgG may be to due to the higher affinity of IgE for its FcεR compared to the affinity of IgG to its FcγR, and therefore, lower amounts of IgE are required to induce a highly tumoricidal effect by immune effector cells. However, the mIgE and chIgG were not tested simultaneously. The inability of chIgE 30.6 to elicit an anti-tumor response was not attributed to a difference in the relative affinity or serum half-life compared to the mIgE 30.6. The lack of efficacy of chIgE 30.6 is not surprising since human IgE does not interact with murine FcεRI [33, 64, 65]; thus there was no activation of an anti-tumor immune response in these mice. Neither the mechanism nor the transient nature of the anti-tumor effect of mIgE is known. However, the transient effect is not due to the loss of antigen expression [67]. It has been suggested that the relevance of the cross-linking of FcεR to release cytokines, such as tumor necrosis factor (TNF) or interleukin-4 (IL-4), from mast cells may be involved in the anti-tumor effect of mIgE 30.6 [67].

7.3.2.4 Mouse/Human Chimeric IgE Specific for Human Folate Binding Protein

Another study has also aimed to compare the anti-tumor effect of cancer-specific antibodies of the IgE and IgG classes. Mouse/human chimeric IgE (MOv18-IgE) and IgG1 (MOv18-IgG1) antibodies specific for the folate binding protein (FBP) have been developed [69]. FBP is expressed at higher densities on the surface of ovarian cancer cells compared to normal cells making it an appropriate target for antibody therapy. In vitro studies demonstrate that MOv18-IgE is able to induce degranulation of human basophils as measured by histamine release [69]. In this assay, both a non-specific IgE and MOv18-IgE induced histamine release from basophils when crosslinked by an anti-human IgE. Importantly, only MOv18-IgE induced histamine release in the presence of IGROV1 (FBP^+) cancer cells, demonstrating a cancer-specific response of the MOv18-IgE. In order to test the in vivo efficacy of the MOv18 antibodies, C.B-17 scid/scid (SCID) mice were subcutaneously challenged with IGROV1 cells followed by an intravenous injection with a mixture of human PBMC and either MOv18-IgE or MOv18-IgG1. Thirty-five days after tumor challenge control mice showed excessive tumor growth (Fig. 7.4). In contrast, both the MOv18-IgE and the MOv18-IgG1 inhibited tumor growth up

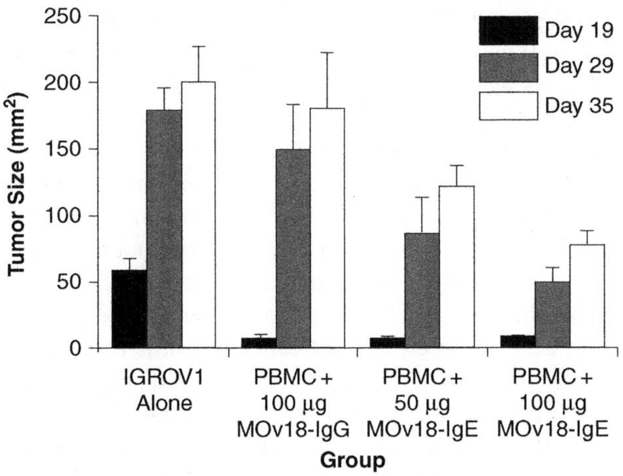

Fig. 7.4 MOv18-IgE inhibits the growth of IGROV1 human ovarian adenocarcinoma cells in vivo in the presence of human PBMC as effectors. A matched variable region set of mouse/human chimeric IgE and IgG1 antibodies specific for FBP was tested for their ability to inhibit the subcutaneous growth of cells in a SCID mouse xenograft model of human ovarian cancer. Mice were treated intraperitoneally with anti-asialo G_{M1} to eliminate host natural killer cells. One day later, mice were challenged subcutaneously with 2×10^6 IGROV1 cells followed by intravenous injection of 2.5×10^6 human PBMC combined with either 100 µg MOv18-IgG1, 100 µg MOv18-IgE or 50 µg MOv18-IgE. The mean tumor size ± the standard error of the mean (SEM) measured on days 19, 29 and 35 are shown ($n = 4$ for all groups). Reproduced with permission from Fig. 4A Gould et al. [69]. Copyright Wiley-VCH Verlag GmbH & Co. KGaA

to day 19; however, MOv18-IgG1 did not demonstrate protection after this time. Only MOv18-IgE (100 µg) was able to prevent tumor growth for an additional 16 days (to day 35) compared to mice treated with the same concentration of MOv18-IgG1, which developed tumors after 19 days. It is also important to note that mice treated with half of the concentration (50 µg) of IgE compared to IgG1 (100 µg) showed 40% inhibition of tumor growth at day 35 (Fig. 7.4). Due to the inability of human IgE to bind murine FcεR, the use of human PBMC was essential for the anti-tumor effect of MOv18-IgE [69]. This demonstrates that human effector cells are required for the IgE-mediated anti-tumor response. It is important to note that the anti-tumor activity of MOv18-IgE may be underestimated in this model since the effectors are limited to human PBMC, which are exogenously administered. In contrast, in humans there would be a permanent supply of the entire effector repertoire including PBMC, and thus, the anti-tumor activity of IgE is expected to be superior compared to that observed in this mouse model. Furthermore, the capacity of the IgE to elicit an adaptive immune response could not be evaluated since immunodeficient mice were used. Despite these drawbacks, this study demonstrates that the anti-cancer effects of MOv18-IgE were superior compared to those of its IgG1 counterpart and that the Fc-mediated effector functions of the antibody are essential.

The anti-cancer effect of MOv18-IgE was confirmed using a different mouse model [70]. Nude mice (nu/nu) were challenged intraperitoneally with human HUA ovarian cancer cells expressing FBP. The following day, human PBMC were injected intraperitoneally alone or in combination with 100 μg MOv18-IgE or MOv18-IgG1. Treatment with PBMC and MOv18-IgE significantly increased survival to 40 days compared to mice treated with the mixture of PBMC and MOv18-IgG1 (22 days) or compared to mice treated with PBS (19 days). MOv18-IgG1 in combination with PBMC in this model did not show a protective effect. Immunohistochemistry analysis of HUA xenografts demonstrated that human monocytes were localized around tumor lesions in MOv18-IgE-treated mice only, suggesting that these effector cells play an important role in the anti-tumor effect of this antibody. This was confirmed using monocyte-depleted PMBC in this tumor model [48].

Further studies have helped to identify the mechanisms of the anti-cancer effects of MOv18-IgE. In vitro assays demonstrated the ability of MOv18-IgE to lyse cancer cells via ADCC by human monocytes [70] or eosinophils [48]. ADCC is an important and relevant mechanism of action of recombinant antibodies approved for cancer immunotherapy [71]. In addition, in vitro analysis demonstrated that MOv18-IgE is able to induce ADCP through the interaction with its low-affinity receptor CD23 expressed on the surface of (IL-4)-activated monocytes [48]. IL-4 was shown to induce the expression of CD23, but not FcεRI, on the surface of monocytes isolated from human PBMC. The role of CD23 in ADCP was confirmed by using an antibody to block the binding of IgE to CD23 in which this ADCP activity was decreased. In contrast, blocking CD23 did not affect the MOv18-IgE-induced ADCC activity, indicating that ADCC is mediated by FcεRI and not by CD23. In addition, primary monocytes pre-stimulated with MOv18-IgE showed an increase of surface FcεRI expression, which correlated with the increase of MOv18-IgE-mediated ADCC, confirming that the high-affinity IgE receptor is required for IgE-mediated ADCC in vitro. These results have also been observed using U-937 (a human monocyte cell line) as effector cells [47]. Galectin-3, a beta-galactosidase-binding lectin that also binds human IgE, was shown not to be relevant for the ADCC and ADCP activities of MOv18-IgE in this model [47]. These studies have helped to define the mechanism of MOv18-IgE-mediated toxicity as well as to shed light on the basic biological function of the FcεRs. Both IgE-mediated ADCC and ADCP are discussed in detail in Chapter 8.

7.3.2.5 Engineered IgE Specific for Human HER2/*neu*

HER2/*neu* (also known as ErbB-2 or HER-2), a member of the epidermal growth factor family, is overexpressed on approximately 25–30% of breast cancers and is associated with poor prognosis [72]. Its overexpression and association with more aggressive disease along with its extracellular accessibility make this antigen attractive for antibody therapy. In fact, the FDA-approved antibody trastuzumab (Herceptin®), a humanized IgG1 specific for HER2/*neu*, can lead to an objective response in some patients with tumors overexpressing HER2/*neu* when used

alone or an even higher response when combined with chemotherapy [73–78]. Unfortunately, most of the patients with advanced breast cancer who achieve an initial response to trastuzumab-based treatment acquire resistance and eventually succumb to the disease [75, 79]. Therefore, as a new treatment for HER2/*neu* expressing tumors, an anti-HER2/*neu* IgE was developed [49]. This humanized IgE was derived using DNA sequences corresponding to the published protein sequences of the heavy and light chains of the trastuzumab variable regions [49]. This IgE was expressed in HEK293 human embryonic kidney cells and its in vitro efficacy was compared to trastuzumab. Both trastuzumab and its IgE homologue exhibited similar direct anti-tumor effects on SK-BR-3 human breast cancer cells in vitro [49]. Both antibodies also induced U-937-mediated killing of a murine colon carcinoma cell line expressing human HER2/*neu* (CT26-HER2/*neu*) as well as SK-BR-3 cells. However, the mechanism of cell killing was found to be different for the two antibodies. Trastuzumab was shown to mediate ADCP of target cells, while the IgE facilitated ADCC. In addition, the IgE antibody stimulated the degranulation of mast cells when crosslinked with HER2/*neu*-positive cancer cells, indicating that an anti-tumor immune response with the characteristics of an allergic reaction can be induced by a cancer-specific IgE.

Our group has also developed a new generation of anti-HER2/*neu* IgE. This antibody is fully human in origin and contains the variable regions of the C6MH3-B1 single-chain Fv (scFv) specific for the extracellular domain of human HER2/*neu* that was originally isolated from a human phage library [80]. This scFv was also previously affinity matured in vitro by sequential mutation of the third complimentary determining region (CDR) in both the variable heavy chain (V_H) and the variable light chain (V_L) regions [81]. The highest affinity mutations of both the V_H and the V_L were selected based on binding to HER2/*neu*. The affinity-matured scFv demonstrated a 1230-fold increase in affinity compared to the parental C6.5 scFv [81]. These affinity-matured V_L and V_H regions were cloned into either the human κ light chain or the human ε heavy chain expression vectors, respectively, to yield a fully human anti-HER2/*neu* IgE [82]. This antibody, expressed in murine myeloma cells, is properly assembled and secreted, binds antigen and binds FcεRI. Although the anti-cancer effect of this antibody is currently being explored, it is important to note that a major advantage is that this molecule is totally of human origin (not chimeric or humanized). In addition, this anti-HER2/*neu* IgE binds a different epitope compared to the FDA-approved anti-HER2/*neu* IgG1 trastuzumab (Herceptin®) [83]. Thus, this IgE antibody could be used in combination (simultaneous or sequential) with trastuzumab to activate a diverse and more potent immune response targeting breast cancer.

7.3.2.6 Chimeric IgE Targeting Human CD20

The anti-CD20 IgG1 antibody rituximab (Rituxan®) is currently being used in the clinic for the treatment of non-Hodgkin's lymphoma (NHL). However, resistance to the antibody occurs in most patients [84, 85] and alternative strategies are still needed. We have developed a novel anti-CD20 antibody composed of the variable

region of rituximab, the human constant κ light chain and the human Fcε constant region (anti-CD20 IgE). This antibody expressed in murine myeloma cells is properly assembled and secreted and exhibits specific binding to the antigen and to the FcεRI. Preliminary studies show that anti-CD20 IgE elicited significant direct cytotoxicity and ADCC activity against human $CD20^+$ NHL cell lines [82, 86]. Moreover, crosslinking of anti-CD20 IgE with lymphoma cells expressing CD20 triggered local cutaneous anaphylaxis in transgenic mice expressing human FcεRIα [86]. We expect that the anti-CD20 IgE, like other antibodies of the IgE class targeting TAA, can be used as a direct anti-tumor agent for passive immunotherapy as well as an adjuvant of cancer vaccines, which may potentially have a significant impact on the treatment of NHL.

7.3.3 Induction of an Endogenous IgE Response via Mimotope Vaccination

The above studies are focused on the development of tumor-specific IgE antibodies and their use for passive immunotherapy of cancer. An alternative strategy is the induction of an endogenous IgE response that targets a TAA [87]. For this purpose, a novel approach was taken to establish a vaccination protocol that would result in the induction of an anti-cancer-specific IgE response in vivo. Using the epitope recognized by trastuzumab (humanized anti-HER2/*neu* IgG1), epitope mimics (mimotopes) were generated [88]. This mimotope consisted of the 1, 12-cyclic peptide C-QMWAPQWGPD-C coupled via its carboxy terminus to a succinimidyl-4-(*N*-maleinimidomethyl) cyclohexane-1-carboxylate-activated immunogenic carrier, keyhole limpet hemocyanin (KLH), through a linker (GPGPG) by *S*-acetyl-thio-acetate ("QMW-KLH"). A non-targeted peptide 1, 12-cyclic C-DGGWLSKGSW-C coupled to KLH in the same manner was used as a negative control ("KLH"). Vaccination using these mimotopes yields the generation of endogenous "trastuzumab-like" antibodies in vivo [87, 88]. Moreover, it has been shown that a specific IgE response can be induced by the combination of oral immunization with the mimotope and antacid treatment that is known to induce food allergy [89, 90].

The above vaccination strategies were combined in BALB/c mice to elicit an endogenous anti-HER2/*neu* IgE response [87] (Fig. 7.5). For the antacid treatment, mice were given omeprazole, a proton pump inhibitor, orally once daily for 2 days prior to vaccination. Mice were also given omeprazole twice on the day of immunization. The mimotopes were administered orally in the protective ulcer medication sucralfate as described previously for the induction of food allergy [89, 90]. This strategy resulted in the induction of a high-titer endogenous IgE response (Fig. 7.6). In addition, the induced IgE recognized the mimicked oral antigen (HER2/*neu*) on the surface of human SK-BR-3 breast cancer cells and resulted in both the degranulation and cytotoxicity of RBL-2H3 rat basophilic leukemia cells expressing the rodent FcεRI [87]. Taken together, these studies show that this unique vaccination strategy can lead to the induction of an endogenous anti-cancer IgE response.

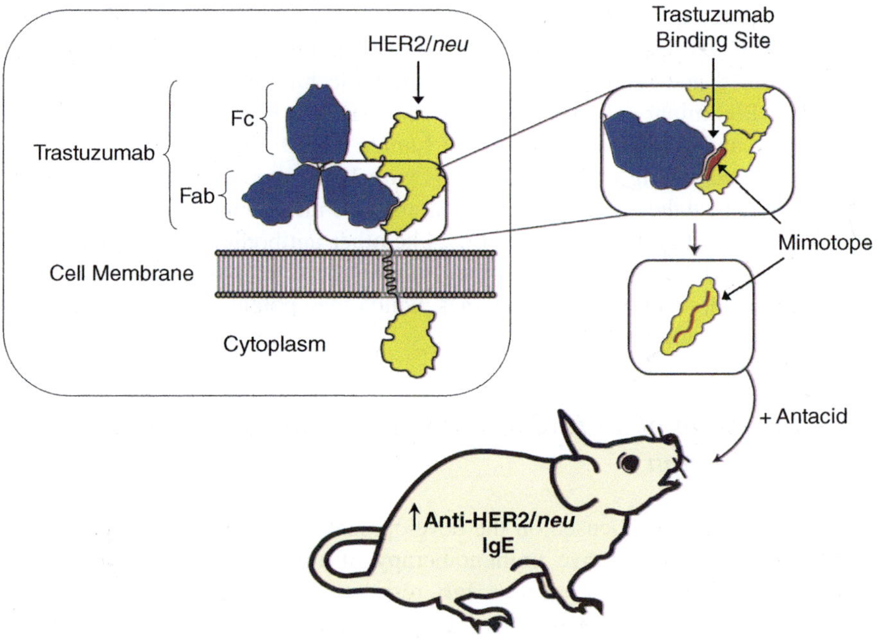

Fig. 7.5 Schematic diagram outlining the strategy for the generation of mimotope peptides and their administration during oral vaccination. HER2/*neu* is a transmembrane receptor consisting of three domains: extracellular, transmembrane and cytoplasmic. The extracellular domain of HER2/*neu* is recognized by the FDA-approved therapeutic antibody trastuzumab (Herceptin®). The region of HER2/*neu* that is recognized by trastuzumab was used to generate a mimotope that when used in combination with an antacid in an oral vaccination setting would lead to the generation of an endogenous anti-HER2/*neu* IgE antibody response in the mouse

7.4 Conclusions

Since the early 1990s the number of antibodies of the IgE class developed for passive immunotherapy of cancer has rapidly increased, and it is expected that this growth will continue. In order to target both epithelial and hematopoietic malignancies, IgE antibodies targeting different TAA such as FBP, HER2/*neu*, and CD20 have been developed. Importantly, these antibodies have demonstrated significant anti-tumor activity in vitro and in some cases in animal models. Moreover, an endogenous IgE response that targets a TAA can be induced by a vaccination strategy. Studies of IgE-mediated anti-tumor immunity have advanced the understanding of IgE biology and uncovered specific roles for its different receptors, FcεRI and FcεRII (CD23). Armed with this knowledge and the tools required to develop tumor-specific IgE antibodies, investigators are focused on addressing the effectiveness of these approaches in light of the success and limitations of IgG-based immunotherapy. These efforts are expected to result in the continued generation of IgE antibodies that can harness the allergic reaction and redirect it to fight the

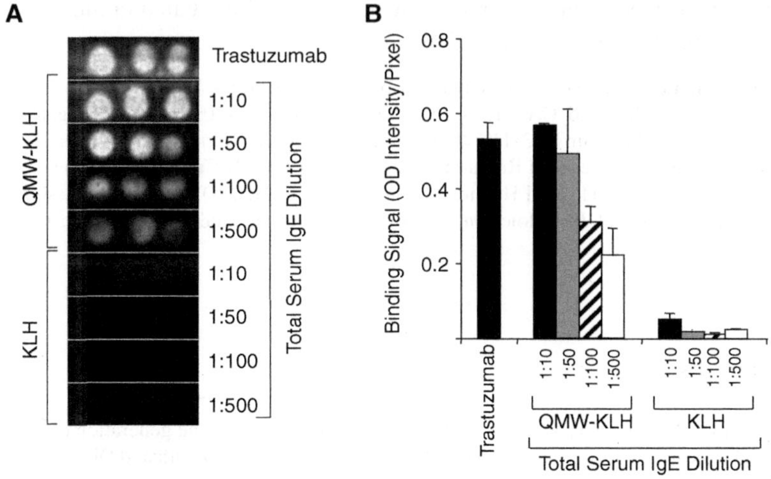

Fig. 7.6 Induction of endogenous antigen-specific IgE is achieved by oral vaccination using a mimotope peptide. BALB/c mice (seven per group) were immunized with the mimotope C-QMWAPQWGPD-C ("QMW-KLH") or the carrier molecule KLH by itself as described in Fig. 7.5. Each animal received 11.6 μg of the proton pump inhibitor omeprazole intravenously on days 1, 2 and 3 of each immunization cycle. Mice were immunized on days 3, 17, 45, 59 and 87. **Panel A**: QMW-specific serum IgE titers determined by DotBlot assay. **Panel B**: Optical density of the DotBlot spots determined by densitometry analysis of a 20 × 20 pixel area from three independent spots along with standard deviations per condition and dilution. Signals from these spots are shown as total optical density per square pixel area. Panel B of this figure was created using the data shown in panel A, which was adapted from Fig. 2 in Riemer et al. [87] with permission from The American Association for Cancer Research

tumor leading to the induction of a potent anti-cancer response capable of reducing tumor burden or even facilitating full tumor rejection with long-term anti-tumor immune memory. However, a limitation in the basic and translational studies of IgE antibodies that have human constant regions has been the lack of appropriate animal models to properly and fully evaluate their efficacy and toxicity. Given the involvement of IgE in anaphylaxis, toxicological studies are critical for the preclinical analysis of these IgE molecules. Advances in the model systems for the study of human IgE are expected to overcome this limitation and expedite the evaluation of IgE immunological functions in vivo. Such advances include the development of FcεRI transgenic animals such as mice expressing the human FcεRIα chain [64, 65]. Transgene expression in these mice parallels the effector cell-specific expression of FcεRI in humans, making this an attractive model to evaluate both efficacy and toxicity. In fact, these "humanized FcεRI" transgenic mice have already been utilized to evaluate PCA in vivo induced by IgE with human Fc fragments [64, 86], and they open the possibility to further evaluate the potential use of human IgE for the treatment of human cancers. Advances in the understanding of IgE-mediated anti-tumor immune responses, protein design, and experimental models help us to better

understand the benefits and potential drawbacks of IgE-mediated immunotherapy of cancer paving the way to clinical trials.

Acknowledgments This work was supported by NIH/NCI grants R01CA107023, R01 supplements CA107023-02S1 and CA57152-13S1, NIH/NCI T32-CA009120, NIH Fogarty AITRP-AIDS Malignancies Program D43-TW000013-S1, the Susan G. Komen Breast Cancer Foundation Basic, Clinical and Translational Research Grant BCTR0706771, Cancer Research Coordinating Committee (CRCC), the Howard Hughes Medical Institute (HHMI) Gilliam Fellowship, and the Whitcome Fellowship of the Molecular Biology Interdepartmental PhD Program (MBIDP) at UCLA.

References

1. Janeway CA, Travers P, Walport M, and Shlomchik M (2005) The generation of lymphocyte antigen receptors. In: Immunobiology: The Immune System in Health and Disease. New York: Garland Science Publishing, pp. 123–154
2. Penichet ML and Morrison SL (2004) Design and engineering of human forms of monoclonal antibodies. Drug Dev Res 61:121–136
3. Arnold JN, Wormald MR, Sim RB, Rudd PM, and Dwek RA (2007) The impact of glycosylation on the biological function and structure of human immunoglobulins. Annu Rev Immunol 25:21–50
4. Stavnezer J, Guikema JE, and Schrader CE (2008) Mechanism and regulation of class switch recombination. Annu Rev Immunol 26:261–292
5. Helguera G, Daniels TR, Rodriguez JA, and Penichet ML (2010) Monoclonal antibodies, human engineered. In: Encyclopedia of Industrial Biotechnology: Bioprocess, Bioseparation, and Cell Technology, M. Flickinger (ed.). New York: John Wiley & Sons, Inc. http://mrw.interscience.wiley.com/emrw/9780470054581/home/
6. Adams GP and Weiner LM (2005) Monoclonal antibody therapy of cancer. Nat Biotechnol 23:1147–1157
7. Reichert JM, Rosensweig CJ, Faden LB, and Dewitz MC (2005) Monoclonal antibody successes in the clinic. Nat Biotechnol 23:1073–1078
8. Wan T, Beavil RL, Fabiane SM, Beavil AJ, Sohi MK, Keown M, Young RJ, Henry AJ, Owens RJ, Gould HJ, and Sutton BJ (2002) The crystal structure of IgE Fc reveals an asymmetrically bent conformation. Nat Immunol 3:681–686
9. Beavil AJ, Young RJ, Sutton BJ, and Perkins SJ (1995) Bent domain structure of recombinant human IgE-Fc in solution by X-ray and neutron scattering in conjunction with an automated curve fitting procedure. Biochemistry 34:14449–14461
10. Janeway CA, Travers P, Walport M, and Shlomchik M. (2005) The humoral immune response. In: Immunobiology: The Immune System in Health and Disease. New York: Garland Science Publishing, pp. 367–406
11. Gould HJ, Sutton BJ, Beavil AJ, Beavil RL, McCloskey N, Coker HA, Fear D, and Smurthwaite L (2003) The biology of IGE and the basis of allergic disease. Annu Rev Immunol 21:579–628
12. Ravetch JV and Kinet JP (1991) Fc receptors. Annu Rev Immunol 9:457–492
13. Davis KG, Glennie M, Harding SE, and Burton DR (1990) A model for the solution conformation of rat IgE. Biochem Soc Trans 18:935–936
14. Zheng Y, Shopes B, Holowka D, and Baird B (1991) Conformations of IgE bound to its receptor Fc epsilon RI and in solution. Biochemistry 30:9125–9132
15. Maenaka K, van der Merwe PA, Stuart DI, Jones EY, and Sondermann P (2001) The human low affinity Fcgamma receptors IIa, IIb, and III bind IgG with fast kinetics and distinct thermodynamic properties. J Biol Chem 276:44898–44904

16. Ishizaka T, Helm B, Hakimi J, Niebyl J, Ishizaka K, and Gould HJ (1986) Biological properties of a recombinant human immunoglobulin epsilon-chain fragment. Proc Natl Acad Sci USA 83:8323–8327
17. Keown MB, Ghirlando R, Mackay GA, Sutton BJ, and Gould HJ (1997) Basis of the 1:1 stoichiometry of the high affinity receptor Fc epsilon RI-IgE complex. Eur Biophys J 25: 471–476
18. Garman SC, Wurzburg BA, Tarchevskaya SS, Kinet JP, and Jardetzky TS (2000) Structure of the Fc fragment of human IgE bound to its high-affinity receptor Fc epsilonRI alpha. Nature 406:259–266
19. Gould HJ and Sutton BJ (2008) IgE in allergy and asthma today. Nat Rev Immunol 8:205–217
20. Conrad DH (1990) Fc epsilon RII/CD23: the low affinity receptor for IgE. Annu Rev Immunol 8:623–645
21. Hibbert RG, Teriete P, Grundy GJ, Beavil RL, Reljic R, Holers VM, Hannan JP, Sutton BJ, Gould HJ, and McDonnell JM (2005) The structure of human CD23 and its interactions with IgE and CD21. J Exp Med 202:751–760
22. McCloskey N, Hunt J, Beavil RL, Jutton MR, Grundy GJ, Girardi E, Fabiane SM, Fear DJ, Conrad DH, Sutton BJ, and Gould HJ (2007) Soluble CD23 monomers inhibit and oligomers stimulate IGE synthesis in human B cells. J Biol Chem 282:24083–24091
23. Sayers I, Housden JE, Spivey AC, and Helm BA (2004) The importance of Lys-352 of human immunoglobulin E in FcepsilonRII/CD23 recognition. J Biol Chem 279:35320–35325
24. Jensen-Jarolim E, Achatz G, Turner MC, Karagiannis S, Legrand F, Capron M, Penichet ML, Rodriguez JA, Siccardi AG, Vangelista L, Riemer AB, and Gould HJ (2008) AllergoOncology: the role of IgE-mediated allergy in cancer. Allergy 63: 1255–1266
25. Fu SL, Pierre J, Smith-Norowitz TA, Hagler M, Bowne W, Pincus MR, Mueller CM, Zenilman ME, and Bluth MH (2008) Immunoglobulin E antibodies from pancreatic cancer patients mediate antibody-dependent cell-mediated cytotoxicity against pancreatic cancer cells. Clin Exp Immunol 153:401–409
26. Matta GM, Battaglio S, Dibello C, Napoli P, Baldi C, Ciccone G, Coscia M, Boccadoro M, and Massaia M (2007) Polyclonal immunoglobulin E levels are correlated with hemoglobin values and overall survival in patients with multiple myeloma. Clin Cancer Res 13: 5348–5354
27. Schulman ES (2001) Development of a monoclonal anti-immunoglobulin E antibody (omalizumab) for the treatment of allergic respiratory disorders. Am J Respir Crit Care Med 164:S6–11
28. Presta LG, Lahr SJ, Shields RL, Porter JP, Gorman CM, Fendly BM, and Jardieu PM (1993) Humanization of an antibody directed against IgE. J Immunol 151:2623–2632
29. Strunk RC and Bloomberg GR (2006) Omalizumab for asthma. N Engl J Med 354:2689–2695
30. Dodig S, Richter D, Cepelak I, and Benko B (2005) Anti-IgE therapy with omalizumab in asthma and allergic rhinitis. Acta Pharm 55:123–138
31. Manz RA, Hauser AE, Hiepe F, and Radbruch A (2005) Maintenance of serum antibody levels. Annu Rev Immunol 23:367–386
32. Preithner S, Elm S, Lippold S, Locher M, Wolf A, da Silva AJ, Baeuerle PA, and Prang NS (2006) High concentrations of therapeutic IgG1 antibodies are needed to compensate for inhibition of antibody-dependent cellular cytotoxicity by excess endogenous immunoglobulin G. Mol Immunol 43:1183–1193
33. Kinet JP (1999) The high-affinity IgE receptor (Fc epsilon RI): from physiology to pathology. Annu Rev Immunol 17:931–972
34. Sukumar S, Conrad DH, Szakal AK, and Tew JG (2006) Differential T cell-mediated regulation of CD23 (Fc epsilonRII) in B cells and follicular dendritic cells. J Immunol 176:4811–4817
35. Delespesse G, Sarfati M, Wu CY, Fournier S, and Letellier M (1992) The low-affinity receptor for IgE. Immunol Rev 125:77–97

36. Clynes RA, Towers TL, Presta LG, and Ravetch JV (2000) Inhibitory Fc receptors modulate in vivo cytoxicity against tumor targets. Nat Med 6:443–446.
37. Nimmerjahn F and Ravetch JV (2007) Antibodies, Fc receptors and cancer. Curr Opin Immunol 19:239–245
38. Weng WK and Levy R (2001) Expression of complement inhibitors CD46, CD55, and CD59 on tumor cells does not predict clinical outcome after rituximab treatment in follicular non-Hodgkin lymphoma. Blood 98:1352–1357
39. Peipp M, Dechant M, and Valerius T (2008) Effector mechanisms of therapeutic antibodies against ErbB receptors. Curr Opin Immunol 20:436–443
40. Hudis CA (2007) Trastuzumab – mechanism of action and use in clinical practice. N Engl J Med 357:39–51
41. Wang SY, Racila E, Taylor RP, and Weiner GJ (2008) NK-cell activation and antibody-dependent cellular cytotoxicity induced by rituximab-coated target cells is inhibited by the C3b component of complement. Blood 111:1456–1463
42. Janeway CA, Travers P, Walport M, and Shlomchik M (2005) Allergy and hypersensitivity. In: Immunobiology: The Immune System in Health and Disease. New York: Garland Science Publishing,. pp. 517–555
43. Bieber T (1997) Fc epsilon RI on human epidermal Langerhans cells: an old receptor with new structure and functions. Int Arch Allergy Immunol 113:30–34
44. Bieber T (1997) Fc epsilon RI-expressing antigen-presenting cells: new players in the atopic game. Immunol Today 18:311–313
45. Maurer D, Ebner C, Reininger B, Fiebiger E, Kraft D, Kinet JP, and Stingl G (1995) The high affinity IgE receptor (Fc epsilon RI) mediates IgE-dependent allergen presentation. J Immunol 154:6285–6290
46. Maurer D, Fiebiger S, Ebner C, Reininger B, Fischer GF, Wichlas S, Jouvin MH, Schmitt-Egenolf M, Kraft D, Kinet JP, and Stingl G (1996) Peripheral blood dendritic cells express Fc epsilon RI as a complex composed of Fc epsilon RI alpha- and Fc epsilon RI gamma-chains and can use this receptor for IgE-mediated allergen presentation. J Immunol 157: 607–616
47. Karagiannis SN, Bracher MG, Beavil RL, Beavil AJ, Hunt J, McCloskey N, Thompson RG, East N, Burke F, Sutton BJ, Dombrowicz D, Balkwill FR, and Gould HJ (2008) Role of IgE receptors in IgE antibody-dependent cytotoxicity and phagocytosis of ovarian tumor cells by human monocytic cells. Cancer Immunol Immunother 57:247–263
48. Karagiannis SN, Bracher MG, Hunt J, McCloskey N, Beavil RL, Beavil AJ, Fear DJ, Thompson RG, East N, Burke F, Moore RJ, Dombrowicz DD, Balkwill FR, and Gould HJ (2007) IgE-antibody-dependent immunotherapy of solid tumors: cytotoxic and phagocytic mechanisms of eradication of ovarian cancer cells. J Immunol 179:2832–2843
49. Karagiannis P, Singer J, Hunt J, Gan SK, Rudman SM, Mechtcheriakova D, Knittelfelder R, Daniels TR, Hobson PS, Beavil AJ, Spicer J, Nestle FO, Penichet ML, Gould HJ, Jensen-Jarolim E, and Karagiannis SN (2009) Characterisation of an engineered trastuzumab IgE antibody and effector cell mechanisms targeting HER2/*neu*-positive tumour cells. Cancer Immunol Immunother 58:915–930
50. Arase N, Arase H, Hirano S, Yokosuka T, Sakurai D, and Saito T (2003) IgE-mediated activation of NK cells through Fc gamma RIII. J Immunol 170:3054–3058
51. Coca AF and Grove EF (1925) Studies in hypersensitiveness: a study of the atopic reagins. J Immunol 10:445–464
52. Stanworth DR (1993) The discovery of IgE. Allergy 48:67–71
53. Bennich HH, Ishizaka K, Johansson SG, Rowe DS, Stanworth DR, and Terry WD (1968) Immunoglobulin E. A new class of human immunoglobulin. Immunochemistry 5:327–328
54. Bartholomaeus WN and Keast D (1972) Reaginic antibody to tumour and alloantigens in mice. Nat New Biol 239:206–207
55. Lynch NR and Salomon JC (1977) Passive local anaphylaxis: demonstration of antitumor activity and complementation of intratumor BCG. J Natl Cancer Inst 58:1093–1098

56. Kohler G and Milstein C (1975) Continuous cultures of fused cells secreting antibody of predefined specificity. Nature 256:495–497
57. Morrison SL, Johnson MJ, Herzenberg LA, and Oi VT (1984) Chimeric human antibody molecules: mouse antigen-binding domains with human constant region domains. Proc Natl Acad Sci USA 81:6851–6855
58. Neuberger MS, Williams GT, Mitchell EB, Jouhal SS, Flanagan JG, and Rabbitts TH (1985) A hapten-specific chimaeric IgE antibody with human physiological effector function. Nature 314:268–270
59. Bruggemann M, Williams GT, Bindon CI, Clark MR, Walker MR, Jefferis R, Waldmann H, and Neuberger MS (1987) Comparison of the effector functions of human immunoglobulins using a matched set of chimeric antibodies. J Exp Med 166:1351–1361
60. Nagy E, Berczi I, and Sehon AH (1991) Growth inhibition of murine mammary carcinoma by monoclonal IgE antibodies specific for the mammary tumor virus. Cancer Immunol Immunother 34:63–69
61. Isaacs JD, Clark MR, Greenwood J, and Waldmann H (1992) Therapy with monoclonal antibodies. An in vivo model for the assessment of therapeutic potential. J Immunol 148:3062–3071
62. Panaccio M, Gillespie MT, Walker ID, Kirszbaum L, Sharpe JA, Tobias GH, McKenzie IF, and Deacon NJ (1987) Molecular characterization of the murine cytotoxic T-cell membrane glycoprotein Ly-3 (CD8). Proc Natl Acad Sci USA 84:6874–6878
63. Kershaw MH, Darcy PK, Trapani JA, and Smyth MJ (1996) The use of chimeric human Fc(epsilon) receptor I to redirect cytotoxic T lymphocytes to tumors. J Leukoc Biol 60: 721–728
64. Fung-Leung WP, De Sousa-Hitzler J, Ishaque A, Zhou L, Pang J, Ngo K, Panakos JA, Chourmouzis E, Liu FT, and Lau CY (1996) Transgenic mice expressing the human high-affinity immunoglobulin (Ig) E receptor alpha chain respond to human IgE in mast cell degranulation and in allergic reactions. J Exp Med 183:49–56
65. Dombrowic, D, Brini AT, Flamand V, Hicks E, Snouwaert JN, Kinet JP, and Koller BH (1996) Anaphylaxis mediated through a humanized high affinity IgE receptor. J Immunol 157: 1645–1651
66. Teng MW, Kershaw MH, Jackson JT, Smyth MJ, and Darcy PK (2006) Adoptive transfer of chimeric FcepsilonRI gene-modified human T cells for cancer immunotherapy. Hum Gene Ther 17:1134–1143
67. Kershaw MH, Darcy PK, Trapani JA, MacGregor D, and Smyth MJ (1998) Tumor-specific IgE-mediated inhibition of human colorectal carcinoma xenograft growth. Oncol Res 10: 133–142
68. Mount PF, Sutton VR, Li W, Burgess J, McKenzie IF, Pietersz GA, and Trapani JA (1994) Chimeric (mouse/human) anti-colon cancer antibody c30.6 inhibits the growth of human colorectal cancer xenografts in scid/scid mice. Cancer Res 54:6160–6166
69. Gould HJ, Mackay GA, Karagiannis SN, O'Toole CM, Marsh PJ, Daniel BE, Coney LR, Zurawski VR Jr, Joseph M, Capron M, Gilbert M, Murphy GF, and Korngold R (1999) Comparison of IgE and IgG antibody-dependent cytotoxicity in vitro and in a SCID mouse xenograft model of ovarian carcinoma. Eur J Immunol 29:3527–3537
70. Karagiannis SN, Wang Q, East N, Burke F, Riffard S, Bracher MG, Thompson RG, Durham SR, Schwartz LB, Balkwill FR, and Gould HJ (2003) Activity of human monocytes in IgE antibody-dependent surveillance and killing of ovarian tumor cells. Eur J Immunol 33: 1030–1040
71. Weng WK and Levy R (2003) Two immunoglobulin G fragment C receptor polymorphisms independently predict response to rituximab in patients with follicular lymphoma. J Clin Oncol 21:3940–3947
72. Slamon DJ, Clark, GM, Wong SG, Levin WJ, Ullrich A, and McGuire WL (1987) Human breast cancer: correlation of relapse and survival with amplification of the HER-2/*neu* oncogene. Science 235:177–182

73. Baselga J, Tripathy D, Mendelsohn J, Baughman S, Benz CC, Dantis L, Sklarin NT, Seidman AD, Hudis CA, Moore J, Rosen PP, Twaddell T, Henderson IC, and Norton L (1996) Phase II study of weekly intravenous recombinant humanized anti-p185HER2 monoclonal antibody in patients with HER2/*neu*-overexpressing metastatic breast cancer. J Clin Oncol 14:737–744
74. Baselga J, Tripathy D, Mendelsohn J, Baughman S, Benz CC, Dantis L, Sklarin NT, Seidman AD, Hudis CA, Moore J, Rosen PP, Twaddell T, Henderson IC, and Norton L. (1999) Phase II study of weekly intravenous trastuzumab (Herceptin) in patients with HER2/*neu*-overexpressing metastatic breast cancer. Semin Oncol 26:78–83
75. Vogel CL, Cobleigh MA, Tripathy D, Gutheil JC, Harris LN, Fehrenbacher L, Slamon DJ, Murphy M, Novotny WF, Burchmore M, Shak S, Stewart SJ, and Press M (2002) Efficacy and safety of trastuzumab as a single agent in first-line treatment of HER2-overexpressing metastatic breast cancer. J Clin Oncol 20:719–726
76. Pegram MD, Lipton A, Hayes DF, Weber BL, Baselga JM, Tripathy D, Baly D, Baughman SA, Twaddell T, Glaspy JA, and Slamon DJ (1998) Phase II study of receptor-enhanced chemosensitivity using recombinant humanized anti-p185HER2/*neu* monoclonal antibody plus cisplatin in patients with HER2/*neu*-overexpressing metastatic breast cancer refractory to chemotherapy treatment. J Clin Oncol 16:2659–2671
77. Pegram MD, Pienkowski T, Northfelt DW, Eiermann W, Patel R, Fumoleau P, Quan E, Crown J, Toppmeyer D, Smylie M, Riva A, Blitz S, Press MF, Reese D, Lindsay MA, and Slamon DJ (2004) Results of two open-label, multicenter phase II studies of docetaxel, platinum salts, and trastuzumab in HER2-positive advanced breast cancer. J Natl Cancer Inst 96:759–769
78. Slamon DJ, Leyland-Jones B, Shak S, Fuchs H, Paton V, Bajamonde A, Fleming T, Eiermann W, Wolter J, Pegram M, Baselga J, and Norton L (2001) Use of chemotherapy plus a monoclonal antibody against HER2 for metastatic breast cancer that overexpresses HER2. N Engl J Med 344:783–792
79. Baselga J, Carbonell X, Castaneda-Soto NJ, Clemens M, Green M, Harvey V, Morales S, Barton C, and Ghahramani P (2005) Phase II study of efficacy, safety, and pharmacokinetics of trastuzumab monotherapy administered on a 3-weekly schedule. J Clin Oncol 23:2162–2171
80. Schier R, Marks JD, Wolf EJ, Apell G, Wong C, McCartney JE, Bookman MA, Huston JS, Houston LL, Weiner LM, and Adams GP (1995) In vitro and in vivo characterization of a human anti-c-erbB-2 single-chain Fv isolated from a filamentous phage antibody library. Immunotechnology 1:73–81
81. Schier R, McCall A, Adams GP, Marshall KW, Merritt H, Yim M, Crawford RS, Weiner LM, Marks C, and Marks JD (1996) Isolation of picomolar affinity anti-c-erbB-2 single-chain Fv by molecular evolution of the complementarity determining regions in the center of the antibody binding site. J Mol Biol 263:551–567
82. Penichet ML. Novel antibodies of IgE class targeting HER2/*neu* and CD20 for the treatment of cancer. Proceedings of the 2nd International AllergoOncology Symposium (Vienna, Austria, April 11–12, 2008) Abstract No. S-10
83. Tang Y, Lou J, Alpaugh RK, Robinson MK, Marks JD, and Weiner LM (2007) Regulation of antibody-dependent cellular cytotoxicity by IgG intrinsic and apparent affinity for target antigen. J Immunol 179:2815–2823
84. Coiffier B (2007) Rituximab therapy in malignant lymphoma. Oncogene 26:3603–3613
85. Smith MR (2003) Rituximab (monoclonal anti-CD20 antibody): mechanisms of action and resistance. Oncogene 22:7359–7368
86. Helguera G, Rodriguez JA, Daniels TR, Ortiz-Sanchez E, Quintero R, Timmerman JM, Wu A, Martinez-Maza O, and Penichet ML. Anti-CD20 IgE: a novel antibody for the treatment of non-Hodgkin's lymphoma. Proceedings of the American Association for Cancer Research Special Conference "Tumor Immunology: An integrated perspective" (Miami, Florida, USA, December 2–5, 2008). Abstract No. B18/PR04
87. Riemer AB, Untersmayr E, Knittelfelder R, Duschl A, Pehamberger H, Zielinski CC, Scheiner O, and Jensen-Jarolim E (2007) Active induction of tumor-specific IgE antibodies by oral mimotope vaccination. Cancer Res 67:3406–3411

88. Riemer AB, Klinger M, Wagner S, Bernhaus A, Mazzucchelli L, Pehamberger H, Scheiner O, Zielinski CC, and Jensen-Jarolim E (2004) Generation of peptide mimics of the epitope recognized by trastuzumab on the oncogenic protein Her-2/*neu*. J Immunol 173:394–401
89. Scholl I, Untersmayr E, Bakos N, Roth-Walter F, Gleiss A, Boltz-Nitulescu G, Scheiner O, and Jensen-Jarolim E (2005) Antiulcer drugs promote oral sensitization and hypersensitivity to hazelnut allergens in BALB/c mice and humans. Am J Clin Nutr 81:154–160
90. Untersmayr E, Scholl I, Swoboda I, Beil WJ, Forster-Waldl E, Walter F, Riemer A, Kraml G, Kinaciyan T, Spitzauer S, Boltz-Nitulescu G, Scheiner O, and Jensen-Jarolim E (2003) Antacid medication inhibits digestion of dietary proteins and causes food allergy: a fish allergy model in BALB/c mice. J Allergy Clin Immunol 112:616–623

Chapter 8
IgE Interacts with Potent Effector Cells Against Tumors: ADCC and ADCP

Sophia N. Karagiannis, Frank O. Nestle, and Hannah J. Gould

Abstract We examine the properties of IgE antibodies which may render them effective against tumors. This may be due to the uniquely high affinity of IgE antibodies for their Fc epsilon (Fcε) receptors and the expression of IgE antibodies on potent effector cells. Owing to these properties, IgE antibodies activate effector cell mechanisms that may be different from and stronger than those mediated by antibodies of other classes, thereby inducing superior anti-tumor responses. In examining the potential of IgE–FcεRI complexes on effector cells to activate effector cells (and describe evidence to-date) we suggest that the interactions of IgE antibodies with tumor-associated antigens on tumor cells and Fc receptors on IgE receptor-bearing cells trigger the association of tumor and effector cells. The outcome of these interactions is effector cell activation and effective tumor cell death by a number of mechanisms including antibody-dependent cellular cytotoxicity (ADCC) and antibody-dependent cellular phagocytosis (ADCP).

8.1 IgE Operates Through Powerful Fc Epsilon Receptors

IgE has two known receptors: the high-affinity receptor FcεRI and the low-affinity receptor CD23 (FcεRII) [1, 2]. FcεRI and CD23 are specific for the Fc epsilon (Fcε) region of the antibody. The IgE-binding molecule galectin-3 binds to oligosaccharides of IgE [3].

8.1.1 The High-Affinity IgE Receptor FcεRI

In humans, FcεRI is found on a variety of immune cells, namely, mast cells, basophils, eosinophils, monocytes, Langerhans cells, dendritic cells (DC) and platelets. There are two forms of FcεRI: the tetrameric form (αβγ2) is expressed

S.N. Karagiannis (✉)
NIHR Biomedical Research Centre at Guy's and St. Thomas's Hospitals and King's College London, Cutaneous Medicine and Immunotherapy, St. John's Institute of Dermatology, Division of Genetics and Molecular Medicine, King's College London School of Medicine, Guy's Hospital, London, UK
e-mail: sophia.karagiannis@kcl.ac.uk

M.L. Penichet, E. Jensen-Jarolim (eds.), *Cancer and IgE*,
DOI 10.1007/978-1-60761-451-7_8,

on mast cells and basophils, and the trimeric form (αγ2) is found on monocytes [4], eosinophils [5–8] and antigen-presenting cells (APC) [9–12]. The IgE α subunit with two immunoglobulin extracellular domains contains the IgE-binding site with a ligand : receptor stoichiometry of 1:1, while the β and γ subunits have no role in binding IgE. The γ-chain, a ubiquitous signal transduction subunit, is shared by a number of immunoreceptors, and notably IgG receptors FcγR [13] and the IgA receptor FcαRI [14] on a range of hematopoietic cells. It is essential for cell surface expression of the receptor complexes and is known to enhance intracellular signaling [15, 16]. The presence of the β-chain serves as an amplifier of IgE-mediated functions both in vitro and in vivo [17, 18], is known to enhance expression of unoccupied receptor on the cell surface [19] and is therefore, at least in part, responsible for the observed high levels of FcεRI expression in mast cells and basophils [20]. Ligation of the receptor by IgE and cross-linking by antigen results in the activation of multiple signaling pathways, leading to a variety of effector cell responses (Fig. 8.1). Unlike humans, mice express only the tetrameric form (αβγ2), and the distribution of FcεRI is restricted to mast cells and basophils [1, 15].

The affinity of IgE for FcεRI ($K_a = 10^8 - 10^{11}\,M^1$) is 2–5 orders of magnitude higher than that of IgGs for their receptors [4, 21] (Table 8.1, Fig. 8.1). The high affinity of the receptor–antibody interaction may have profound implications for both the potency of IgE-mediated effector functions and the longevity of IgE-mediated immune responses. Due to the high affinity of the IgE–FcεRI complex,

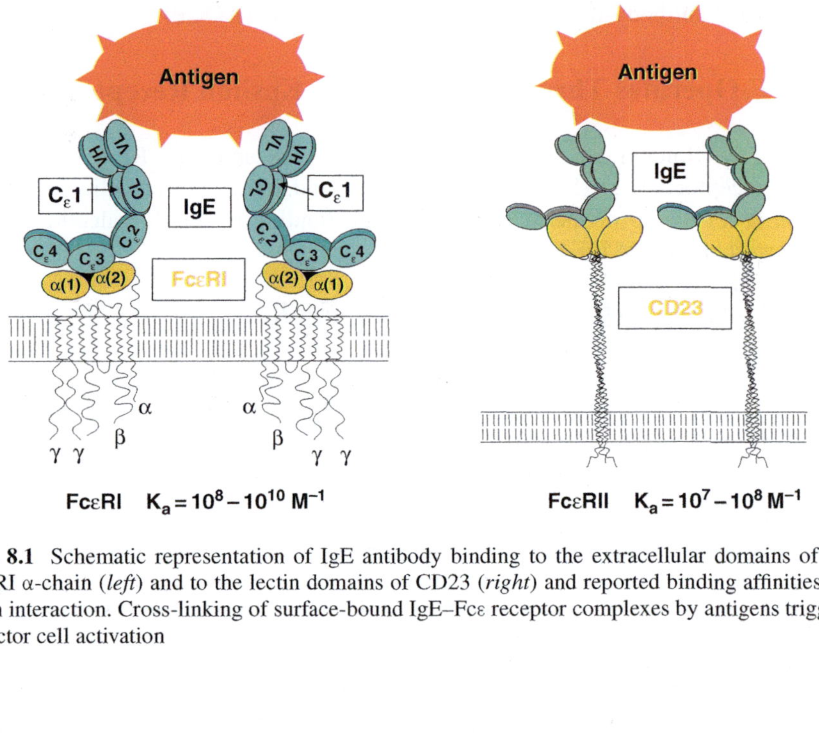

Fig. 8.1 Schematic representation of IgE antibody binding to the extracellular domains of the FcεRI α-chain (*left*) and to the lectin domains of CD23 (*right*) and reported binding affinities for each interaction. Cross-linking of surface-bound IgE–Fcε receptor complexes by antigens triggers effector cell activation

Table 8.1 Binding affinities of Immunoglobulins for their Fc receptors

Fc receptor	Ig ligand	Affinity (K_a)	References
FcαR	IgA	$10^6\ M^{-1}$	Wines et al. [130]
FcεRI	IgE	10^8–$10^{11}\ M^{-1}$	Gould et al. [1]
FcεRII (CD23)	IgE	10^7–$10^8\ M^{-1}$	Gould et al. [1]
FcγRI (CD64)	IgG	10^8–$10^9 M^{-1}$	Ravetch and Kinet [4]
FcγRII (CD32)	IgG	$<10^7 M^{-1}$	Maenaka et al. [21]
FcγRIII (CD16)	IgG	$10^5\ M^{-1}$	Maenaka et al. [21]

IgE is the only antibody class that can be strongly retained by effector cells in the absence of antigen. The high affinity of IgE for FcεRI may account for the long half-life of IgE in tissues (around 2 weeks measured in skin), which is longer than that measured for IgG (2–3 days). The relative retentions of each antibody class in tissues are proportional to the affinity constants [1, 4]. The high affinity of the IgE–FcεRI complex may suggest the potential of IgE to engage FcεRI in superior anti-tumor cell responses in tissues compared to those mediated by IgG and its receptors. This may be because FcεRI on the surface of effector cells recruited into tissues may sequester IgE.

A number of studies on the emerging protective role of IgE in parasitic infections implicate the requirement for FcεRI expressed on the surface of mast cells to mediate the inflammatory cascades that confer protection against parasites [22–24]. The roles FcεRI play in allergic responses, both in the "early phase," involving mast cell activation and degranulation, and the "late phase," involving recruitment and activation of inflammatory cells, have been extensively studied [25]. FcεRI-expressing tissue mast cells and blood basophils bind antigen-specific IgE and on cross-linking by multivalent antigen release potent inflammatory mediators, such as histamine, leukotrienes, proteases and a variety of Th2-type cytokines, initiating and enhancing the recruitment and activation of T cells, monocytes, eosinophils, basophils and APC to the site of antigen challenge (Fig. 8.1). The resulting inflammatory response may also serve to activate and perpetrate immune effector functions in situ. In addition, local or recruited IgE-sensitized APC promote IgE production by B cells, thus maintaining mast-cell and APC sensitization and long-term immunologic memory and immune surveillance both in situ and systemically.

IgG receptors on the surface of effector cells are capable of mediating anti-tumor responses. FcγRIII (CD16), which is the nearest IgG receptor homologue to FcεRI, containing the ligand-binding α-chain with the closest homology to the α-chain of FcεRI, and which has a very low affinity for IgG ($K_a = 10^5 M^{-1}$) [21] (Table 8.1), has been shown to participate in IgG antibody-dependent T-cell-, natural killer (NK) cell- and macrophage-mediated tumor cell cytotoxicity [antibody-dependent cellular cytotoxicity (ADCC)] [4, 26–28]. FcγRIII has also been reported to engender macrophage-mediated tumor cell phagocytosis [antibody-dependent cellular phagocytosis (ADCP)] [29]. The high-affinity IgG receptor, FcγRI or CD64, with affinity for IgG ($K_a = 10^8 M^{-1}$) two orders of magnitude lower than that measured for

the IgE–FcεRI complex [4], can mediate both ADCC and ADCP of tumor cells [30–33]. Since FcγRs confer anti-tumor responses, it is likely that the potency of engaging IgE with FcεRI in parasitic infections and allergies may also be harnessed to combat cancer cells. The high-affinity of IgE–FcεRI complexes implies that strategies aimed at engaging IgE–FcεRI against tumor cells may confer superior anti-tumor cell responses in tissues compared to those mediated by IgG and its receptors.

8.1.2 The Low-Affinity IgE Receptor (CD23)

The human low-affinity IgE receptor, CD23 a type II integral membrane protein, is different from all other immunoglobulin receptors in that it belongs to the C-type lectin superfamily. Its two splice variants, CD23a and CD23b, differ in their first six (CD23b) or seven (CD23a) amino acids at the cytoplasmic N-terminus and contain different signaling motifs that determine their functions [34]. Human CD23a is expressed only on antigen-activated B cells prior to differentiation into antibody-secreting plasma cells and is involved in IgE antibody-dependent antigen presentation and regulation of IgE synthesis. The expression of human CD23b is induced by IL-4 on various inflammatory cells, for example, T cells, eosinophils, platelets, monocytes, B cells, DC and epithelial cells [1, 35]. Engagement of CD23b by IgE–antigen complexes promotes monocyte/macrophage activation, induces nitric oxide synthase (iNOS) and generates pro-inflammatory cytokines [36, 37] (Fig. 8.1). These processes are thought to play a role in clearance of parasitic infections through the release of TNF-α and nitric oxide (NO) [38, 39]. A natural function for human CD23b is IgE antibody-dependent cellular ADCP of hapten-coated red cells by monocytes/macrophages [35, 40], suggesting that CD23 may mediate this function against tumor cells.

In humans, IgE binds to CD23 with relatively high affinity ($K_a = 10^7 - 10^8\,M^{-1}$), as high as that of IgG for its high-affinity receptor FcγRI [1, 4] (Table 8.1, Fig. 8.1). Numerous studies now describe the functions of CD23 inducing inflammatory and memory responses in response to allergens and parasitic infections. There are also reports that tumor-associated macrophages (TAMs) express CD23 in a number of human cancers [41]. Furthermore, the soluble fragments of CD23 (sCD23) have also been associated with blood-borne cancers. Increased sCD23 levels are associated with poorer patient survival in chronic lymphocytic leukemia [42]. It is conceivable that sCD23 may be elevated in certain malignancies, resulting in blocking the formation of IgE–FcεRII complexes on the surface of effector cells, thereby interfering with IgE-mediated anti-tumoral responses. However, a potential role for CD23 in tumor killing is only starting to emerge [43, 44]. The effector cell functions mediated by CD23 in the context of allergies and parasitic infections, coupled with its comparatively high affinity for IgE, may make it a potentially effective IgE receptor for mediating tumor cell targeting and killing.

8.1.3 Galectin-3

Galectin-3, also known as the beta-galactoside-binding lectin galectin-3, epsilon-binding protein (e-BP), IgE-binding protein or Mac-2, binds specifically to oligosaccharide structures with a terminal β-galactose through a lectin–carbohydrate interaction [45]. It recognizes both IgE and FcεRI and can activate immune responses [3, 46]. Due to its ability to form pentameric complexes with oligosaccharides, it can crosslink FcεRI or receptor-bound IgE on the surface of mast cells and basophils [47, 48]. Despite its potential to enhance mast cell activation and mediate the phagocytotic properties of monocytes, increased expression of galectin-3 has been associated with poor prognosis in thyroid and pancreatic cancers, whereas reduced levels of the protein were detected in colon, ovarian, breast, endometrium and skin cancers, compared to normal tissues [49]. Galectin-3 expression in malignancies may have a bearing on the immunogenic nature of the tumor, but this has not yet been fully explored. Although expressed in monocytic cells, at least in one in vitro study, galectin-3 did not appear to mediate tumor cell death [43]. To-date, there is no evidence linking galectin-3 to IgE antibody-dependent tumor cell killing although further research may shed more light on potential mechanisms that may link galectin-3 to IgE-mediated immune cell activation signals against cancer cells.

8.2 What is Known About IgE Effector Cells in Cancer? Missing Activation Signals May Tip the Balance in Favor of Tumor Growth

The relationship between tumor cells and the immune system is vastly complex. The dialog between tumor cells and the immune system in cancer results in inflammation and tumor regression but has also been associated with tumor growth, angiogenesis, invasion and metastasis. Patient prognoses for some cancers also appear to be dependent on the nature of the immune responses elicited in the tumor microenvironment; positive and negative correlations between immune infiltrate and clinical outcome have been reported. It is well established that solid tumors are associated with inflammatory responses resulting in infiltration of mast cells, B and T lymphocytes, neutrophils, NK cells, DC, macrophages and eosinophils [50]. These cells are recruited by a variety of cytokines and chemokines expressed by local inflammatory cells that bind to upregulated adhesion molecules and cell surface receptors in situ. Tumor cells also secrete cytokines and chemokines that contribute to this process; often, this promotes angiogenesis, tumor growth and metastasis [51].

Most of the inflammatory cell infiltrates are IgE effector cells. These cells have the potential to direct strong anti-tumor activities in situ that may tip the balance

against tumor growth and invasion. Herewith, we describe the relationship between these effector cells and cancer tissues and how effector cell activities are influenced by tumor cells.

8.2.1 Mast Cells and Basophils

Tryptase-positive mast cells infiltrate the invasive fronts in greater numbers than in any other area of malignant tumor lesions, but their contribution to cancer growth and spread has been controversial [52]. In breast cancer the presence of mast cells in the peritumoral areas has correlated with a favorable clinical prognosis [53, 54]. Hodgkin's lymphoma, endometrial cancer and melanoma patients with higher numbers of mast cells in tumor lesions have a worse prognosis, whereas mast cell numbers in lymph nodes do not correlate with clinical outcomes in Hodgkin's lymphoma [55–57]. Increased mast cell numbers in breast cancer lesions and lymph nodes with metastases have been reported compared to those from benign lesions and from lymph nodes clear of metastatic disease [58–60].

Mast cell activation and degranulation promotes the destruction of local tissue architecture, tissue remodeling and angiogenesis, and this is thought to assist tumor cell growth and metastasis [61]. A number of factors may also contribute to the inability of resident mast cells to mount effective immune responses against tumors. One reason may be the location of mast cells in the invasive fronts, away from the core of solid tumors, suggesting that mast cells may respond to tumor cell stimuli and may be recruited to assist tumor growth and invasion. Another factor may be the production of tryptase, this may result in the loss of local tissue architecture that promotes tumor invasion but also in stimulating proliferation of vascular endothelial cells, promoting tumor-associated neovascularization. The production of angiogenic factors and cytokines by mast cells in response to tumors (VEGF, TGF-β, FGF-2, IL-8, TNF-α, MMP-9) appears to tip the balance in favor of tumor growth and metastasis [62–66]. It has been suggested that the intensity of mast cell activation/response in the absence of antigenic stimuli may be a contributing factor in this process [61, 67]. Since mast cells are potent IgE effector cells, it is therefore tempting to consider that treatment with tumor antigen-specific IgE antibodies may stimulate mast cells against cancer cells and help redress the balance in favor of immune activation and IgE-mediated anti-tumoral responses.

The role of basophils in cancer has not been extensively elucidated. One notable exception is perhaps blood malignancies such as chronic myeloid leukemia, where basophil numbers are increased in later stages of the disease and basophil markers are used for diagnostic but also prognostic evaluations [68]. Basophils have also been observed in the inflammatory infiltrate in experimental tumors. They may be recruited into tumor areas by in situ expression of cytokines such as IL-4 and in response to chemoattractant signals like VCAM-1 and MCP-1 [69] and are thought to be associated with tumor regression. Their potential IgE-mediated anti-tumor functions are yet to be explored.

8.2.2 Monocytes/Macrophages

TAMs are found in virtually all types of tumors and can comprise more than 50% of the total tumor mass in both primary and metastatic lesions [70]. Blood monocytes are constantly recruited to the tumor sites by chemokines and cytokines released by tumor cells (CSF-1, CC chemokines) and neighboring endothelial cells (VEGF). Evidence suggests that TAMs switch off anti-tumor immunity and are associated with poor clinical outcomes [71]. Once in tumor sites, TAMs can function by promoting tumor growth and metastasis, producing angiogenic factors and metalloproteinases [72, 73]. Macrophage infiltration of various tumors such as melanoma, stomach and colorectal cancers has been correlated with immunogenicity but also inversely correlated with metastatic potential, while also the opposite has been reported for cancers of the breast, prostate and endometrium.

Macrophages from normal and infected tissues have been shown to lyse tumor cells, present tumor-associated antigens to T cells and express co-stimulatory factors that enhance T cell and NK cell anti-tumor functions [74]. On the contrary, TAMs are generally thought to be immature in their phenotype and this may be partly due to their in situ exposure to tumor cell and immune cell-secreted cytokines such as IL-4, IL-10 TGF-β1 and prostaglandin E2. It has been proposed that these signals polarize macrophages into the alternatively activated type II or M2 macrophage phenotype. M2 TAMs constitutively express high levels of IL-1β and IL-6 and low levels of TNF-α. They are thought to have impaired antigen-presenting capacity, can suppress activation of T cells, induce T cell apoptosis, switch off DC maturation through secretion of IL-10 and engage in tissue repair and remodeling in favor of tumor growth, angiogenesis and invasion [73, 75].

TAMs accumulate in hypoxic tumor regions where they produce iNOS-derived NO, which can induce tumor cell apoptosis. However, it has been suggested that cytotoxic mediators, such as NOs that are produced by monocytes/macrophages in cancer tissues, are modulated by tumor cells. Arginase expression by TAM is thought to be a tumor-induced mechanism preventing formation of sufficient NO concentrations that are cytotoxic to tumors [76]. This may ensure that iNOS expression and/or activity are reduced, leading to lower levels of NO production than required for tumor cell cytotoxicity. Tumor-induced modulation of NO production is also potentially anti-apoptotic and/or pro-angiogenic. Thus, in tumors the balance of NO production appears tipped in favor of tumor growth [77, 78].

Although TAMs are known to be "conditioned" by tumor cells in situ to tumor growth, they also harbor the potential to become activated to kill tumor cells and release tumorigenic, pro-apoptotic and angiostatic compounds [79–82]. There are on-going studies evaluating targeted therapies aimed at exploring the plastid nature of these cells to this effect [83, 84].

So could TAMs be primed by IgE antibodies to turn against tumor cells? Immunohistochemical studies in breast cancer confirm the presence of CD23 on the surface of TAMs and the ability of this receptor to mediate expression of iNOS in human macrophages [36, 41, 85, 86]. Engaging CD23 by IgE and antigen on the surface of monocytic cells induces production of inflammatory mediators such

as TNF-α and iNOS in inflammatory responses in allergies and parasitic infections [85–88]. It is therefore conceivable that tumor antigen-specific IgE-mediated signals could target circulating monocytes and TAMs, enhance their tumor killing mechanisms and induce an allergy-like anti-tumor response in situ. Numerous findings now suggest that macrophages associated with tumors may be activated by IgE antibodies to kill tumors and that the pro-tumor growth signals may not be an inevitable fate of monocytes/macrophages. Future studies may help elucidate the potential of IgE antibodies in providing crucial signals that recondition TAMs to target immune responses against tumor cells.

8.2.3 Eosinophils

Infiltrating eosinophils are associated with a significantly better prognosis in some malignancies (esophageal squamous cell carcinoma, gastric cancer, head and neck cancer and colorectal carcinoma) [89–92]. Eosinophils contain cytotoxic granule proteins, such as major basic protein (MBP), eosinophil peroxidase, eosinophil cationic protein and eosinophil-derived neurotoxin, which are capable of inducing tissue damage and dysfunction [93], enhancing local inflammation and immune responses. Some, like eosinophil-derived neurotoxin, can induce tumor cell apoptosis and have been considered as potential treatments for cancer [94]. Eosinophil-derived cytotoxic mediators could therefore be harnessed to kill tumor cells. Several studies indicate that cytokines such as IL-4 or chemokines such as eotaxin-1 are associated with the inhibition of tumor cell growth and tumor cell killing [95, 96].

A number of experimental models have demonstrated that eosinophil infiltration in solid tumors is correlated with tumor eradication and evidence suggests that eosinophils participate in tumor cell killing in vitro and also in anti-tumor immune surveillance in vivo [97, 98]. It is also of great importance that eosinophils can exert potent anti-tumor activities in Th2 cytokine-rich environments, normally associated with immune tolerance in cancer. In a recent study of mouse melanoma, eosinophils were seen to be concentrated in necrotic areas and capsule regions of the tumors, where evidence of eosinophil MBP suggested extensive degranulation and eosinophil participation in tumor necrosis [99]. Eosinophil recruitment was a dynamic and an on-going process that occurred independently of Th2-dependent immune responses, implying that these cells can perform potent anti-tumoral functions in situ. In a separate study of CTL-resistant mouse melanoma, regression of tumor metastases was directly associated with tumor-associated eosinophil activation via STAT6, degranulation and secretion of eotaxin-1 and clearance of lung and visceral metastases [100].

Although eosinophils express exceedingly small numbers of IgE receptors on their cell surfaces [7, 101, 102], engagement of receptors with IgE has been shown to activate these cells to kill tumor cells [44]. The role of these cells in protecting against parasitic infections by ADCC mechanisms has also been reported

[103]. Eosinophils may also co-operate with other IgE effector cells such as monocytes/macrophages in tumor clearance, and this has been demonstrated in a number of in vivo studies [97, 104, 105]. The anti-tumoral potential of these potent IgE effector cells is yet to be fully realized. It certainly appears that the cells possess tumor-killing potential in situ, which may further be enhanced by implementation of IgE antibody therapies for cancer.

8.2.4 Natural Killer Cells

As essential effector cells of the innate response, NK cells have been associated with successful defenses in vivo, tumor cell killing capacity ex vivo and better patient prognosis in a number of cancers such as multiple myelomas, breast and non-small cell lung cancers [106–108]. NK cell anti-tumoral activities are also thought to form part of the clinical benefits conferred by therapeutic antibodies such as trastuzumab in breast cancer patients [109]. FcεRI expression has not been detected in NK cells, and IgE-mediated anti-tumoral activities may not be mediated via this receptor. However, NK cells are able to mediate ADCC through engagement of Fc receptors by antibodies; indeed, it has been demonstrated that FcR gamma subunit-deficient mice exhibit loss of phagocytic and ADCC functions, suggesting the potential for antibodies to activate NK cells against cancer cells [110]. NK cells in breast cancer tissues can secrete enhanced levels of IL-4, compared to those secreted by NK cells from patient blood. Increased levels of tumor-associated IL-4 would upregulate CD23b on resident and tumor-infiltrating monocytes/macrophages [111], possibly enhancing their tumor-targeting and killing potential. The potential effects of tumor antigen-specific IgE antibodies on NK cell anti-tumor activities still remain to be elucidated.

8.2.5 Antigen-Presenting Cells

APC such as B lymphocytes, monocytes/macrophages, Langerhans cells and DC in tumor infiltrates express CD23 and/or FcεRI. It has been proposed that one of the immune escape mechanisms of tumor cells is the pathway inducing defective differentiation and maturation of APC, thereby reducing adaptive immune responses against tumor antigens. IL-6 secreted by tumor cells and resident TAMs in tumor microenvironments is thought to inhibit the differentiation of CD34+ cells into mature DC and thus reduce their antigen-presenting capacity. It has also been demonstrated that immature DC can be activated by locally secreted lymphokines in the tumor microenvironments, such as IL-4, IL-13 or IFN-γ; these have been shown to rescue maturation of DCs known to be blocked by tumors [112, 113].

Engagement of IgE with the high-affinity IgE receptor FcεRI on the surface of DC increases the efficiency of antigen uptake and presentation by 100- to 1,000-fold [114]. This may be significant in the context of IgE therapy against tumors,

since even small amounts of IgE on the surface of DCs may be sufficient to lead to an efficient activation of autologous T-cells and thus provoke powerful anti-tumoral adaptive immunity. Furthermore, expression of CD23 has been detected at different stages of DC maturation and CD23 expression has also been detected, albeit at lower levels, under immunosuppressive conditions induced by tumor cells [113]. This suggests that DCs harbor the potential to engage IgE via CD23, leading to antigen presentation. Although the outcome of the antigen presentation depends on the local environment, tumor antigen-specific IgE antibodies may contribute to enhance maturation of DC as well as stimulate effective adaptive immune responses against cancers [115–118].

The role of B lymphocytes in cancer has been controversial. In some in vivo models of colon carcinoma and melanoma, B cells possess tumor growth-promoting functions, possibly through secretion of immunomodulatory cytokines such as IL-6 and IL-10 [119–121]. It is conceivable however, that even within the immunosuppressive environments of tumors, tumor antigen-specific IgE antibodies may tip the balance against tumor growth by exploiting the potent mechanisms of B-cell activation, antigen presentation and induction of adaptive immunity, associated thus far with IgE in allergic diseases and immune responses against parasites.

8.3 Evidence for IgE and Effector Cell-Mediated Anti-Tumoral Responses

Is IgE a possible missing link with potential to "re-educate" immune effector cells against cancer? The benefits of IgE-mediated effector functions against tumor cells have been emerging in a number of in vivo and in vitro systems. Mounting evidence also points at the importance and pivotal role of IgE effector cells in mediating IgE inflammatory responses against tumors and a possible role for IgE in promoting adaptive immunity. Exciting insights into mechanisms of effector cell activation and tumor cell targeting and killing are also being elucidated.

8.3.1 Evidence for PBMC and Monocyte Activities in IgE-Mediated Anti-Tumoral Responses

Tumor killing effector functions mediated by antibodies have been previously evaluated in ADCC assays using human peripheral blood mononuclear cells (PBMC) to target tumor cells. IgE-mediated anti-tumoral effector cell functions have also been studied in similar assays and in some cases in direct comparison to corresponding IgG antibodies. Evidence now suggests that primary monocytes/macrophages and monocytic cells engaged with tumor antigen-specific IgE have the potential to kill tumor cells. We describe what has been learned about PBMC and monocyte/macrophage anti-tumoral activities mediated by IgE.

8.3.2 Chimeric Ovarian Carcinoma Antigen-Specific MOv18 IgE – Efficacy and Effector Cells

The potency of effector functions activated by tumor antigen-specific IgE has been explored in a series of studies on chimeric antibodies (with human constant regions and mouse variable regions) MOv18 IgE and MOv18 IgG1. These antibodies were engineered from the original MOv18 clone against a tumor-specific antigen, folate-binding protein (FBP), expressed in 80% of ovarian cancers. IgE and IgG were compared in two disparate human xenograft models of ovarian carcinoma grown in immunodeficient mice. Treatment with IgE afforded superior protection than the equivalent IgG1 antibodies in both systems [122, 123].

In one human ovarian carcinoma xenograft model, grown subcutaneously in severe combined immunodeficiency (SCID) mice, intravenous treatment of the mice with MOv18 IgE combined with human PBMC, added as effector cells, had a superior and longer-lasting effect in restricting tumor growth than the same treatment with IgG1 [122]. IgE-mediated effects on tumor growth were only observed when antibodies were combined with human PBMC, and as the human Fcε region of the chimeric IgE is not recognized by mouse Fcε receptors, it became apparent that the human IgE effector cells were necessary for the anti-tumoral functions of IgE. Histological examination of tumor sections from mice treated with MOv18 IgE exhibited larger areas of tumor necrosis, compared to controls, further suggesting that anti-tumoral effector cell functions were activated in response to IgE treatment. This study clearly pointed at the potentially superior effector functions of IgE as a cancer therapeutic.

Subsequent studies in a patient-derived human ovarian carcinoma model, grown orthotopically (intraperitoneally) in nude mice, demonstrated that intraperitoneal administration with MOv18 IgE and human PBMC gave significantly greater protection than PBMC alone, while MOv18 IgG1 with human PBMC offered no survival advantage (Fig. 8.2A) [123]. Immunohistochemical studies of tumor sections showed infiltration of human monocytes/macrophages (CD68+) into tumor lesions, while no human macrophage infiltrates were found in tumors from mice treated with human PBMC alone (Fig. 8.3). Monocyte/macrophage infiltration correlated with significantly enhanced survival of mice given tumor antigen-specific IgE. Immunohistochemical studies examining the presence of other human PBMC effector cells in xenograft tumor areas failed to identify any infiltrating (CD3+) T cell, (CD19+ and CD20+) B cell or (CD56+) NK cell populations associated with tumors. These observations suggested that human macrophages may be important IgE effector cells that are recruited by tumor antigen-specific IgE in tumor areas and their presence may contribute to tumor growth arrest in this in vivo model.

More recent studies utilizing the ovarian carcinoma xenograft model confirm a vital role of monocytes as IgE effector cells in anti-folate receptor IgE antibody responses in vivo [43, 44]. Depletion of monocytes from PBMC abrogated the survival advantage conferred by MOv18 IgE, while reconstitution of monocytes in the PBMC treatments restored IgE-mediated enhanced survival of mice (Fig. 8.2B,

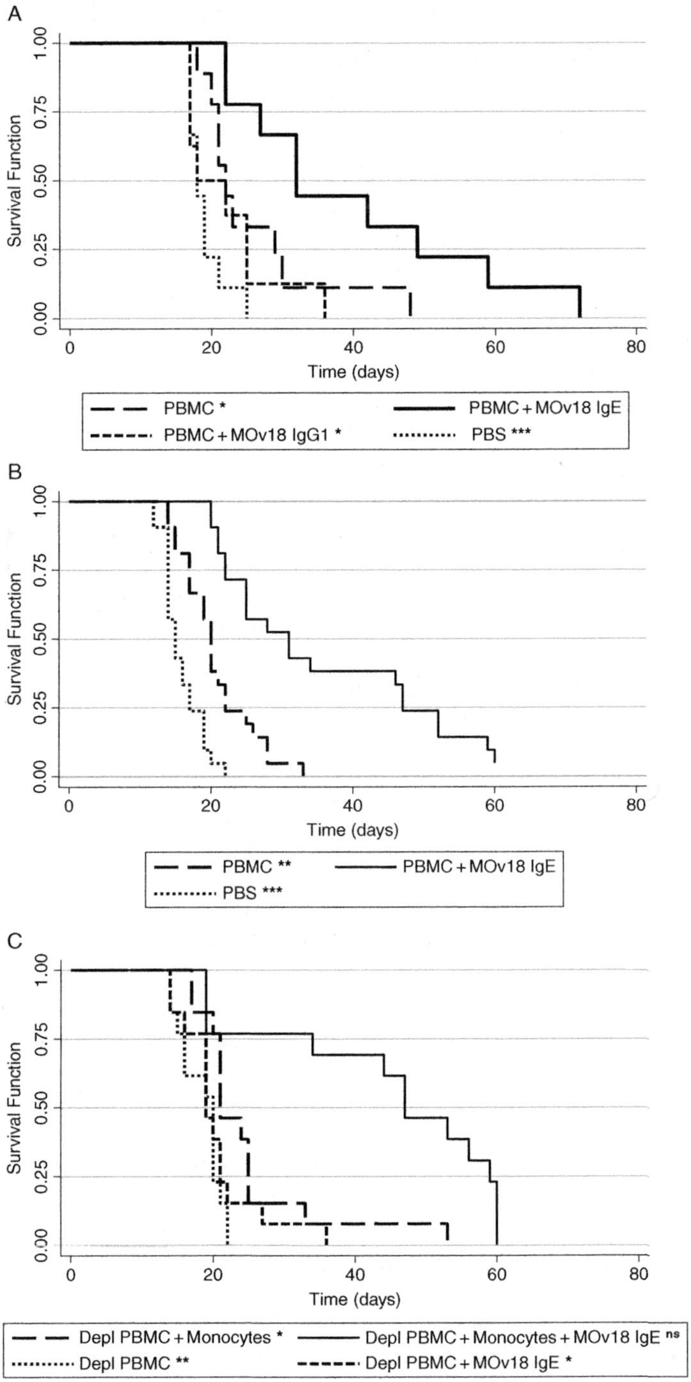

Fig. 8.2 (continued)

8.2C) [44]. In a separate study, U937 monocytic cells, which express FcεRI and low levels of CD23, when administered in combination with MOv18 IgE prolonged the survival of ovarian carcinoma-bearing mice compared to controls [43]. These findings confirmed that monocytes are important effector cells in tumor antigen-specific IgE-mediated responses in vivo.

8.3.3 Lessons on the MOv18 IgE-Mediated Tumor Killing Mechanisms – ADCC

The above data demonstrating tumor infiltration by monocytes and their significant involvement in prolonging survival of tumor-bearing mice were complemented by in vitro assays examining the interactions between monocytes and tumor cells mediated by IgE. A number of these studies not only implicated monocytes as IgE effector cells but also gave valuable insights into the mechanisms of IgE-mediated tumor targeting and killing.

In preliminary in vitro ^{51}Cr-release (ADCC) assays examining MOv18 IgE-mediated effector functions, MOv18 IgG and human PBMC conferred superior ADCC of FBP-expressing IGROV1 ovarian tumor cells compared to those of MOv18 IgE and PBMC [122]. In a subsequent study, using two ADCC assay systems, levels of IgE-mediated ADCC of tumor cells by PBMC were 50% lower compared to those measured with the corresponding IgG1 [123]. These data were in stark contrast to the clear superiority of MOv18 IgE over IgG1 in two human ovarian carcinoma xenograft models in vivo. A number of important findings and insights arose from these observations:

a) Long retention of IgE–FcεRI complexes in tissues: The intrinsic affinity of IgE–FcεRI is at least 10^2 higher than that of IgG–FcγR complexes, reflected in prolonged half-life of IgE (~14 days) in tissues compared to IgG (~2–3 days). This may be translated to recruitment and retention of antibody in tumor areas and may contribute to the superior efficacy of IgE in vivo. The opposite is true

Fig. 8.2 (**A**) Survival of ovarian carcinoma human xenograft-bearing nude mice: survival (days) of nude mice injected with a patient-derived intraperitoneal xenograft is enhanced following treatment with chimeric folate receptor-specific antibody MOv18 IgE together with human PBMC (*solid line*). Survival is plotted for each of nine animals treated as shown. Data from Karagiannis et al. [123]. Copyright Wiley-VCH Verlag GmbH, and Co. KGaA. Reproduced with permission. (**B**) Effect of monocytes and MOv18 IgE antibody on survival of human ovarian carcinoma xenograft-bearing mice. Survival is superior in animals treated with the combination of MOv18 IgE and human PBMC. Survival is plotted for each of 13 animals treated as shown. (**C**) Impaired efficacy using PBMC depleted of monocytes can be salvaged by reconstituting PBMC with monocytes, implying that monocytes are necessary and sufficient for therapeutic IgE-mediated folate receptor targeting. Survival is plotted for each of 21 animals in each group, studied in the same experiment shown in (**B**). Data reproduced with permission from Karagiannis et al. [44]. Significance of values compared with samples given PBMC + MOv18 IgE by the Student's *t* test. n/s, $p > 0.05$; $^{*}p < 0.05$; $^{**}p < 0.005$; $^{***}p < 0.0005$

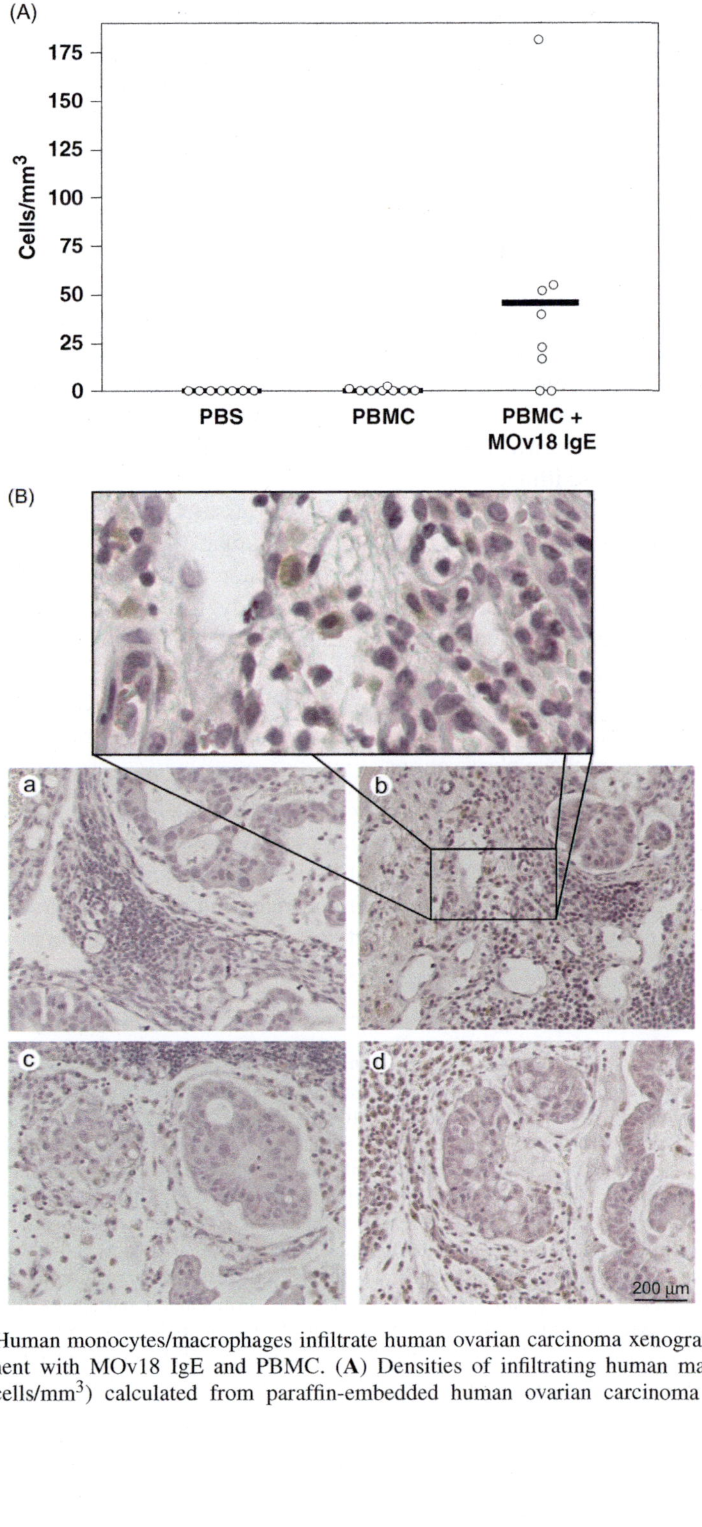

Fig. 8.3 Human monocytes/macrophages infiltrate human ovarian carcinoma xenografts following treatment with MOv18 IgE and PBMC. (**A**) Densities of infiltrating human macrophages (CD68+ cells/mm^3) calculated from paraffin-embedded human ovarian carcinoma xenograft

for IgE in circulation (half-life ~2 days) compared to IgG (~20 days) and may be reflected in the lower tumor killing capacity of IgE compared to IgG in vitro.

b) Effects of Fcε receptor density on tumor killing by monocytes: The nature and density of Fc receptors expressed on the surface of human peripheral blood monocytes were examined. No CD23 expression was detected and the abundance of FcεRI on monocytes (~2,900 molecules/cell) is about 100 times lower than that on mast cells or basophils and 50–100 times lower than that of FcγR receptors on monocytes (~200,000 molecules/cell). FcγRIII is the IgG receptor with the closest homology to FcεRI and is also the Fcγ receptor implicated in IgG ADCC. Despite the 50-fold reduction in abundance of FcεRI than FcγRIII on monocytes, MOv18 IgE was half as active in ADCC as MOv18 IgG1 in vitro [123], and this is most likely due to the high affinity of the IgE–FcεRI interaction.
c) Effect of Fcε receptor occupancy on tumor killing by monocytes: Another significant observation was that human PBMC from allergic donors were less effective than those from non-allergic individuals in mediating IgE ADCC. Studies on occupancy of IgE receptors on monocytes demonstrated that levels of ADCC were proportional to the numbers of free IgE receptors on the surface of monocytes. These findings implicated FcεRI in the mechanism of IgE-mediated tumor killing by ADCC.
d) Role of FcεRI in tumor cell ADCC by monocytes: Purified human monocytes were able to kill tumor cells by ADCC in vitro. Since freshly purified blood monocytes were found to express low levels of FcεRI, but no CD23, this further implicated the high-affinity receptor in IgE tumor death by ADCC.

8.3.4 MOv18 IgE-Mediated Tumor Killing Mechanisms – ADCP

Early microscopical observations of effector–tumor cell interactions gave the first clue of another potential tumor killing mechanism not detected by ADCC assays [123]. Time course examinations of IgE-mediated effects of PBMC–tumor cell contact revealed that tumor cells and monocytes, but not T cells, B cells or NK cells

Fig. 8.3 (continued) sections of nude mice following i.p. tumor transplant and treatment with MOv18 IgE and human PBMC. Horizontal bars indicate the mean values. (**B**) Immunohistological examination of human and mouse macrophage infiltrates in sections of ovarian carcinoma xenografts grown in nude mice treated with MOv18 IgE and human PBMC. Human macrophages were rarely observed in ovarian carcinoma xenografts from mice treated with PBMC alone (**a**) compared with those treated with PBMC and MOv18 IgE (**b**). Human macrophages are mostly seen in stromal areas adjacent to tumor islands (**b**). Mouse macrophages are abundant in stromal areas surrounding tumor as well as in tumor islands whether mice were treated with PBMC alone (**c**) or PBMC and MOv18 IgE (**d**). Figure from Karagiannis et al. [123], copyright Wiley-VCH Verlag GmbH, and Co. KGaA. Reproduced with permission

from PBMC, engaged in physical contact in the presence of MOv18 IgE. Monocyte–tumor cell contact and tumor cell death were observed as early as 20 min in culture and contact was maintained up to 3 h. ADCP of tumor cells by monocytes was evident from 90 min in cultures and always associated with loss of viability and/or membrane integrity of tumor cells.

These observations prompted a series of experiments aimed at measuring ADCP as well as elucidating the mechanisms underlying IgE-mediated ADCP of tumor cells. A new three-color flow cytometric (ADCC/ADCP) assay was developed to simultaneously measure cytotoxicity and phagocytosis of tumor cells (Fig. 8.4) [124]. There were already indications that the high-affinity IgE receptor, FcεRI, mediated ADCC of tumor cells, and further experiments confirmed this function (Fig. 8.5A). There were also enough data to suggest that the low-affinity IgE receptor, CD23b, which can be expressed in response to IL-4 on the surface of monocytes/macrophages, is capable of mediating ADCP and that it mediates IgE effector functions in allergic diseases and parasitic infections. Stimulation of monocytes by IL-4 induces expression of CD23. Expression of CD23 by monocytes enhanced their tumor killing capacity (from 25 to 30% without CD23 to up to 70% tumor cell death in vitro), and this increase in tumor cell death was attributed to tumor cell ADCP (Fig. 8.5B). Microscopical observations confirmed these findings and demonstrated that induction of CD23 expression resulted in enhanced monocyte–tumor cell contact and extensive phagocytosis of tumor cell material, which validates the findings of the ADCC/ADCP assays and the role of CD23 in tumor cell killing by ADCP [44]. A further hint of an anti-tumoral role for CD23 in vivo was provided by evidence that enhanced CD23 expression on the surface of monocytic cells in combination with MOv18 IgE was associated with increased

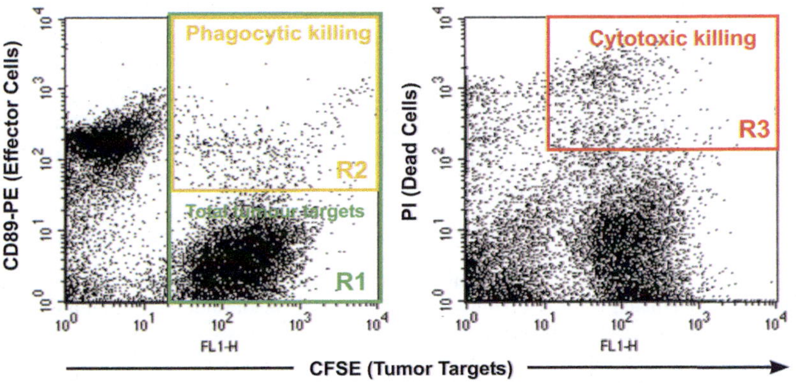

Fig. 8.4 A three-color flow cytometric assay can simultaneously measure ADCC and ADCP of tumor cells by effector cells. Dot plots of mixed monocyte effector and IGROV1 ovarian tumor target cells from which calculations were made. Region 1 (R1) represents total $CFSE^+$ tumor cell targets. Region 2 (R2) depicts the $CFSE^+$ tumor cells present within PE-stained monocytes ($CFSE^+/PE^+$), depicting ADCP. Region 3 (R3) contains tumor cells killed externally by effector cells (ADCC) ($CFSE^+/PI^+$). Data reproduced with permission from Karagiannis et al. [44].

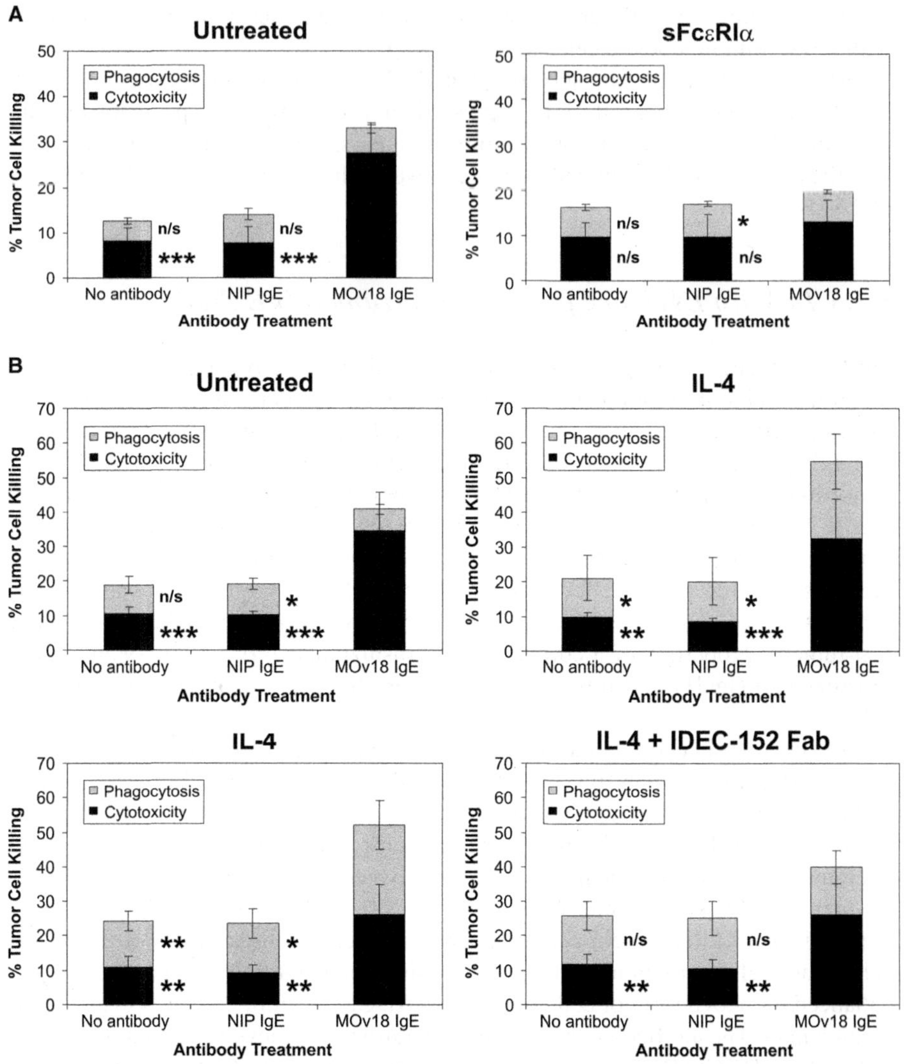

Fig. 8.5 (**A**) Monocytes can be activated by MOv18 IgE to kill tumor cells in vitro. The addition of MOv18 IgE to monocytes and IGROV1 tumor cells results in increased ADCC, compared to background levels measured with hapten-specific antibody (NIP IgE) or with no antibody controls (*left*). Blocking of MOv18 IgE binding to the IgE receptor, FcεRI, with soluble IgE receptor, correlated with loss of IgE-mediated killing of tumor cells (*right*). (**B**) CD23 role in MOv18 IgE-mediated ADCP of ovarian tumor cells. MOv18 IgE-mediated killing of IGROV1 tumor cells by untreated (*top left*) monocytes results in cytotoxic killing of tumor cells. Stimulation of monocytes with IL-4 enhanced the expression of CD23 (*top right*) and resulted in enhanced tumor killing capacity and killing by ADCP. ADCP killing of tumor cells by IL-4-stimulated primary monocytes (*bottom left*) was blocked by an anti-CD23 antibody Fab (*bottom right*), confirming a role for CD23 in tumor cell killing by ADCP. ADCC, *black bars*; ADCP, *gray bars*. Results shown are means ± SD of six independent experiments. Significance of values compared with samples given MOv18 IgE by the Student's *t* test. n/s, $p > 0.05$; $^{*}p < 0.05$; $^{**}\ p < 0.005$; $^{***}p < 0.0005$. Reproduced with permission from Karagiannis et al. [44].

survival of human ovarian carcinoma xenograft-bearing mice compared to treatment with CD23-dim monocytic cells and MOv18 IgE .

From the volume of data showing that CD23-expressing monocytic cells accumulate in tumors where IL-4 is expressed, it is tempting to speculate that the "missing signal" in the form of a tumor antigen-specific IgE antibody may activate these cells to kill tumor cells and help reverse the tumor growth-promoting role of TAMs.

8.3.5 *In Vitro Evidence from a Trastuzumab IgE Study*

Further evidence that IgE antibodies are capable of activating monocytic cells to target and kill tumor cells was presented in a recent study examining the functional properties of an engineered IgE homologue to trastuzumab (trastuzumab-like IgE) against the human epidermal growth factor receptor 2 (HER2/neu), a tumor-associated antigen expressed in approximately 30% of breast carcinomas [125]. Trastuzumab (Herceptin®), a humanized IgG1, is the main antibody in clinical use for the treatment of early and metastatic breast cancers. Based on previous research on the effects of the chimeric MOv18 IgE in activating effector cells to kill tumors, and the clinical efficacy of trastuzumab, the potential anti-tumoral properties of a corresponding trastuzumab IgE merited examination. Trastuzumab (IgG1) and trastuzumab IgE were therefore compared in functional assays.

Trastuzumab-like IgE retained the well-characterized tumor cell growth arrest properties of trastuzumab (IgG1), independently of effector cells. Both trastuzumab and trastuzumab-like IgE could activate monocytic cells to kill tumor cells, and the levels of tumor death mediated by each antibody were comparable. However, they operated by different mechanisms: trastuzumab mediated tumor cell ADCP, whereas trastuzumab IgE killed tumor cells by ADCC after 2.5 h in culture. These distinct mechanisms of killing were confirmed by microscopic observations of monocytic cell–tumor cell interactions. Addition of trastuzumab and trastuzumab IgE induced enhanced monocytic-tumor cell contact, and ADCP of tumor cells was evident with trastuzumab. The antibody concentrations required to achieve maximum tumor cell killing by ADCC/ADCP were the same for trastuzumab (IgG1) and trastuzumab-like IgE in these assays. Trastuzumab-like IgE concentrations required for killing of breast cancer cells by effector cells were also 10-fold lower than the optimum found for MOv18 IgE killing of ovarian tumor cells in the same in vitro assay system. This implies that lower levels of trastuzumab-like IgE, compared to MOv18 IgE, may be required to achieve in vivo tumor growth arrest. In vitro tumor cell viability assays confirmed that like trastuzumab, trastuzumab-like IgE without effector cells can also mediate tumor growth arrest after 24 and 48 h in culture, suggesting that trastuzumab-like IgE retains the ability to block vital tumor cell growth signals through engagement of the HER2/neu receptor.

As trastuzumab-like IgE functioned with similar potency, but through mechanisms different from those of trastuzumab (IgG1), in vivo studies in clinically

relevant tumor models may help further elucidate efficacy and effector cell functions of IgE therapies against breast cancer. Furthermore, in light of different effector cell mechanisms potentiated by each antibody, examining whether a combination of trastuzumab and trastuzumab IgE could have potential synergistic anti-tumor effects is warranted.

8.3.6 Experimental Evidence Supporting Stimulation of Mast Cells, Basophils and Eosinophils by IgE

Mast cells are well-known activators and perpetrators of IgE responses in allergic diseases. Emerging evidence suggests that these powerful immunostimulatory effector cells can also become activated in response to tumor antigen-specific IgE. Human peripheral blood basophils release histamine in response to engagement of surface FcεRI with a chimeric antibody MOv18 IgE against the ovarian carcinoma antigen FBP when cross-linked by either polyclonal antibodies or FBP-expressing tumor cells [122]. In vitro microscopical studies of human PBMC incubated with FBP-expressing ovarian carcinoma cells and MOv18 IgE demonstrated basophils in frequent contact with tumor cells, engaging in targeted exocytosis of basophil granule contents [123]. This observation was significant as basophils are rare (less than 2%) in PBMC populations and the expected ratio of basophil effector : tumor target cell would be less than 1:1. This suggested that tumor antigen-specific IgE can recruit and activate basophils to contact and target antigen-expressing tumor cells. Recent studies of an engineered trastuzumab-like IgE antibody against the human breast cancer antigen HER2/neu demonstrated that trastuzumab IgE–FcεRI complexes on the surface of mast cells can be cross-linked by HER2/neu-expressing tumor cells to trigger mast cell degranulation in an antigen-specific manner [125].

These data are in agreement with growing evidence in favor of possible anti-tumoral functions of mast cells and basophils in vivo [126, 127] (see Noelle R., Chapter 6). It is tempting to speculate that these powerful IgE effector cells can be primed by tumor antigen-specific IgE antibodies to activate downstream immune responses against cancer cells; these responses may resemble inflammatory mechanisms well known in allergic diseases and parasitic infections.

A role for eosinophils as effector cells in IgE-mediated tumor targeting and killing has also been demonstrated [44, 128] (see Parish C., Chapter 11). In an in vitro assay examining the functions of the chimeric MOv18 IgE antibody specific for the ovarian carcinoma antigen FBP (MOv18 IgE), it was demonstrated that IgE could activate blood eosinophils to specifically kill tumor cells by ADCC in vitro; light and fluorescent microscopical observations revealed degranulating eosinophils associated with tumor cells in response to treatment with MOv18 IgE leading to tumor cell death (Fig. 8.6) [44]. In agreement, evidence by ADCC and proliferation studies using spleen-derived T lymphocytes from IgE-inoculated mice as effector cells confirmed the tumor cell killing (ADCC) capacity of cytotoxic T cells and

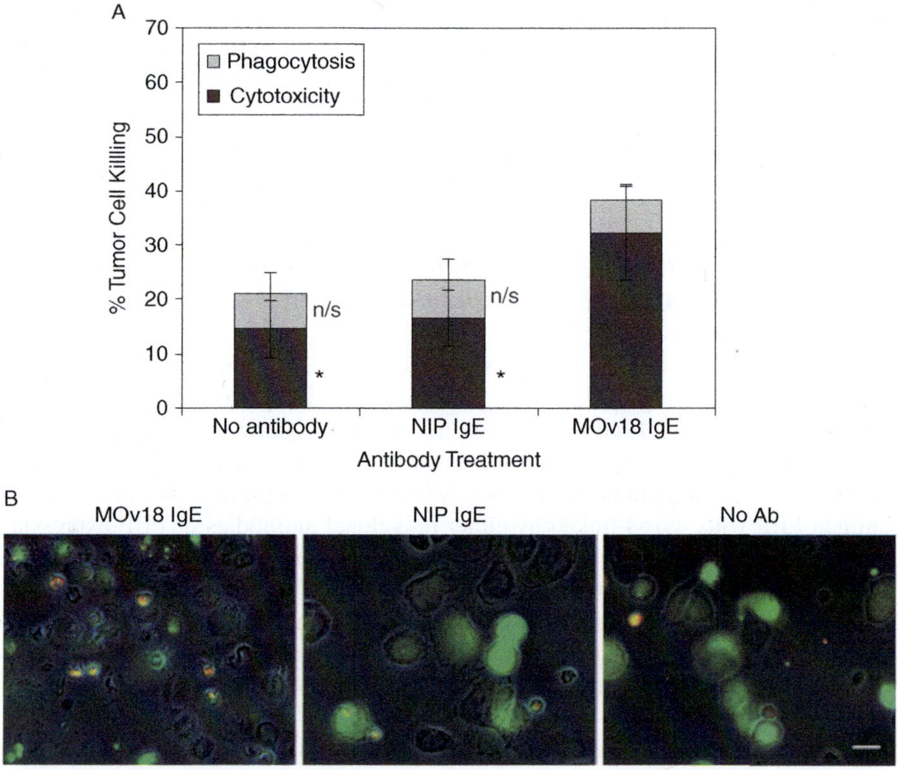

Fig. 8.6 Anti-folate-receptor antibody MOv18 IgE can activate human eosinophils to kill tumor cells. (**A**) MOv18 IgE-mediated ovarian carcinoma IGROV1 cell killing of tumor cells by primary eosinophils. ADCC, *black bars*; ADCP, *gray bars*. Results are means ± SD of four independent experiments. Significance was compared with samples given MOv18 IgE by the Student's *t* test. n/s, $p > 0.05$; $^{*}p < 0.05$; $^{**}p < 0.005$; $^{***}p < 0.0005$. (**B**) Superimposed bright-field and fluorescent images of IGROV1–eosinophil interactions. CFSE-stained IGROV1 tumor cells (*green*) and CD49d-PE-labeled eosinophils (*red*) were incubated with IgE antibodies for 2.5 h. Treatment with MOv18 IgE resulted in frequent contact between eosinophils and tumor cells; tumor cell destruction was evident (*left*). Eosinophil-IGROV1 cell contact was observed less frequently in samples given control NIP IgE (*middle*) or no antibody (*right*). Original magnification, ×400. Scale bars, 20 μm. Reproduced with permission from Karagiannis et al. [44]

proliferative capacity of spleen-derived CD4+ T cells following antigenic tumor peptide stimuli. Eosinophil depletion eliminated IgE-mediated tumor growth arrest, suggesting induction of IgE-induced anti-tumoral immunological and inflammatory responses [128] (see Vangelista L. and Siccardi A., Chapter 9).

It appears, therefore, that the ingredients for the induction of an IgE-mediated response characteristic of allergic or inflammatory diseases are in place in human malignant diseases. These come in the form of resident and infiltrating mast cells and eosinophils in tumor regions and their capacity to induce potent inflammatory responses by IgE-mediated engagement of tumor cells in situ.

8.3.7 IgEs Against Pancreatic Cancer – A Case for Patient-Derived IgE Antibodies and Their Effector Functions

The presence of IgE antibodies in patients with pancreatic cancer and their tumor cell killing potential was investigated in a recent report, giving value to IgE as a potential therapeutic approach and confirming that naturally expressed IgE antibodies possess the ability to stimulate effector cells to kill cancer cells [129]. Fu et al. demonstrated that IgE and levels of soluble CD23 were uniquely elevated in pancreatic cancer patient sera, while levels of other immunoglobulin classes did not differ between patient and control groups. Pancreatic patient serum IgEs, but not IgEs from normal blood sera, could recognize a 50-kDa unidentified tumor antigen in pancreatic tumor cell lysates. Importantly, IgEs purified from patient sera killed pancreatic tumor cells only when combined with human PBMC in ADCC assays.

The presence of sCD23 in patient sera was not further examined in this report and levels of IgE and sCD23 were not correlated to clinical outcomes for the patients, but further examination of the role of sCD23 in IgE-mediated tumor cell killing may provide vital clues of how IgE effector functions are modulated in cancer patients. Finally, this study raises the potential that patient-derived tumor antigen-specific IgEs can direct inflammatory and immune cells against tumor cells and may be considered as future cancer therapeutics.

8.4 Conclusion

The mechanisms by which IgE antibodies exert their anti-tumor effects against cancer cells are now starting to emerge. IgE antibodies can engage both cell surface IgE receptors, FcεRI and CD23, and activate several lines of effector cells against tumor cells in vitro and in vivo employing a range of anti-tumoral activities. Research into the anti-tumoral functions of IgE antibodies demonstrate that the tumor-promoting roles of inflammatory cells in cancer may not be their only anticipated fate and that the fine balance between tumor growth-inducing inflammation and tumor targeting may be redressed in cancer therapy by IgE antibodies. Monocytes/macrophages, eosinophils, mast cells and basophils, either resident in tumor areas or recruited from the circulation, may be directed by tumor antigen-specific IgE antibodies to contribute to potent anti-tumoral responses. IgE may also activate APC to stimulate adaptive immune responses; these mechanisms still remain to be elucidated.

A number of biological/immunological questions facing the research community in the cancer immunology arena remain: (a) What are the immunological signals that down-regulate effective IgE immune responses against tumor cells in cancer and which parts of these networks may be amenable to therapeutic interventions? (b) Could IgE antibodies, and their Fcε receptors, either in their membrane-bound or soluble forms (such as various fragments of sCD23) be used as biomarkers in malignancies and could their presence have diagnostic or prognostic value? (c) What

are the effector cell mechanisms/pathways that will determine/predict the efficacy of IgE antibodies as cancer therapeutics? (d) What are the pivotal model systems that will predict the safety of cancer-specific IgE antibodies for clinical applications? (e) IgEs against tumor antigens have shown considerable promise for cancer therapy in various in vitro and in vivo systems. The question still remains whether antibodies of the IgE class can fulfill their potential in translational medicine and help us win the battle against cancer.

Acknowledgments The authors acknowledge financial support from the Department of Health via the National Institute for Health Research (NIHR) comprehensive Biomedical Research Centre award to Guy's, and St Thomas' NHS Foundation Trust in partnership with King's College London and King's College Hospital NHS Foundation Trust. The authors thank Dr. James Spicer for his support and helpful comments, Professor Andrew P. Grieve for advice on statistical evaluations and Dr. Rebecca Beavil and Ms. Kate Kirwan for expert assistance with the figures.

References

1. Gould HJ, Sutton BJ, Beavil AJ, Beavil RL, McCloskey N, Coker HA, Fear D, and Smurthwaite L (2003) The biology of IGE and the basis of allergic disease. *Annu Rev Immunol* 21, 579–628
2. Zhang M, Murphy RF, and Agrawal DK (2007) Decoding IgE Fc receptors. *Immunol Res* 37, 1–16
3. Liu FT, Hsu DK, Zuberi RI, Hill PN, Shenhav A, Kuwabara I, and Chen SS (1996) Modulation of functional properties of galectin-3 by monoclonal antibodies binding to the non-lectin domains. *Biochemistry* 35, 6073–6079
4. Ravetch JV and Kinet JP (1991) Fc receptors. *Annu Rev Immunol* 9, 457–492
5. Gounni AS, Lamkhioued B, Delaporte E, Dubost A, Kinet JP, Capron A, and Capron M (1994) The high-affinity IgE receptor on eosinophils: from allergy to parasites or from parasites to allergy? *J Allergy Clin Immunol* 94, 1214–1216
6. Gounni AS, Lamkhioued B, Ochiai K, Tanaka Y, Delaporte E, Capron A, Kinet JP, and Capron M (1994) High-affinity IgE receptor on eosinophils is involved in defence against parasites. *Nature* 367, 183–186
7. Sihra BS, Kon OM, Grant JA, and Kay AB (1997) Expression of high-affinity IgE receptors (Fc epsilon RI) on peripheral blood basophils, monocytes, and eosinophils in atopic and nonatopic subjects: relationship to total serum IgE concentrations. *J Allergy Clin Immunol* 99, 699–706
8. Ying S, Barata LT, Meng Q, Grant JA, Barkans J, Durham SR, and Kay AB (1998) High-affinity immunoglobulin E receptor (Fc epsilon RI)-bearing eosinophils, mast cells, macrophages and Langerhans' cells in allergen-induced late-phase cutaneous reactions in atopic subjects. *Immunology* 93, 281–288
9. Wang B, Rieger A, Kilgus O, Ochiai K, Maurer D, Fodinger D, Kinet JP, and Stingl G (1992) Epidermal Langerhans cells from normal human skin bind monomeric IgE via Fc epsilon RI. *J Exp Med* 175, 1353–1365
10. Bieber T, de la Salle H, Wollenberg A, Hakimi J, Chizzonite R, Ring J, Hanau D, and de la Salle C (1992) Human epidermal Langerhans cells express the high affinity receptor for immunoglobulin E (Fc epsilon RI). *J Exp Med* 175, 1285–1290
11. Maurer D, Fiebiger S, Ebner C, Reininger B, Fischer GF, Wichlas S, Jouvin MH, Schmitt-Egenolf M, Kraft D, Kinet JP, and Stingl G (1996) Peripheral blood dendritic cells express Fc epsilon RI as a complex composed of Fc epsilon RI alpha- and Fc epsilon RI gamma-chains and can use this receptor for IgE-mediated allergen presentation. *J Immunol* 157, 607–616

12. Maurer D, Fiebiger E, Reininger B, Wolff-Winiski B, Jouvin MH, Kilgus O, Kinet JP, and Stingl G (1994) Expression of functional high affinity immunoglobulin E receptors (Fc epsilon RI) on monocytes of atopic individuals. *J Exp Med* 179, 745–750
13. Scholl PR and Geha RS (1993) Physical association between the high-affinity IgG receptor (Fc gamma RI) and the gamma subunit of the high-affinity IgE receptor (Fc epsilon RI gamma). *Proc Natl Acad Sci USA* 90, 8847–8850
14. Morton HC, van den Herik-Oudijk IE, Vossebeld P, Snijders A, Verhoeven AJ, Capel PJ, and van de Winkel JG (1995) Functional association between the human myeloid immunoglobulin A Fc receptor (CD89) and FcR gamma chain. Molecular basis for CD89/FcR gamma chain association. *J Biol Chem* 270, 29781–29787
15. Kinet JP (1999) The high-affinity IgE receptor (Fc epsilon RI): from physiology to pathology. *Annu Rev Immunol* 17, 931–972
16. Kraft S and Kinet JP (2007) New developments in FcepsilonRI regulation, function and inhibition. *Nat Rev Immunol* 7, 365–378
17. Dombrowicz D, Lin S, Flamand V, Brini AT, Koller BH, and Kinet JP (1998) Allergy-associated FcRbeta is a molecular amplifier of IgE- and IgG-mediated in vivo responses. *Immunity* 8, 571–529
18. Lin S, Cicala C, Scharenberg AM, and Kinet JP (1996) The Fc(epsilon)RIbeta subunit functions as an amplifier of Fc(epsilon)RIgamma-mediated cell activation signals. *Cell* 85, 985–995
19. Donnadieu E, Jouvin MH, and Kinet JP (2000) A second amplifier function for the allergy-associated Fc(epsilon)RI-beta subunit. *Immunity* 12, 515–523
20. Kraft S, Rana S, Jouvin MH, and Kinet JP (2004) The role of the FcepsilonRI beta-chain in allergic diseases. *Int Arch Allergy Immunol* 135, 62–72
21. Maenaka K, van der Merwe PA, Stuart DI, Jones EY, and Sondermann P (2001) The human low affinity Fcgamma receptors IIa, IIb, and III bind IgG with fast kinetics and distinct thermodynamic properties. *J Biol Chem* 276, 44898–44904
22. Matsuda H, Fukui K, Kiso Y, and Kitamura Y (1985) Inability of genetically mast cell-deficient W/Wv mice to acquire resistance against larval Haemaphysalis longicornis ticks. *J Parasitol* 71, 443–448
23. Matsuda H, Nakano T, Kiso Y, and Kitamura Y (1987) Normalization of anti-tick response of mast cell-deficient W/Wv mice by intracutaneous injection of cultured mast cells. *J Parasitol* 73, 155–160
24. Matsuda H, Watanabe N, Kiso Y, Hirota S, Ushio H, Kannan Y, Azuma M, Koyama H, and Kitamura Y (1990) Necessity of IgE antibodies and mast cells for manifestation of resistance against larval Haemaphysalis longicornis ticks in mice. *J Immunol* 144, 259–262
25. Gould HJ and Sutton BJ (2008) IgE in allergy and asthma today. *Nat Rev Immunol* 8, 205–217
26. Tokuyama H, Hagi T, Mattarollo SR, Morley J, Wang Q, Fai-So H, Moriyasu F, Nieda M, and Nicol AJ (2008) V gamma 9 V delta 2 T cell cytotoxicity against tumor cells is enhanced by monoclonal antibody drugs–rituximab and trastuzumab. *Int J Cancer* 122, 2526–2534
27. Clynes RA, Towers TL, Presta LG, and Ravetch JV (2000) Inhibitory Fc receptors modulate in vivo cytoxicity against tumor targets. *Nat Med* 6, 443–446
28. Dyall R, Vasovic LV, Clynes RA, and Nikolic-Zugic J (1999) Cellular requirements for the monoclonal antibody-mediated eradication of an established solid tumor. *Eur J Immunol* 29, 30–37
29. Munn DH, McBride M, and Cheung NK (1991) Role of low-affinity Fc receptors in antibody-dependent tumor cell phagocytosis by human monocyte-derived macrophages. *Cancer Res* 51, 1117–1123
30. Kudo T, Suzuki M, Katayose Y, Shinoda M, Sakurai N, Kodama H, Ichiyama M, Takemura S, Yoshida H, Saeki H, Saijyo S, Takahashi J, Tominaga T, and Matsuno S (1999) Specific targeting immunotherapy of cancer with bispecific antibodies. *Tohoku J Exp Med* 188, 275–288

31. Rouard H, Tamasdan S, Moncuit J, Moutel S, Michon J, Fridman WH, and Teillaud JL (1997) Fc receptors as targets for immunotherapy. *Int Rev Immunol* 16, 147–185
32. Watanabe M, Wallace PK, Keler T, Deo YM, Akewanlop C, and Hayes DF (1999) Antibody dependent cellular phagocytosis (ADCP) and antibody dependent cellular cytotoxicity (ADCC) of breast cancer cells mediated by bispecific antibody, MDX-210. *Breast Cancer Res Treat* 53, 199–207
33. Bevaart L, Goldstein J, Vitale L, Russoniello C, Treml J, Zhang J, Graziano RF, Leusen JH, van de Winkel JG, and Keler T (2006) Direct targeting of genetically modified tumour cells to Fc gammaRI triggers potent tumour cytotoxicity. *Br J Haematol* 132, 317–325
34. Yokota A, Kikutani H, Tanaka T, Sato R, Barsumian EL, Suemura M, and Kishimoto T (1988) Two species of human Fc epsilon receptor II (Fc epsilon RII/CD23): tissue-specific and IL-4-specific regulation of gene expression. *Cell* 55, 611–618
35. Yokota A, Yukawa K, Yamamoto A, Sugiyama K, Suemura M, Tashiro Y, Kishimoto T, and Kikutani H (1992) Two forms of the low-affinity Fc receptor for IgE differentially mediate endocytosis and phagocytosis: identification of the critical cytoplasmic domains. *Proc Natl Acad Sci USA* 89, 5030–5034
36. Mossalayi MD, Paul-Eugene N, Ouaaz F, Arock M, Kolb JP, Kilchherr E, Debre P, and Dugas B (1994) Involvement of Fc epsilon RII/CD23 and L-arginine-dependent pathway in IgE-mediated stimulation of human monocyte functions. *Int Immunol* 6, 931–934
37. Paul-Eugene N, Mossalayi D, Sarfati M, Yamaoka K, Aubry JP, Bonnefoy JY, Dugas B, and Kolb JP (1995) Evidence for a role of Fc epsilon RII/CD23 in the IL-4-induced nitric oxide production by normal human mononuclear phagocytes. *Cell Immunol* 163, 314–318
38. Mossalayi MD, Arock M, Mazier D, Vincendeau P, and Vouldoukis I (1999) The human immune response during cutaneous leishmaniasis: NO problem. *Parasitol Today* 15, 342–345
39. Vouldoukis I, Riveros-Moreno V, Dugas B, Ouaaz F, Becherel P, Debre P, Moncada S, and Mossalayi MD (1995) The killing of Leishmania major by human macrophages is mediated by nitric oxide induced after ligation of the Fc epsilon RII/CD23 surface antigen. *Proc Natl Acad Sci USA* 92, 7804–7808
40. Spittler A, Oehler R, Goetzinger P, Holzer S, Reissner CM, Leutmezer F, Rath V, Wrba F, Fuegger R, Boltz-Nitulescu G, and Roth E (1997) Low glutamine concentrations induce phenotypical and functional differentiation of U937 myelomonocytic cells. *J Nutr* 127, 2151–2157
41. Schoppmann SF, Birner P, Stockl J, Kalt R, Ullrich R, Caucig C, Kriehuber E, Nagy K, Alitalo K, and Kerjaschki D (2002) Tumor-associated macrophages express lymphatic endothelial growth factors and are related to peritumoral lymphangiogenesis. *Am J Pathol* 161, 947–956
42. Saka B, Aktan M, Sami U, Oner D, Sanem O, and Dincol G (2006) Prognostic importance of soluble CD23 in B-cell chronic lymphocytic leukemia. *Clin Lab Haematol* 28, 30–35
43. Karagiannis SN, Bracher MG, Beavil RL, Beavil AJ, Hunt J, McCloskey N, Thompson RG, East N, Burke F, Sutton BJ, Dombrowicz D, Balkwill FR, and Gould HJ (2008) Role of IgE receptors in IgE antibody-dependent cytotoxicity and phagocytosis of ovarian tumor cells by human monocytic cells. *Cancer Immunol Immunother* 57, 247–263
44. Karagiannis SN, Bracher MG, Hunt J, McCloskey N, Beavil RL, Beavil AJ, Fear DJ, Thompson RG, East N, Burke F, Moore RJ, Dombrowicz DD, Balkwill FR, and Gould HJ (2007) IgE-antibody-dependent immunotherapy of solid tumors: cytotoxic and phagocytic mechanisms of eradication of ovarian cancer cells. *J Immunol* 179, 2832–2843
45. Liu FT (2005) Regulatory roles of galectins in the immune response. *Int Arch Allergy Immunol* 136, 385–400
46. Frigeri LG and Liu FT (1992) Surface expression of functional IgE binding protein, an endogenous lectin, on mast cells and macrophages. *J Immunol* 148, 861–867
47. Zuberi RI, Hsu DK, Kalayci O, Chen HY, Sheldon HK, Yu L, Apgar JR, Kawakami T, Lilly CM, and Liu FT (2004) Critical role for galectin-3 in airway inflammation

and bronchial hyperresponsiveness in a murine model of asthma. *Am J Pathol* 165, 2045–2053

48. Ahmad N, Gabius HJ, Andre S, Kaltner H, Sabesan S, Roy R, Liu B, Macaluso F, and Brewer CF (2004) Galectin-3 precipitates as a pentamer with synthetic multivalent carbohydrates and forms heterogeneous cross-linked complexes. *J Biol Chem* 279, 10841–10847
49. van den Brule F, Califice S, and Castronovo V (2004) Expression of galectins in cancer: a critical review. *Glycoconj J* 19, 537–542
50. Brigati C, Noonan DM, Albini A, and Benelli R (2002) Tumors and inflammatory infiltrates: friends or foes? *Clin Exp Metastasis* 19, 247–258
51. Lin EY and Pollard JW (2004) Role of infiltrated leucocytes in tumour growth and spread. *Br J Cancer* 90, 2053–2058
52. Crivellato E, Nico B, and Ribatti D (2008) Mast cells and tumour angiogenesis: new insight from experimental carcinogenesis. *Cancer Lett* 269, 1–6
53. Dabiri S, Huntsman D, Makretsov N, Cheang M, Gilks B, Bajdik C, Gelmon K, Chia S, and Hayes M (2004) The presence of stromal mast cells identifies a subset of invasive breast cancers with a favorable prognosis. *Mod Pathol* 17, 690–695
54. Aaltomaa S, Lipponen P, Papinaho S, and Kosma VM (1993) Mast cells in breast cancer. *Anticancer Res* 13, 785–788
55. Glimelius I, Edstrom A, Fischer M, Nilsson G, Sundstrom C, Molin D, Amini RM, and Enblad G (2005) Angiogenesis and mast cells in Hodgkin lymphoma. *Leukemia* 19, 2360–2362
56. Molin D, Edstrom A, Glimelius I, Glimelius B, Nilsson G, Sundstrom C, and Enblad G (2002) Mast cell infiltration correlates with poor prognosis in Hodgkin's lymphoma. *Br J Haematol* 119, 122–124
57. Ribatti D, Ennas MG, Vacca A, Ferreli F, Nico B, Orru S, and Sirigu P (2003) Tumor vascularity and tryptase-positive mast cells correlate with a poor prognosis in melanoma. *Eur J Clin Invest* 33, 420–425
58. Ribatti D, Finato N, Crivellato E, Guidolin D, Longo V, Mangieri D, Nico B, Vacca A, and Beltrami CA (2007) Angiogenesis and mast cells in human breast cancer sentinel lymph nodes with and without micrometastases. *Histopathology* 51, 837–842
59. Kankkunen JP, Harvima IT, and Naukkarinen A (1997) Quantitative analysis of tryptase and chymase containing mast cells in benign and malignant breast lesions. *Int J Cancer* 72, 385–388
60. Thoresen S, Thorsen T, and Hartveit F (1982) Does progesterone receptor in human breast cancer reflect the mast-cell content of the tumour tissue? *Br J Cancer* 45, 618–620
61. Ribatti D, Crivellato E, Roccaro AM, Ria R, and Vacca A (2004) Mast cell contribution to angiogenesis related to tumour progression. *Clin Exp Allergy* 34, 1660–1664
62. Norrby K (2000) Oral administration of a nitric oxide synthase inhibitor enhances de novo mammalian angiogenesis mediated by TNF-alpha, saline and mast-cell secretion. *APMIS* 108, 496–502
63. Grutzkau A, Kruger-Krasagakes S, Kogel H, Moller A, Lippert U, and Henz BM (1997) Detection of intracellular interleukin-8 in human mast cells: flow cytometry as a guide for immunoelectron microscopy. *J Histochem Cytochem* 45, 935–945
64. Grutzkau A, Kruger-Krasagakes S, Baumeister H, Schwarz C, Kogel H, Welker P, Lippert U, Henz BM, and Moller A (1998) Synthesis, storage, and release of vascular endothelial growth factor/vascular permeability factor (VEGF/VPF) by human mast cells: implications for the biological significance of VEGF206. *Mol Biol Cell* 9, 875–884
65. Qu Z, Liebler JM, Powers MR, Galey T, Ahmadi P, Huang XN, Ansel JC, Butterfield JH, Planck SR, and Rosenbaum JT (1995) Mast cells are a major source of basic fibroblast growth factor in chronic inflammation and cutaneous hemangioma. *Am J Pathol* 147, 564–573
66. Blair RJ, Meng H, Marchese MJ, Ren S, Schwartz LB, Tonnesen MG, and Gruber BL (1997) Human mast cells stimulate vascular tube formation. Tryptase is a novel, potent angiogenic factor. *J Clin Invest* 99, 2691–2700

67. Crivellato E, Beltrami CA, Mallardi F, and Ribatti D (2004) The mast cell: an active participant or an innocent bystander? *Histol Histopathol* 19, 259–270
68. Valent P, Agis H, Sperr W, Sillaber C, and Horny HP (2008) Diagnostic and prognostic value of new biochemical and immunohistochemical parameters in chronic myeloid leukemia. *Leuk Lymphoma* 49, 635–638
69. Di Carlo E, Modesti A, Coletti A, Colombo MP, Giovarelli M, Forni G, Diodoro MG, and Musiani P (1998) Interaction between endothelial cells and the secreted cytokine drives the fate of an IL4- or an IL5-transduced tumour. *J Pathol* 186, 390–397
70. Leek RD, Lewis CE, Whitehouse R, Greenall M, Clarke J, and Harris AL (1996) Association of macrophage infiltration with angiogenesis and prognosis in invasive breast carcinoma. *Cancer Res* 56, 4625–4629
71. Lewis CE and Pollard JW (2006) Distinct role of macrophages in different tumor microenvironments. *Cancer Res* 66, 605–612
72. Bingle L, Brown NJ, and Lewis CE (2002) The role of tumour-associated macrophages in tumour progression: implications for new anticancer therapies. *J Pathol* 196, 254–265
73. Mantovani A, Sozzani S, Locati M, Allavena P, and Sica A (2002) Macrophage polarization: tumor-associated macrophages as a paradigm for polarized M2 mononuclear phagocytes. *Trends Immunol* 23, 549–555
74. Leek RD and Harris AL (2002) Tumor-associated macrophages in breast cancer. *J Mammary Gland Biol Neoplasia* 7, 177–189
75. Elgert KD, Alleva DG, and Mullins DW (1998) Tumor-induced immune dysfunction: the macrophage connection. *J Leukoc Biol* 64, 275–290
76. Weigert A and Brune B (2008) Nitric oxide, apoptosis and macrophage polarization during tumor progression. *Nitric Oxide* 19, 95–102
77. Keller R, Geiges M, and Keist R (1990) L-arginine-dependent reactive nitrogen intermediates as mediators of tumor cell killing by activated macrophages. *Cancer Res* 50, 1421–1425
78. Xie K, Huang S, Dong Z, Juang SH, Gutman M, Xie QW, Nathan C, and Fidler IJ (1995) Transfection with the inducible nitric oxide synthase gene suppresses tumorigenicity and abrogates metastasis by K-1735 murine melanoma cells. *J Exp Med* 181, 1333–1343
79. Masztalerz A, Van Rooijen N, Den Otter W, and Everse LA (2003) Mechanisms of macrophage cytotoxicity in IL-2 and IL-12 mediated tumour regression. *Cancer Immunol Immunother* 52, 235–242
80. Dirkx AE, Oude Egbrink MG, Wagstaff J, and Griffioen AW (2006) Monocyte/macrophage infiltration in tumors: modulators of angiogenesis. *J Leukoc Biol* 80, 1183–1196
81. Houghton AM, Grisolano JL, Baumann ML, Kobayashi DK, Hautamaki RD, Nehring LC, Cornelius LA, and Shapiro SD (2006) Macrophage elastase (matrix metalloproteinase-12) suppresses growth of lung metastases. *Cancer Res* 66, 6149–6155
82. Huang Y, Lee C, Borgstrom P, and Gjerset RA (2007) Macrophage-mediated bystander effect triggered by tumor cell apoptosis. *Mol Ther* 15, 524–533
83. Hagemann T, Lawrence T, McNeish I, Charles KA, Kulbe H, Thompson RG, Robinson SC, and Balkwill FR (2008) "Re-educating" tumor-associated macrophages by targeting NF-kappaB. *J Exp Med* 205, 1261–1268
84. Colombo N, Peccatori F, Paganin C, Bini S, Brandely M, Mangioni C, Mantovani A, and Allavena P (1992) Anti-tumor and immunomodulatory activity of intraperitoneal IFN-gamma in ovarian carcinoma patients with minimal residual tumor after chemotherapy. *Int J Cancer* 51, 42–46
85. Thomsen LL and Miles DW (1998) Role of nitric oxide in tumour progression: lessons from human tumours. *Cancer Metastasis Rev* 17, 107–118
86. Dugas B, Mossalayi MD, Damais C, and Kolb JP (1995) Nitric oxide production by human monocytes: evidence for a role of CD23. *Immunol Today* 16, 574–580
87. Perlmann P, Perlmann H, ElGhazali G, and Blomberg MT (1999) IgE and tumor necrosis factor in malaria infection. *Immunol Lett* 65, 29–33

88. Fremeaux-Bacchi V, Aubry JP, Bonnefoy JY, Kazatchkine MD, Kolb JP, and Fischer EM (1998) Soluble CD21 induces activation and differentiation of human monocytes through binding to membrane CD23. *Eur J Immunol* 28, 4268–4274
89. Iwasaki K, Torisu M, and Fujimura T (1986) Malignant tumor and eosinophils. I. Prognostic significance in gastric cancer. *Cancer* 58, 1321–1327
90. Samoszuk M (1997) Eosinophils and human cancer. *Histol Histopathol* 12, 807–812
91. Ishibashi S, Ohashi Y, Suzuki T, Miyazaki S, Moriya T, Satomi S, and Sasano H (2006) Tumor-associated tissue eosinophilia in human esophageal squamous cell carcinoma. *Anticancer Res* 26, 1419–1424
92. Fernandez-Acenero MJ, Galindo-Gallego M, Sanz J, and Aljama A (2000) Prognostic influence of tumor-associated eosinophilic infiltrate in colorectal carcinoma. *Cancer* 88, 1544–1548
93. Gleich GJ and Adolphson CR (1986) The eosinophilic leukocyte: structure and function. *Adv Immunol* 39, 177–253
94. Newton DL and Rybak SM (1998) Unique recombinant human ribonuclease and inhibition of Kaposi's sarcoma cell growth. *J Natl Cancer Inst* 90, –1791
95. Ellyard JI, Simson L, and Parish CR (2007) Th2-mediated anti-tumour immunity: friend or foe? *Tissue Antigens* 70, 1–11
96. Furbert-Harris PM, Laniyan I, Harris D, Dunston GM, Vaughn T, Abdelnaby A, Parish-Gause D, and Oredipe OA (2003) Activated eosinophils infiltrate MCF-7 breast multicellular tumor spheroids. *Anticancer Res* 23, 71–78
97. Tepper RI, Pattengale PK, and Leder P (1989) Murine interleukin-4 displays potent anti-tumor activity in vivo. *Cell* 57, 503–512
98. Rothenberg ME, Luster AD, and Leder P (1995) Murine eotaxin: an eosinophil chemoattractant inducible in endothelial cells and in interleukin 4-induced tumor suppression. *Proc Natl Acad Sci USA* 92, 8960–8964
99. Cormier SA, Taranova AG, Bedient C, Nguyen T, Protheroe C, Pero R, Dimina D, Ochkur SI, O'Neill K, Colbert D, Lombari TR, Constant S, McGarry MP, Lee JJ, and Lee NA (2006) Pivotal advance: eosinophil infiltration of solid tumors is an early and persistent inflammatory host response. *J Leukoc Biol* 79, 1131–1139
100. Mattes J, Hulett M, Xie W, Hogan S, Rothenberg ME, Foster P, and Parish C (2003) Immunotherapy of cytotoxic T cell-resistant tumors by T helper 2 cells: an eotaxin and STAT6-dependent process. *J Exp Med* 197, 387–393
101. Kayaba H, Dombrowicz D, Woerly G, Papin JP, Loiseau S, and Capron M (2001) Human eosinophils and human high affinity IgE receptor transgenic mouse eosinophils express low levels of high affinity IgE receptor, but release IL-10 upon receptor activation. *J Immunol* 167, 995–1003
102. Dombrowicz D, Quatannens B, Papin JP, Capron A, and Capron M (2000) Expression of a functional Fc epsilon RI on rat eosinophils and macrophages. *J Immunol* 165, –1271
103. Nutten S, Papin JP, Woerly G, Dunne DW, MacGregor J, Trottein F, and Capron M (1999) Selectin and Lewis(x) are required as co-receptors in antibody-dependent cell-mediated cytotoxicity of human eosinophils to Schistosoma mansoni schistosomula. *Eur J Immunol* 29, 799–808
104. Tepper RI, Coffman RL, and Leder P (1992) An eosinophil-dependent mechanism for the antitumor effect of interleukin-4. *Science* 257, 548–551
105. Pericle F, Giovarelli M, Colombo MP, Ferrari G, Musiani P, Modesti A, Cavallo F, Di Pierro F, Novelli F, and Forni G (1994) An efficient Th2-type memory follows CD8+ lymphocyte-driven and eosinophil-mediated rejection of a spontaneous mouse mammary adenocarcinoma engineered to release IL-4. *J Immunol* 153, 5659–5673
106. Esendagli G, Bruderek K, Goldmann T, Busche A, Branscheid D, Vollmer E, and Brandau S (2008) Malignant and non-malignant lung tissue areas are differentially populated by natural killer cells and regulatory T cells in non-small cell lung cancer. *Lung Cancer* 59, 32–40

107. Gu T, Kilinc MO, and Egilmez NK (2008) Transient activation of tumor-associated T-effector/memory cells promotes tumor eradication via NK-cell recruitment: minimal role for long-term T-cell immunity in cure of metastatic disease. *Cancer Immunol Immunother* 57, 997–1005
108. Jurisic V, Srdic T, Konjevic G, Markovic O, and Colovic M (2007) Clinical stage-depending decrease of NK cell activity in multiple myeloma patients. *Med Oncol* 24, 312–317
109. Arnould L, Gelly M, Penault-Llorca F, Benoit L, Bonnetain F, Migeon C, Cabaret V, Fermeaux V, Bertheau P, Garnier J, Jeannin JF, and Coudert B (2006) Trastuzumab-based treatment of HER2-positive breast cancer: an antibody-dependent cellular cytotoxicity mechanism? *Br J Cancer* 94, 259–267
110. Miyajima I, Dombrowicz D, Martin TR, Ravetch JV, Kinet JP, and Galli SJ (1997) Systemic anaphylaxis in the mouse can be mediated largely through IgG1 and Fc gammaRIII. Assessment of the cardiopulmonary changes, mast cell degranulation, and death associated with active or IgE- or IgG1-dependent passive anaphylaxis. *J Clin Invest* 99, 901–914
111. Lorenzen J, Lewis CE, McCracken D, Horak E, Greenall M, and McGee JO (1991) Human tumour-associated NK cells secrete increased amounts of interferon-gamma and interleukin-4. *Br J Cancer* 64, 457–462
112. Menetrier-Caux C, Montmain G, Dieu MC, Bain C, Favrot MC, Caux C, and Blay JY (1998) Inhibition of the differentiation of dendritic cells from CD34(+) progenitors by tumor cells: role of interleukin-6 and macrophage colony-stimulating factor. *Blood* 92, 4778–4791
113. Menetrier-Caux C, Thomachot MC, Alberti L, Montmain G, and Blay JY (2001) IL-4 prevents the blockade of dendritic cell differentiation induced by tumor cells. *Cancer Res* 61, 3096–3104
114. Bieber T (1997) Fc epsilon RI on human epidermal Langerhans cells: an old receptor with new structure and functions. *Int Arch Allergy Immunol* 113, 30–34
115. Luiten RM, Fleuren GJ, Warnaar SO, and Litvinov SV (1996) Target-specific activation of mast cells by immunoglobulin E reactive with a renal cell carcinoma-associated antigen. *Lab Invest* 74, 467–475
116. Luiten RM, Warnaar SO, Schuurman J, Pasmans SG, Latour S, Daeron M, Fleuren GJ, and Litvinov SV (1997) Chimeric immunoglobulin E reactive with tumor-associated antigen activates human Fc epsilon RI bearing cells. *Hum Antibodies* 8, 169–180
117. Sapino A, Cassoni P, Ferrero E, Bongiovanni M, Righi L, Fortunati N, Crafa P, Chiarle R, and Bussolati G (2003) Estrogen receptor alpha is a novel marker expressed by follicular dendritic cells in lymph nodes and tumor-associated lymphoid infiltrates. *Am J Pathol* 163, 1313–1320
118. Dadabayev AR, Sandel MH, Menon AG, Morreau H, Melief CJ, Offringa R, van der Burg SH, Janssen-van Rhijn C, Ensink NG, Tollenaar RA, van de Velde CJ, and Kuppen PJ (2004) Dendritic cells in colorectal cancer correlate with other tumor-infiltrating immune cells. *Cancer Immunol Immunother* 53, 978–986
119. Shah S, Divekar AA, Hilchey SP, Cho HM, Newman CL, Shin SU, Nechustan H, Challita-Eid PM, Segal BM, Yi KH, and Rosenblatt JD (2005) Increased rejection of primary tumors in mice lacking B cells: inhibition of anti-tumor CTL and TH1 cytokine responses by B cells. *Int J Cancer* 117, 574–586
120. Barbera-Guillem E, Nelson MB, Barr B, Nyhus JK, May KF, Jr., Feng L, and Sampsel JW (2000) B lymphocyte pathology in human colorectal cancer. Experimental and clinical therapeutic effects of partial B cell depletion. *Cancer Immunol Immunother* 48, 541–549
121. Tan TT and Coussens LM (2007) Humoral immunity, inflammation and cancer. *Curr Opin Immunol* 19, 209–216
122. Gould HJ, Mackay GA, Karagiannis SN, O'Toole CM, Marsh PJ, Daniel BE, Coney LR, Zurawski VR, Jr., Joseph M, Capron M, Gilbert M, Murphy GF, and Korngold R (1999) Comparison of IgE and IgG antibody-dependent cytotoxicity in vitro and in a SCID mouse xenograft model of ovarian carcinoma. *Eur J Immunol* 29, 3527–3537

123. Karagiannis SN, Wang Q, East N, Burke F, Riffard S, Bracher MG, Thompson RG, Durham SR, Schwartz LB, Balkwill FR, and Gould HJ (2003) Activity of human monocytes in IgE antibody-dependent surveillance and killing of ovarian tumor cells. *Eur J Immunol* 33, 1030–1040
124. Bracher M, Gould HJ, Sutton BJ, Dombrowicz D, and Karagiannis SN (2007) Three-colour flow cytometric method to measure antibody-dependent tumour cell killing by cytotoxicity and phagocytosis. *J Immunol Methods* 323, 160–171
125. Karagiannis P, Singer J, Hunt J, Gan SK, Rudman SM, Mechtcheriakova D, Knittelfelder R, Daniels TR, Hobson PS, Beavil AJ, Spicer J, Nestle FO, Penichet ML, Gould HJ, Jensen-Jarolim E, and Karagiannis SN (2009) Characterisation of an engineered trastuzumab IgE antibody and effector cell mechanisms targeting HER2/neu-positive tumour cells. *Cancer Immunol Immunother* 58, 915–930
126. Nagy E, Berczi I, and Sehon AH (1991) Growth inhibition of murine mammary carcinoma by monoclonal IgE antibodies specific for the mammary tumor virus. *Cancer Immunol Immunother* 34, 63–69
127. Kershaw MH, Darcy PK, Trapani JA, MacGregor D, and Smyth MJ (1998) Tumor-specific IgE-mediated inhibition of human colorectal carcinoma xenograft growth. *Oncol Res* 10, 133–142
128. Reali E, Greiner JW, Corti A, Gould HJ, Bottazzoli F, Paganelli G, Schlom J, and Siccardi AG (2001) IgEs targeted on tumor cells: therapeutic activity and potential in the design of tumor vaccines. *Cancer Res* 61, 5517–5522
129. Fu SL, Pierre J, Smith-Norowitz TA, Hagler M, Bowne W, Pincus MR, Mueller CM, Zenilman ME, and Bluth MH (2008) Immunoglobulin E antibodies from pancreatic cancer patients mediate antibody-dependent cell-mediated cytotoxicity against pancreatic cancer cells. *Clin Exp Immunol* 153, 401–409
130. Wines BD, Hulett MD, Jamieson GP, Trist HM, Spratt JM, and Hogarth PM (1999) Identification of residues in the first domain of human Fc alpha receptor essential for interaction with IgA. J *Immunol* 162, 2146–2153

Chapter 9
IgE as Adjuvant in Tumor Vaccination

Elisa A. Nigro, Antonio G. Siccardi, and Luca Vangelista

Abstract Activation of the antigen-IgE-FcεRI axis results in a potent inflammatory state. The redirection of this IgE-mediated activation of the immune system from allergic reactions toward tumors is the main theme of the new AllergoOncology field. Our particular approach has been to employ IgE as an adjuvant in anti-tumor vaccination. IgE-coated tumor cells can protect against tumor challenge, an observation that supports the involvement of IgE in anti-tumor immunity. The adjuvant effect of IgE was shown to result from eosinophil-dependent priming of the T-cell-mediated adaptive immune response. Moreover, the role of FcεRI in IgE anti-tumor adjuvanticity has been recently demonstrated. The interaction of tumor cell-bound IgE with receptors triggers the release of mediators with following recruitment of effector cells, cell killing and tumor antigen cross-priming. Starting from these evidences, several improvements toward a simple and universal use of IgE in anti-tumor cellular vaccines have been accomplished. In view of narrowing the gap between experimental models and therapeutic applications, the field is now shifting toward a humanized systems, employing human IgE and human FcεRIα transgenic mice.

9.1 Introduction

The powerful immunological IgE role exerted physiologically against intestinal parasites and pathologically during allergic reactions is determined by its dual capacity to cause acute and to promote late inflammatory reactions. The molecular basis of IgE strength is provided by its high binding affinity to FcεRI. The activation of the antigen–IgE–FcεRI axis profoundly affects the immune system both in its cellular orchestration and programming, resulting in a potent inflammatory state [1]. Redirection of the IgE-mediated inflammatory state toward tumors is part of the new field of AllergoOncology [2]. With this view in mind, an attempt on using IgE as a potent adjuvant in anti-tumor vaccination has been undertaken.

L. Vangelista (✉)
Department of Biology and Genetics, University of Milan and San Raffaele Scientific Institute, Milan, Italy
e-mail: vangelista.luca@hsr.it

M.L. Penichet, E. Jensen-Jarolim (eds.), *Cancer and IgE*, DOI 10.1007/978-1-60761-451-7_9,

9.2 Mouse IgE is Responsible for Decreased Tumor Growth and Improved Mice Survival

IgE activates innate immunity by inducing mast-cell and basophil degranulation with release of cytokines and mediators of allergic and inflammatory reactions. This IgE-driven activation of innate immunity could ideally be exploited and redirected against tumors. To this aim, a tumor could be disguised as a parasite or an allergen by loading IgE on the surface of tumor cells. Hence, IgE should affect tumor immunogenicity by initiating an immune response at tumor site. IgE targeting onto tumor cells can be performed through a three-step strategy based on biotin–avidin interactions, a system that has already showed its therapeutic efficacy in targeting cytotoxic molecules [3, 4], cytotoxic cells [5, 6] or radioisotopes [7] on tumor cells. Therefore, the three-step strategy allows the targeting of different effector molecules on the surface of tumor cells. During the first step, a systemic administration of a biotinylated monoclonal antibody (mAb) directed against a tumor-associated antigen (TAA) is performed. Then, the second step involves avidin or streptavidin administration. Avidin binds the tumor-bound biotinylated mAb with high affinity ($K_D = 10^{-15}$) and removes the unbound antibody by liver clearance. A biotinylated effector molecule, administered as third and last step, docks selectively at tumor sites via avidin bridging. In addition, the 1:4 stoichiometry ratio between avidin and biotin enables signal amplification [8].

The three-step strategy can be used to target IgE on the surface of TAA-expressing tumor cells, employing biotinylated soluble murine IgE (or control biotinylated murine IgG) as the effector of the third step. Immunocompetent C57BL/6 mice implanted (3 days before the three-step) with MC38-CEA-2, a syngenic adenoma cancer cell line stably transfected to express the human carcinoembryonic antigen (CEA) as TAA [9], showed a decreased tumor progression compared to control mice (treated with biotinylated IgG instead of IgE). The survival curves were also significantly different, and there were even cases of tumor rejection [10]. As for the in vivo tumor cell loading with biotinylated IgE, also the in vitro IgE loading (through avidin-biotin bridges) before cell inoculation, significantly affected tumor growth rate and mice survival. Moreover, re-challenge of tumor-rejecting mice failed to cause tumor development, indicating that a protective immunity was induced [10]. The use of the parental (CEA negative) MC38 cell line for re-challenge demonstrates that the protection mechanism was not due to an anti-CEA response, or at least not exclusively. Mice inoculated with tumor cells loaded with either IgG or heat-inactivated IgE developed tumors of similar volumes, suggesting that the Fc portion of IgE is likely to be essential for immune cell recruitment and activation. Another proof for the protective immunity elicited by targeting IgE on tumor cells came from the evidence that mice inoculated with IgE-loaded tumor cells at suboptimal quantities (not sufficient to induce tumor development) induced tumor protection. Indeed, these mice did not develop tumors after a challenge with parental tumor cells. On the contrary, using suboptimal doses of IgG-loaded tumor cells all challenged mice developed tumors. The IgE-treated mice did not develop

tumors even when challenged a second time with the CEA-negative parental cell line MC38.

The IgE-dependent tumor growth delay, decrease in rate of tumor progression and induction of protective immunity against subsequent challenges was observed not only with the weakly immunogenic MC38 colon adenocarcinoma cell line but also with the immunogenic Rauscher-induced rapidly growing RMA lymphoma cell line. In order to provide a target to the first biotinylated agent of the three-step strategy, RMA cells were stably transfected with the Thy 1.1 antigen [10]. This second tumor cell system provided an additional demonstration that the anti-tumor effect observed in these experimental setups is not tumor- or TAA-dependent, rather it is attributable to the presence of IgE on the surface of tumor cells.

9.2.1 Cell Types Involved in IgE-Induced Tumor Protection

Anti-tumor immunity acquired via IgE loading of tumor cells depends on mechanisms involving different cells of the immune system that need to be defined in detail. Specific cell-type depletion studies highlighted the contribution of eosinophils, $CD4^+$ and $CD8^+$ T lymphocytes in the inhibition of tumor growth. Cell depletion was attained by treating mice intraperitoneally (i.p.) with antibodies against IL-5 (eosinophil depletion), $CD4^+$ or $CD8^+$ (T-lymphocyte depletion), in separate experiments. Indeed, the significant inhibition of tumor growth observed in wild-type mice in presence of IgE was completely abrogated upon eosinophil and T-lymphocyte depletion [10]. Eosinophils are likely to play a role in the initial phase of the IgE-driven inhibition of tumor growth, whereas tumor-specific T-cell priming should determine the cellular adaptive immunity. The anti-tumor protection against subsequent tumor challenges is therefore attributable to the establishment of a memory T-cell response.

In order to define the mechanisms involved in the protective immunity, tumor-specific CTL responses in cultured spleen cells have been studied. Spleen cells derived from IgE-primed tumor-rejecting mice were stimulated in vitro with irradiated tumor cells. A remarkably higher cytotoxic activity was detected as compared to control spleen cells derived from tumor-bearing mice. This is a strong indication that the induction of anti-tumor CTL responses is a consequence of the presence of IgE. In addition, proliferation of tumor-specific $CD4^+$ T-cells has been observed in cultures of spleen cells derived from mice immunized with IgE-loaded tumor cells [10].

Future studies need to be performed to better understand the cellular mechanisms involved in the IgE-driven anti-tumor effect. Preliminary data confirm the implication of dendritic cells as antigen-presenting cells (APC) needed to transfer the tumor antigen information in order to establish an anti-tumor immunity. Cytofluorimetric analysis of draining lymph nodes from mice vaccinated with

irradiated IgE-loaded or not loaded tumor cells, labeled with a fluorescent membrane probe, shows the presence of probe-positive dendritic cells. The significantly higher fraction of probe-positive dendritic cells derived from IgE-vaccinated mice remarks the APC role of these cells in the IgE-driven inflammatory reaction accounting for the establishment of an anti-tumor immune response (unpublished data).

9.2.2 IgE is an Adjuvant in Tumor Vaccination

The induction of an anti-tumor protection against subsequent tumor challenges upon immunization with suboptimal doses of IgE-loaded tumor cells, together with the cell depletion studies, strongly suggests the establishment of a memory T-cell response. According to these evidences, a possible exploitation of the IgE-driven anti-tumor immunity for preventive, or even curative, immunization has been envisaged. To this aim, cellular vaccines have been prepared with IgE- or IgG-loaded irradiated tumor cells. As in the tumor growth studies, the IgE targeting or IgG targeting on MC38-CEA-2 and RMA-Thy 1.1 tumor cell lines has been performed through the three-step method. Mice vaccinated twice (15 days apart) with IgE-loaded irradiated tumor cells showed anti-tumor protection with significant delay in tumor growth after a challenge with parental tumor cells [10]. The anti-tumor protection can be appreciated by vaccinating mice with different doses of the IgE cellular vaccine. The IgE-loaded irradiated cells are highly effective at really low doses (around 10^3 cells subcutaneously (s.c.)/mouse). Conversely, protective immunity can be achieved by vaccination with irradiated IgG-loaded cells at doses 100-fold higher than that with the IgE cellular vaccine. Anti-TAAs serum antibodies can be detected only in mice vaccinated with the highest dose of IgE or IgG cellular vaccines, demonstrating that IgE does not induce an increase in the tumor-specific antibody response [10].

IgE loading on tumor cells by the three-step strategy is effective and does not require the construction of a TAA-specific monoclonal IgE antibody, allowing the use of available biotinylated TAA-specific monoclonal IgG antibodies. Despite these advantageous features, the presence of a TAA-expressing tumor cell line is required for recognition by the biotinylated mAb at the first step. To overcome this need, two faster and easier targeting strategies, as effective as the three-step approach, have been developed. The first strategy is a simplified version of the three-step, involving the biotinylation of the tumor cell surface as first step. As in the original method, the second and third steps consist in the creation of the avidin bridge with IgE. In the second strategy, the tumor cell surface is chemically functionalized with haptens (haptenization) that can be recognized by hapten-specific monoclonal IgE antibodies. Both strategies prevent the need for a TAA-expressing tumor cell line, making the loading strategy suitable for many different tumors, including the poorly immunogenic ones or those not characterized for their TAAs.

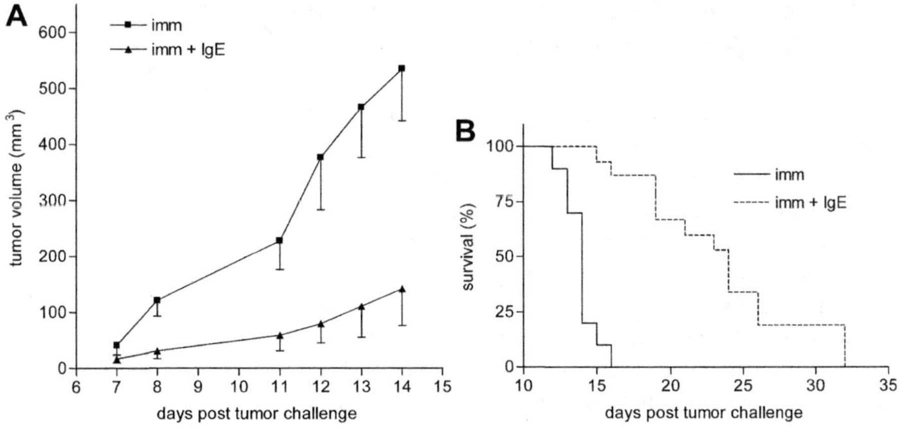

Fig. 9.1 Anti-tumor IgE adjuvanticity in C57BL/6 mice. (**A**) Tumor growth of mice immunized s.c. twice (15 days apart) with 1×10^5 irradiated MC38 cells previously haptenized with DNP and loaded with anti-DNP IgE. Challenge with 3×10^5 parental tumor cells was performed 15 days after the last immunization. Mice immunized with IgE-loaded MC38 cells (15 mice, triangles, imm + IgE) and IgE-free MC38 cells (10 mice, squares, imm). The statistical difference between the two groups was highly significant ($P < 0.001$), evaluated by the Student's *t*-test. (**B**) Mice survival plot: dotted line, mice treated with IgE-loaded cells; continuous line, mice treated in absence of IgE. Statistical analysis on survival data was performed by the Kaplan–Meier method. The difference in survival was highly significant ($P < 0.001$)

Cell haptenization and IgE targeting have been adapted to attain IgE cellular vaccines. As with the three-step approach, mice vaccinated with a double injection of irradiated IgE-loaded tumor cells showed a delay in tumor growth. As depicted in Fig. 9.1, differences in tumor growth can be estimated after tumor challenge in mice vaccinated with IgE-loaded or IgE-free MC38 cells. The rate of tumor growth in the IgE group versus the control group is significantly lower and reflects the difference in mice survival. All mice of the control group died in the first 2 weeks after challenge while the last mice of the IgE group died 32 days post-tumor injection.

Clearly, the evidence for an adjuvant effect exerted by IgE in anti-tumor vaccination represents an important immunological insight and, at the same time, an innovative source for new approaches in cancer therapy. Unknown aspects of IgE cell biology and biochemistry have been discovered and applied to a possible new way to combat cancer. Aside the in vivo studies, a full set of in vitro tests have been developed to monitor and assure the quality of the cellular vaccine preparations. These tests consist mainly in (i) the evaluation of IgE tumor cell loading via cytofluorimetry and (ii) the verification of the IgE cellular vaccine activity toward FcεRI via $FcεRI^+$ cell mediator release assays modified from classic assays to allow detection of mediators in a cell-to-cell contact mode [11]. Moreover, this and the following paragraphs present an overview on how our anti-tumor IgE system has been refined to increase safety and allow the use of human IgE, pointing toward human health.

9.2.3 *Vaccinia Virus and MVA as Cell Killing Agents Coupled to IgE Loading*

Vaccinia virus (VV) is a large, enveloped virus belonging to the Orthopoxvirus genus, widely used for smallpox vaccination until 1980 when the Assembly of the World Health Organization declared smallpox eradicated and recommended the discontinuation of vaccination. In the same year, the application of the recombinant DNA technology to VV marked the birth of genetically engineered poxviruses [12], developed as expression vectors. The strong immunogenicity of VV, together with the homologous recombination that spontaneously takes place during its replication inside infected cells, allows its wide use as expression vector and candidate vaccine against unrelated infectious diseases [13]. Recombinant poxviruses have been used for protectively immunizing animals against diseases of veterinary importance. Examples include the recombinant VV expressing the rabies virus glycoprotein for immunization of wild animals that greatly reduced incidence of rabies as demonstrated in large field tests in Belgium [14]. The ability of poxviruses to induce strong CTL-mediated immune responses has led to consideration of their use as cancer vaccines. Recombinant VVs that express viral antigens or cellular TAAs have provided prophylactic and therapeutic effects against experimental tumors [13].

In the field of IgE anti-tumor adjuvanticity, the replacement of irradiation with VV infection of tumor cells represents a first step toward the construction of a viral vector-based anti-tumor vaccine. VV guarantees cell death by killing tumor cells in few days. IgE adjuvanticity acts in a concerted manner with VV strong immunogenicity, and as a result, a single immunization is sufficient to empower the anti-tumor effect. Conversely, the irradiated IgE-loaded cellular vaccine is able to exert tumor protection only after two immunizations. In the VV vaccination protocol, soluble IgE are targeted through haptenization on the surface of VV-infected tumor cells. As represented in Fig. 9.2, at 14-days post-tumor challenge, all mice vaccinated with VV-infected IgE-loaded tumor cells are tumor-free, whereas all controls (vaccinated with infected tumor cells without IgE) present a huge tumor growing in the site of injection on the animal's flank. The survival curve shows that only one mouse vaccinated with IgE-loaded tumor cells developed the tumor in the following month.

Despite its effectiveness, the use of VV in standard laboratory conditions is hampered by restrictions due to its infectivity. In search for an alternative and more flexible viral system for the anti-tumor vaccination protocol, VV was substituted with the modified vaccinia virus Ankara (MVA) (an attenuated VV derivative, unable to replicate in mammalian cells). The IgE adjuvant effect and its synergy with virus immunogenicity were maintained although the anti-tumor protection was less striking. As obtained with VV infection, the IgE effect is established after a single vaccination, but the almost complete protection observed with the VV protocol cannot be observed using MVA. Using MVA-infected IgE-loaded tumor cells the majority of vaccinated mice present tumor development. However, the tumor growth rate was significantly lower compared to controls. A double immunization with MVA-infected tumor cells decreases the tumor growth rate even in absence

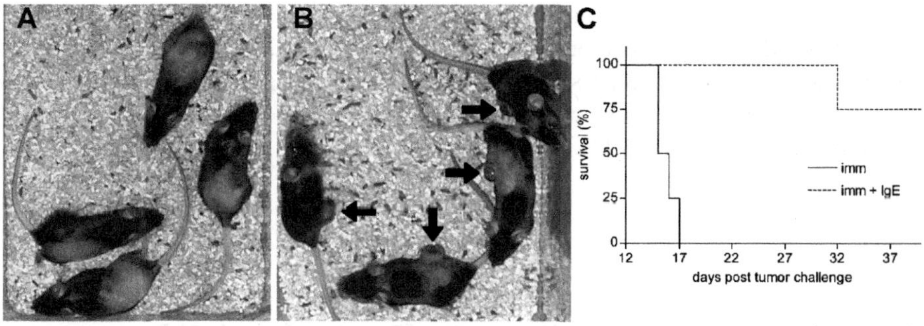

Fig. 9.2 Anti-tumor protection of VV-infected IgE-loaded RMA cells. C57BL/6 mice (four mice per group) were vaccinated s.c. with 10^5 IgE-loaded (**A**) or not loaded (**B**) VV-infected RMA cells at day −15. At day 0 mice received a s.c. tumor challenge of 7×10^4 RMA living cells. The images are representative of one out of three experiments yielding similar results and were taken 14 days after challenge. Mice vaccinated with IgE-loaded cells did not develop tumors (**A**) while all the controls did (B, see *arrows*). (**C**) Mice survival plot: dotted line, mice treated with IgE-loaded cells; continuous line, mice treated in the absence of IgE. Statistical analysis on survival data was performed by the Kaplan–Meier method. The difference in survival was highly significant ($P < 0.001$)

of IgE. As already stated, a single immunization in the presence of IgE confers a powerful anti-tumor immune response, demonstrating the MVA-IgE synergy [15]. In perspective, the MVA-IgE anti-tumor vaccination system is particularly important, as it gives plenty of possibilities for its evolution into a fully engineered viral system.

9.2.4 MVA as a Resource for Human Therapy and Recombinant Protein Expression

MVA is a highly attenuated and severely host-restricted viral vector derived from over 570 serial passages of the parental VV strain in chicken embryo fibroblasts [16]. As a result, MVA, characterized by six major genome deletions [17], is unable to multiply in humans and in most mammalian cell lines. Yet, MVA retains a high expression level of viral and heterologous genes in non-permissive cells [18]. Most importantly, MVA is safer than VV because it is non-pathogenic for humans, even in immuno-compromised patients, such as those with hematologic malignancies or those undergoing chemotherapy treatment [19]. The elicitation of humoral and cellular adaptive immune responses, together with the properties mentioned above, make recombinant MVA an ideal vector for both prophylactic and therapeutic vaccination, as demonstrated by its wide use in ongoing clinical trials [20, 21]. Recombinant MVA viruses expressing both infection disease antigens [22–24] and TAAs [20] have been produced. Different strategies have been developed in order to obtain rMVAs expressing heterologous antigens. An initial method for rMVA production required visual selection and manual picking of infected cell foci [18],

followed by selection strategies based on antibiotic resistances and by a 'Transient Host Range Selection' method [25, 26]. The recently developed 'Red-to-Green gene swapping' method represents a fast and easy strategy for rMVA production in which a fluorescence-enhanced visual selection simplifies greatly the isolation of recombinant MVA clones [27].

9.2.5 Use of Transgenic Mice as Tools to Explore IgE Receptor Involvement and Implement Human IgE

The IgE adjuvant effect could depend upon IgE interaction with its high-affinity receptor, FcεRI (present in mouse on the surface of mast cells and basophils), or with its low-affinity receptor, CD23. Eventually, FcεRI activation would lead to cellular degranulation with mediator release and effector cell recruitment. This cascade should cause a potent local inflammation at the tumor site. The role of the receptors involved in the IgE-driven anti-tumor effect could therefore be investigated using FcεRI$\alpha^{-/-}$ [28] and CD23$^{-/-}$ mice [29]. Knock-out mice, in which one or more genes are turned off through gene knock out, are important animal models for studying the role of the targeted genes. By knocking out a specific gene and observing phenotypic, functional or morphological differences from wild-type conditions, a function for the targeted gene can be often inferred. Recruitment of IgE receptor mice knock outs in our experimental anti-tumor vaccines should be likely to provide information about which receptor is involved in IgE adjuvanticity. In addition, the use of a transgenic FcεRI$\alpha^{-/-}$ hFcεRIα^{+} mouse, in which the α-chain of mouse FcεRI is substituted with the human counterpart, should help in understanding whether human IgE could exert an anti-tumor effect similar to mouse IgE. Thus, the establishment of a human IgE model system in mouse would represent a fundamental resource for future development in the IgE anti-tumor vaccination strategy, moving the field closer to the clinics. All transgenic mice described above and employed in our studies were generated in a BALB/c background; therefore the BALB/c mammary adenocarcinoma cell line TS/A-LACK (*Leishmania* receptor for activated C kinase) [30] has been used to reproduce in BALB/c mice the IgE-driven anti-tumor protection observed in the C57BL/6 model [15]. As expected, BALB/c mice, vaccinated once or twice (15 days apart) with MVA-infected IgE-loaded TS/A-LACK cells, exhibited a tumor protection after challenge very similar to that reported for the C57BL/6 model. Indeed, the IgE adjuvant effect is obtained after a single immunization in mice vaccinated by MVA-infected IgE-loaded TS/A-LACK cells. Conversely, after two immunizations, also the MVA-infected cells (in absence of IgE) induced anti-tumor protection [15]. The successful induction of an IgE-driven anti-tumor effect using a BALB/c tumor cell line in a BALB/c mouse demonstrates that the IgE adjuvanticity is not confined to a specific tumor model, rather it is potentially applicable to different tumors. Particularly interesting is the

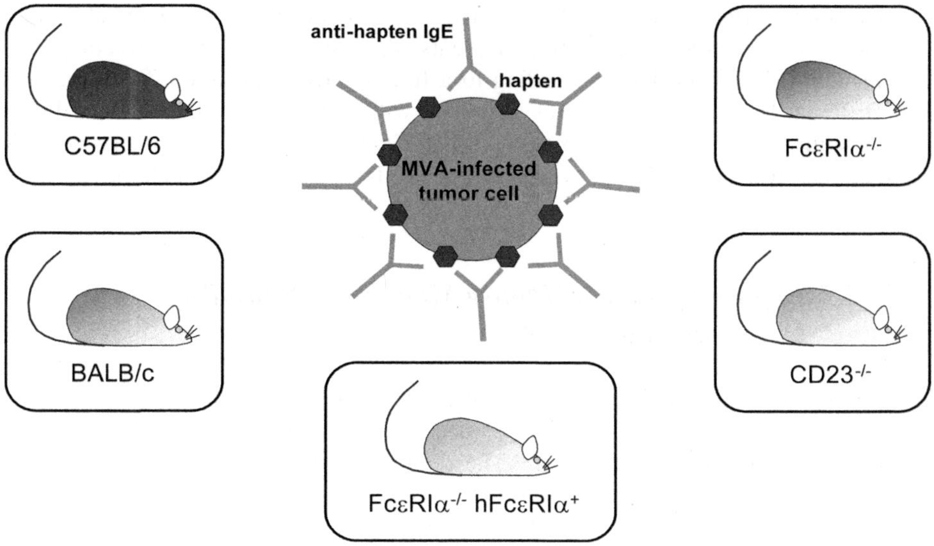

Fig. 9.3 Schematics of mice and MVA-based cell vaccination systems. Cellular anti-tumor vaccines are based on MVA infection and IgE loading via haptenization. The mice model system shifted from C57BL/6 to BALB/c given the availability of several transgenic models in the BALB/c background

fact that TS/A cells have been reported as a poorly immunogenic tumor [31], confirming the power of IgE adjuvanticity. A schematic view of the mice and cell systems described above is represented in Fig. 9.3.

9.2.6 FcεRI is Crucial for IgE Adjuvanticity in Tumor Vaccination

It is conceivable that the IgE-adjuvant effect observed in the anti-tumor vaccination would consist in an immune response due to the instauration of a powerful inflammation at the tumor site, similar to that induced during an allergic manifestation. The availability of FcεRIα$^{-/-}$ mouse [28] permits to understand the role played by the IgE high-affinity receptor in the IgE-adjuvant effect. FcεRIα$^{-/-}$ mice vaccinated in presence of IgE did not show any anti-tumor protection, demonstrating the crucial role played in vivo by FcεRI in the IgE adjuvant effect [15]. In parallel, similar experiments conducted with CD23$^{-/-}$ mice [29] demonstrated that the low-affinity receptor CD23 is not involved in the IgE adjuvant effect, as CD23$^{-/-}$ mice vaccinated in the presence of IgE presented tumor protection similar to wild-type mice. Indeed, CD23$^{-/-}$ mice do express FcεRI; thus, as suggested by the lack of IgE adjuvanticity in FcεRIα$^{-/-}$ mice, these data reinforce the hypothesis that FcεRI is the primary (or unique) mediator of IgE activity in anti-tumor vaccination [15]. The demonstration of a dominant role played by FcεRI in the in vivo IgE-dependent

anti-tumor effect based on IgE adjuvanticity on a vaccination is extremely important as it implies an orchestration of events, starting from a simple protein–protein recognition (IgE-FcεRI) and ending to a full adaptive anti-tumor T-cell memory. Different from other approaches described within this book, not involving IgE as an adjuvant but as a direct tumor cell killer, CD23 did not prove to intervene in the cellular crosstalk promoted by the presence of IgE in tumor vaccination.

9.2.7 Implementation of Mouse Membrane-Bound IgE by Recombinant MVA

Despite the encouraging and promising anti-tumor effect of the IgE-based vaccine, the use of soluble IgE in the vaccination protocol could carry the risk of unwanted anaphylactic reactions. The demonstration of a functional interaction between human membrane-bound IgE (mIgE) and FcεRI [11] provides a mean to the development of a safer protocol for IgE-mediated tumor vaccination. In fact, embedding IgE molecules into the surface of tumor cells eliminates the presence of these potentially dangerous proteins from the bloodstream. In other words, unwanted anaphylactic reactions could in theory derive from unexpected antigen recognition by soluble IgE molecules (or by soluble IgE bound to FcεRI). These immune complexes could then aggregate FcεRI on the surface of mast cells and basophils, triggering potent cell degranulation, ultimately leading to systemic anaphylaxis. Although remote, these events should be prevented when using IgE as a drug or as a vaccine component.

Different from human mIgE [11, 32], mouse mIgE needs to be associated with the Igα–Igβ heterodimer to reach the cell surface [33]. The construction of a chimeric mouse mIgE variant is thus needed to obtain a suitable recombinant protein for the anti-tumor vaccination project. As for human mIgE, mouse mIgG2a can be transported to the cell surface also in absence of Igα–Igβ heterodimers [33]. Considering that a truncated version of human mIgE has been engineered and provided full capacity to activate FcεRI in a cell-to-cell contact [11], a truncated mouse mIgE chimeric construct (deprived of IgE Fabs and containing only the Fc Cε3-Cε4 domains) in which the portion C-terminal to IgE Cε4 was replaced by the corresponding mIgG2a moiety (i.e., the extracellular membrane-proximal domain, the transmembrane domain and the cytoplasmic domain) has been designed and cloned. The construct has been transfected in cell lines and characterized for the ability to activate rodent FcεRI. The truncated chimeric mouse mIgE/IgG2a construct was then subcloned and a recombinant MVA produced and used to infect cells. Despite expression, proper assembly (disulphide bonded dimers) and cell surface export (tested by cytofluorimetry, western blot and surface biotinylation), the truncated chimeric mouse mIgE/IgG2a did not induce mediator release when infected cells contacted a rat basophilic cell line. This may imply a significant FcεRI binding site difference between human and mouse IgE. Therefore, a second chimeric protein in which the mouse IgE Fc portion comprises also the Cε2 domain has been

constructed and is currently being tested for its function. Once an active mouse mIgE construct is obtained, a new vector-based vaccination protocol should become available. rMVA-mIgE-infected tumor cells should then express the truncated membrane form of IgE on their surface creating a new IgE-mediated vaccine. Tumor growth will then be studied in wild-type, FcεRIα$^{-/-}$ and CD23$^{-/-}$ mice, likely reproducing the results obtained in the MVA-infected IgE-loaded tumor cell vaccination protocol, getting closer to the construction of a safe and simplified IgE-based vaccine.

9.2.8 FcεRI Humanized Mice Allow the Use of Human IgE in Tumor Vaccination

FcεRI cellular distribution in humans (mast cells, basophils, dendritic cells, eosinophils, neutrophils, monocytes, macrophages and platelets) is more ubiquitary than in mice (mast cells and basophils); therefore, the output of the human IgE–FcεRI interaction on the anti-tumor vaccination efficiency cannot be predicted. In order to verify whether human secretory IgE targeting on tumor cells exerts anti-tumor protection similar to that observed with mouse secretory IgE, the IgE-based vaccination protocol has been performed in FcεRIα$^{-/-}$ hFcεRIα^{+} mice [34]. FcεRIα$^{-/-}$ hFcεRIα^{+} mice present a cellular FcεRI expression similar to that found in humans [34–36], a very useful model to predict the efficiency of the system in the perspective to translate it to the clinic.

As in the wild-type model with mouse IgE, also in the humanized model, two immunizations guaranteed an anti-tumor protection, regardless of human IgE presence. On the contrary, with a single immunization, human IgE showed an adjuvant effect, mediating an anti-tumor protection comparable to that obtained with two immunizations. Mice immunized only once with MVA-infected cells in absence of IgE were not protected from tumor growth, showing a tumor development comparable to that of non-immunized control mice [15]. Wild-type mice (thus expressing mouse FcεRI), immunized with human IgE-loaded MVA-infected TS/A-LACK cells, are not protected from tumor development, showing a tumor growth comparable to that observed in non-immunized mice [15]. This result was expected and is attributable to the lack of human IgE binding to mouse FcεRI [37]. The reconstitution of the IgE effect in FcεRIα$^{-/-}$ hFcεRIα^{+} mice demonstrates the anti-tumor adjuvanticity of human IgE.

Since human mIgE variants are capable of activating human FcεRI in an antigen-independent manner [11], the transfer of this knowledge to the anti-tumor vaccination strategy (using FcεRIα$^{-/-}$ hFcεRIα^{+} mice) has been immediate. Hence, a rMVA expressing a truncated human mIgE (tmIgE), previously reported to be able to activate FcεRI [11], has been constructed and characterized. Since cells infected with the rMVA-tmIgE present expression of human tmIgE on the cell surface and activate human FcεRI in a rat basophilic leukemia (RBL) cell-based mediator release assay [11], there is a high likelihood to observe anti-tumor IgE adjuvanticity

as in the case of human secretory IgE-targeted on tumor cells. Moreover, human tmIgE should reveal no anti-tumor protection when tested on wild-type mice, in line with the results obtained using human-soluble IgE.

With the aim to produce vector-based tumor vaccines, recombinant MVA capable to realize a further molecular evolution of the mIgE–FcεRI interaction concept are being generated. In other words, a safe and simple MVA-based system should allow expression of mIgE on the surface of tumor cells, providing all the necessary requirements for the IgE adjuvant effect. Furthermore, the construction of rMVAs with multiple gene insertions should disclose the possibility to exploit IgE adjuvanticity together with specific TAA (e.g., HER2/*neu* or CEA) or other adjuvant molecules. Potential candidates are genes encoding for immunomodulatory cytokines (IL-2 or GM-CSF) or co-stimulatory molecules (B7.1 or B7.2) [38]. The co-insertion of one of these genes in rMVA would augment the immune system boosting driven by IgE, likely providing a more robust and long-lasting anti-tumor protection.

9.3 Conclusion

A schematic representation of the mechanisms behind IgE adjuvanticity in anti-tumor vaccination is represented in Fig. 9.4. The presence of IgE on the surface of tumor cells allows binding with FcεRI on FcεRI$^+$ cells in a cell-to-cell contact. In order to express IgE on the surface of tumor cells, different strategies are being developed: starting from the original three-step-mediated IgE-loading strategy [10], followed by cell haptenization and anti-hapten IgE [15], to the engineering of rMVA capable to express truncated mIgE on the surface of infected tumor cells. IgE-FcεRI recognition leads to receptor activation with killing of tumor cells by FcεRI$^+$ effector cells (mast cells and basophils) and/or by other specialized killer cells (eosinophils and cytotoxic T cells), recruited as a consequence of the initial mast-cell and basophil release of pro-inflammatory mediators. The inflammatory reaction at tumor site and the consequent cell killing should result in tumor cells debris release. TAAs present in tumor cell debris should then be available to immature highly phagocytic dendritic cells of the peripheral tissues. Activated dendritic cells should therefore migrate via lymphatic vessels to the regional lymph nodes. Mature dendritic cells would stimulate a strong T-cell response by priming and cross-priming of tumor-specific CD4$^+$ and CD8$^+$ T cells. The consequent establishment of an anti-tumor-immune response is followed by the constitution and consolidation of a tumor-specific immune memory.

Finally and most intriguingly, the IgE adjuvant effect observed and characterized for tumor vaccine engineering might tell us that the power of the IgE-FcεRI system could be extended to other pathologies in which effective or enhanced vaccination strategies are still awaited. This perspective may reveal extremely innovative and promising approaches to improve human health, providing a novel view on an otherwise deleterious molecule, IgE.

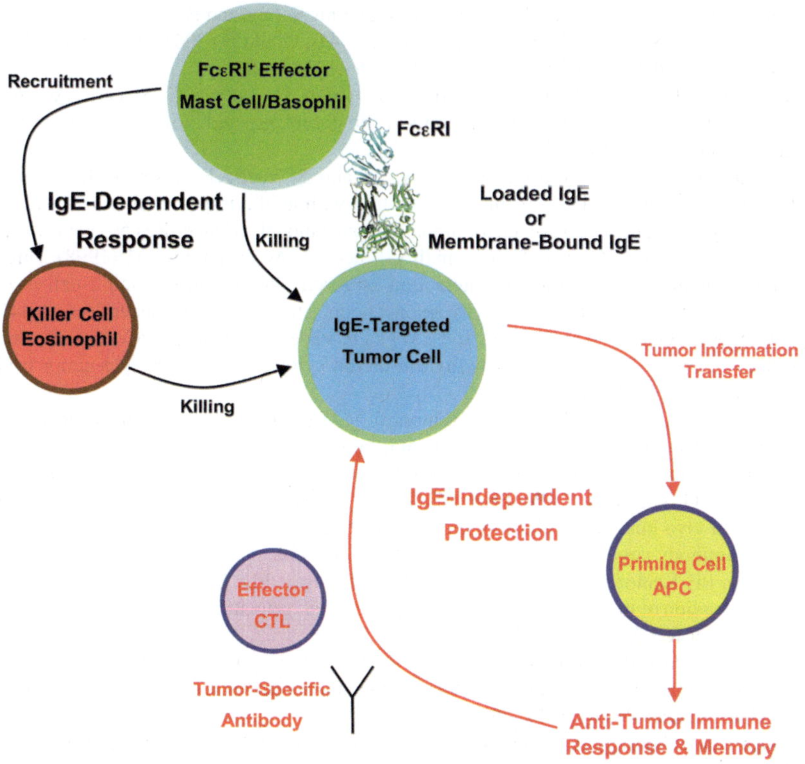

Fig. 9.4 Overview on the mechanisms behind IgE adjuvanticity in anti-tumor vaccination. The crystal structure of the complex between FcεRI α-chain D1D2 and IgE Cε3Cε4 domains [39] is shown to visualize the IgE–FcεRI interaction occurring between tumor cells and $Fc\varepsilon RI^+$ cells, regardless of the IgE targeting approach (i.e., cell loading using complete IgE or cell expression of a truncated version of membrane IgE). The 3D representation was prepared using the program PyMol on the pdb coordinates 1f6a. The interaction between IgE (on tumor cells) and FcεRI (on effector cells) is the central event leading to an IgE-dependent response, ultimately resulting in tumor cell killing, either directly by mast cells and/or basophils or upon recruitment of professional killer cells such as eosinophils. Tumor cell disruption causes cell debris to be collected by professional antigen-presenting cells that in turn transfer tumor antigen information to specialized immune districts for the establishment of an adaptive anti-tumor immune response and memory. The resulting tumor-specific T lymphocytes and antibodies build an IgE-independent tumor protection, the basis for IgE adjuvanticity

Acknowledgments We wish to thank Anna Brini, David Dombrowicz and Elisa Soprana for excellent help and assistance with various aspects of the experimental systems presented here. This work was supported by the Italian MURST Cofin 2004, 2005 and 2007.

References

1. Gould HJ, Sutton BJ, Beavil AJ, Beavil RL, McCloskey N, Coker HA, Fear D, Smurthwaite L (2003) The biology of IGE and the basis of allergic disease. Annu Rev Immunol 21:579–628

2. Jensen-Jarolim E, Achatz G, Turner MC, Karagiannis S, Legrand F, Capron M, Penichet ML, Rodríguez JA, Siccardi AG, Vangelista L, Riemer AB, Gould H (2008) AllergoOncology: the role of IgE-mediated allergy in cancer. Allergy 63:1255–1266
3. Moro M, Pelagi M, Fulci G, Paganelli G, Dellabona P, Casorati G, Siccardi AG, Corti A (1997) Tumor cell targeting with antibody-avidin complexes and biotinylated tumor necrosis factor alpha. Cancer Res 57:1922–1928
4. Gasparri A, Moro M, Curnis F, Sacchi A, Pagano S, Veglia F, Casorati G, Siccardi AG, Dellabona P, Corti A (1999) Tumor pretargeting with avidin improves the therapeutic index of biotinylated tumor necrosis factor alpha in mouse models. Cancer Res 59:2917–2923
5. Guidi F, Spagnoli GC, Neri G, Paganelli G, Siccardi AG, Guttinger M (1998) Three-step tumor targeting via biotin-avidin interaction as a versatile system to elicit T-cell-mediated, non-MHC-restricted cytotoxic activity against neoplastic cells. Int J Cancer 76:443–447
6. Guttinger M, Guidi F, Chinol M, Reali E, Veglia F, Viale G, Paganelli G, Corti A, Siccardi AG (2000) Adoptive immunotherapy by avidin-driven cytotoxic T lymphocyte-tumor bridging. Cancer Res 60:4211–4215
7. Paganelli G, Grana C, Chinol M, Cremonesi M, De Cicco C, De Braud F, Robertson C, Zurrida S, Casadio C, Zoboli S, Siccardi AG, Veronesi U (1999) Antibody-guided three-step therapy for high grade glioma with yttrium-90 biotin. Eur J Nucl Med 26:348–357
8. Siccardi AG, Paganelli G, Pontiroli AE, Pelagi M, Magnani P, Viale G, Faglia G, Fazio F (1996) In vivo imaging of chromogranin A-positive endocrine tumours by three-step monoclonal antibody targeting. Eur J Nucl Med 23:1455–1459
9. Robbins PF, Kantor JA, Salgaller M, Hand PH, Fernsten PD, Schlom J (1991) Transduction and expression of the human carcinoembryonic antigen gene in a murine colon carcinoma cell line. Cancer Res 51:3657–3662
10. Reali E, Greiner JW, Corti A, Gould HJ, Bottazzoli F, Paganelli G, Schlom J, Siccardi AG (2001) IgEs targeted on tumor cells: therapeutic activity and potential in the design of tumor vaccines. Cancer Res 61:5517–5522
11. Vangelista L, Soprana E, Cesco-Gaspere M, Mandiola P, Di Lullo G, Fucci RN, Codazzi F, Palini A, Paganelli G, Burrone OR, Siccardi AG (2005) Membrane IgE binds and activates Fc epsilon RI in an antigen-independent manner. J Immunol 174:5602–5611
12. Wittek R, Moss B (1980) Tandem repeats within the inverted terminal repetition of vaccinia virus DNA. Cell 21:277–284
13. Moss B (1996) Genetically engineered poxviruses for recombinant gene expression, vaccination, and safety. Proc Natl Acad Sci USA 93:11341–11348
14. Brochier B, Costy F, Pastoret PP (1995) Elimination of fox rabies from Belgium using a recombinant vaccinia-rabies vaccine: an update. Vet Microbiol 46:269–279
15. Nigro EA, Brini AT, Soprana E, Ambrosi A, Dombrowicz D, Siccardi AG, Vangelista L (2009) Antitumor IgE Adjuvanticity: Key Role of FcεRI. J Immunol 183:4530–4536
16. Mayr A, Hochstein-Mintzel V, Stickl H (1975) Abstammung, eigenschaften und Verwendung des attenuierten Vaccinia-Stammes MVA. Infection 3:6–16
17. Meyer H, Sutter G, Mayr A (1991) Mapping of deletions in the genome of the highly attenuated vaccinia virus MVA and their influence on virulence. J Gen Virol 72(Pt5): 1031–1038
18. Sutter G, Moss B (1992) Nonreplicating vaccinia vector efficiently expresses recombinant genes. Proc Natl Acad Sci USA 89:10847–10851
19. Mayr A, Danner K (1978) Vaccination against pox diseases under immunosuppressive conditions. Dev Biol Stand 41:225–234
20. Acres B, Bonnefoy JY (2008) Clinical development of MVA-based therapeutic cancer vaccines. Expert Rev Vaccines 7:889–893
21. Liu M, Acres B, Balloul JM, Bizouarne N, Paul S, Slos P, Squiban P (2004) Gene-based vaccines and immunotherapeutics. Proc Natl Acad Sci USA 101(Suppl 2):14567–14571
22. McConkey SJ, Reece WH, Moorthy VS, Webster D, Dunachie S, Butcher G, Vuola JM, Blanchard TJ, Gothard P, Watkins K, Hannan CM, Everaere S, Brown K, Kester KE,

Cummings J, Williams J, Heppner DG, Pathan A, Flanagan K, Arulanantham N, Roberts MT, Roy M, Smith GL, Schneider J, Peto T, Sinden RE, Gilbert SC, Hill AV (2003) Enhanced T-cell immunogenicity of plasmid DNA vaccines boosted by recombinant modified vaccinia virus Ankara in humans. Nat Med 9:729–735
23. Gilbert SC, Moorthy VS, Andrews L, Pathan AA, McConkey SJ, Vuola JM, Keating SM, Berthoud T, Webster D, McShane H, Hill AV (2006) Synergistic DNA-MVA prime-boost vaccination regimes for malaria and tuberculosis. Vaccine 24:4554–4561
24. Mwau M, Cebere I, Sutton J, Chikoti P, Winstone N, Wee EG, Beattie T, Chen YH, Dorrell L, McShane H, Schmidt C, Brooks M, Patel S, Roberts J, Conlon C, Rowland-Jones SL, Bwayo JJ, McMichael AJ, Hanke T (2004) A human immunodeficiency virus 1 (HIV-1) clade A vaccine in clinical trials: stimulation of HIV-specific T-cell responses by DNA and recombinant modified vaccinia virus Ankara (MVA) vaccines in humans. J Gen Virol 85:911–919
25. Staib C, Drexler I, Ohlmann M, Wintersperger S, Erfle V, Sutter G (2000) Transient host range selection for genetic engineering of modified vaccinia virus Ankara. BioTechniques 28:1137–1142, 1144–1146, 1148
26. Staib C, Lowel M, Erfle V, Sutter G (2003) Improved host range selection for recombinant modified vaccinia virus Ankara. BioTechniques 34:694–696, 698, 700
27. Di Lullo G, Soprana E, Panigada M, Palini A, Erfle V, Staib C, Sutter G, Siccardi AG (2009) Marker gene swapping facilitates recombinant Modified Vaccinia Virus Ankara production by host-range selection. J Virol Methods 156:37–43
28. Dombrowicz D, Flamand V, Brigman KK, Koller BH, Kinet JP (1993) Abolition of anaphylaxis by targeted disruption of the high affinity immunoglobulin E receptor alpha chain gene. Cell 75:969–976
29. Yu P, Kosco-Vilbois M, Richards M, Kohler G, Lamers MC (1994) Negative feedback regulation of IgE synthesis by murine CD23. Nature 369:753–756
30. Benigni F, Zimmermann VS, Hugues S, Caserta S, Basso V, Rivino L, Ingulli E, Malherbe L, Glaichenhaus N, Mondino A (2005) Phenotype and homing of CD4 tumor-specific T-cells is modulated by tumor bulk. J Immunol 175:739–748
31. Rosato A, Zoso A, Milan G, Macino B, Dalla Santa S, Tosello V, Di Carlo E, Musiani P, Whalen RG, Zanovello P (2003) Individual analysis of mice vaccinated against a weakly immunogenic self tumor-specific antigen reveals a correlation between CD8 T-cell response and antitumor efficacy. J Immunol 171:5172–5179
32. Vangelista L (2003) Current progress in the understanding of IgE-Fc epsilon RI interaction. Int Arch Allergy Immunol 131:222–233
33. Venkitaraman AR, Williams GT, Dariavach P, Neuberger MS (1991) The B-cell antigen receptor of the five immunoglobulin classes. Nature 352:777–781
34. Dombrowicz D, Brini AT, Flamand V, Hicks E, Snouwaert JN, Kinet JP, Koller BH (1996) Anaphylaxis mediated through a humanized high affinity IgE receptor. J Immunol 157: 1645–1651
35. Dombrowicz D, Lin S, Flamand V, Brini AT, Koller BH, Kinet JP (1998) Allergy-associated FcR beta is a molecular amplifier of IgE- and IgG-b in vivo responses. Immunity 8:517–529
36. Kayaba H, Dombrowicz D, Woerly G, Papin JP, Loiseau S, Capron M (2001) Human eosinophils and human high affinity IgE receptor transgenic mouse eosinophils express low levels of high affinity IgE receptor, but release IL-10 upon receptor activation. J Immunol 167:995–1003
37. Kinet JP (1999) The high-affinity IgE receptor (Fc epsilon RI): from physiology to pathology. Annu Rev Immunol 17:931–972
38. Hodge JW, Higgins J, Schlom J (2009) Harnessing the unique local immunostimulatory properties of modified vaccinia Ankara (MVA) virus to generate superior tumor-specific immune responses and antitumor activity in a diversified prime and boost vaccine regimen. Vaccine 27:4475–4482
39. Garman SC, Wurzburg BA, Tarchevskaya SS, Kinet JP, Jardetzky TS (2000) Structure of the Fc fragment of human IgE bound to its high-affinity receptor Fc epsilonRI alpha. Nature 406:259–266

Chapter 10
The Targets of IgE: Allergen-Associated and Tumor-Associated Molecular Patterns

Erika Jensen-Jarolim, Diana Mechtcheriakova, and Isabella Pali-Schoell

Abstract The most studied targets of IgE immunoglobulins are termed allergens and mostly represent protein antigens from plant or animal origin. However, it has been revealed that also pathogens and self-antigens can be recognized by IgE. Thus, besides a detrimental role in allergy, IgE may exert defense and surveillance functions. Here, we discuss the display of rigid epitope patterns as a common key feature of antigens leading to both formation of high-affinity IgE antibodies by B lymphocytes and IgE-mediated triggering of effector cells. In analogy to the principle of pathogen-associated patterns as danger signals, we introduce here the terms allergen-associated molecular patterns (AAMPs) for the repetitive epitopes exposed by allergens and tumor-associated molecular patterns (TAMPs) in settings when molecular epitope patterns are displayed through overexpressed tumor antigens.

10.1 Background: IgE and the Anaphylactic Reaction

As already discussed in the previous chapters, IgE antibodies have several unique features which enable them to induce highly specific biological responses. Taken together, major features of IgE are (i) high binding strength to their target epitopes through unique affinity maturation program of the IgE-producing B lymphocytes (epsilon B lymphocytes) in an appropriate milieu of cytokine and danger signals [1–3]; (ii) high-affinity interaction of their Fc epsilon (Fcε) domain with specialized FcεRI receptors on a distinct panel of mostly cytotoxic and phagocytic effector cells conferring antibody-dependent cell-mediated cytotoxicity (ADCC) or antibody-dependent cell-mediated phagocytosis (ADCP) functions to them [4–6]; (iii) moderate affinity interactions with specific IgE receptors of the CD23 C-lectin type enabling IgE to participate in antigen uptake, transport and presentation by classical antigen-presenting cells (APCs) including dendritic cells (DCs) and B lymphocytes, as well as non-classical APCs like epithelial cells [7, 8]. Depending on the

E. Jensen-Jarolim (✉)
IPP – Department of Pathophysiology, Center of Pathophysiology, Infectiology and Immunology, Medical University Vienna, Vienna, Austria
e-mail: erika.jensen-jarolim@meduniwien.ac.at

M.L. Penichet, E. Jensen-Jarolim (eds.), *Cancer and IgE*,
DOI 10.1007/978-1-60761-451-7_10,

time point, duration and repetition of antigen contact IgE will either induce reactions of the immediate anaphylactic type or nourish chronic Th2-type inflammation [9–11]. In any circumstances, an ongoing IgE-mediated response will be hard to turn off, symbolic for the sensitization state of the individual and characterized by "tissue memory" of IgE [12], prolonging the survival rate of its effector cells. To counterbalance an undesired IgE response toward actually harmless allergens, today's allergen immunotherapy aims at inducing a tolerant state in the patient [13, 14]. This immune tolerance is supported by the production of immunomodulating cytokines and the induction of non- or anti-inflammatory blocking IgG antibodies which interact with FcγRIIb receptors on epsilon B lymphocytes and on FcεRI-positive effector cells and thus are able to downregulate IgE levels [15]. In this process, immunomoduloatory cytokines IL-10 and TGF-beta are driving forces [16]. Both cytokines are, however, also produced by some tumor types and may participate in undesired tolerance phenomena in cancer diseases [17]. On the other hand, it has been reported that epithelial tumors are the source of typical Th2 cytokines as IL-4 and IL-13 [18, 19] which are directly involved in IgE class switch [20]. Anecdotic reports on natural IgE present in tumor tissues indicate that they may have pathophysiological significance in tumor surveillance and attack [21, 22]. Systematic allergooncological approaches to study the prevalence of natural antitumor IgE are at this time point missing [23]. Nevertheless, the advanced knowledge derived from the studies on allergic diseases may help to understand the function of IgE in malignancies. For this, a comparison of the possible target structures of IgE on allergens and on self-antigens like tumor antigens has been undertaken in this chapter.

10.2 Crosslinking of Antigens – A Biological Tool for Immunoregulation

Antibodies, when expressed by B lymphocytes as membrane immunoglobulins (mIg; also termed B-cell receptor, BCR) and in their secreted form, represent homodimeric molecules, thus being principally equipped with two identical antigen binding sites called paratopes [24]. The paratopes are opposed to the epitopes of an antigen which represent exposed molecular surface plains, covering a relative flat area between 600 and 1,000 Å^2 [25, 26]. Some B-cell epitopes may be cryptic, meaning normally not accessible to the immune system, and might be exposed after physical, chemical or enzymatic processing of an antigen.

The cognition that several short, discontinuous stretches of an antigenic protein chain together form the 3D antibody epitopes [27] has rendered multiple efforts using structural mimics of epitopes, that is mimotopes, as a circumvention strategy for 3D epitope definition [28, 29]. (Such mimotopes can also be applied for epitope-specific vaccination and are suitable for induction of tumoricidic IgE when applied by the oral route; see also [30, 31] and Chapter 7 of this book.)

However, linear sub-epitopes in the range between 8 and 12 amino acids could be as well mapped recently with high accuracy using an antibody- based proteomics

approach [32]. On the membrane of a resting B cell the distance of BCRs has been determined to be approximately 40 nm [33]. The phenomenon that properly spaced multiple copies of an epitope are needed to turn on or turn off a B lymphocyte rendered the cognition that antigens may act as immunoregulators [34]. The collected evidence concerns predominantly the formation of IgM and, consecutively, IgG antibodies by B lymphocytes [35]. Similarly, direct isotype switch from IgM to IgE can occur [36], but depending on the antigen, IgE switch may even occur in an IgM-independent fashion [37]. Chapter 3 of this book gives a comprehensive overview on this topic, also with respect to the effects on affinities of different IgE species.

During the last four decades numerous studies have focused on the evaluation of the epitope requirements for B-lymphocyte activation. Already early immunization studies have indicated that some antigens per se rather induced tolerance, whereas others were prone to act immunogenic. This was systematically analyzed in vitro using conjugates of flagellin as a carrier with different hapten density on it [38]. Within the same series of chapters, Feldmann specified this observation by stating that antigen molecules in a monomeric fashion or with few epitopes never induced tolerance, whereas highly dense display of epitopes did [39]. He concluded that "a tolerance-inducing antigen must bind more avidly to B-cell membranes than an immunogen..." [39]. Obviously, the dense display of epitopes on the body's own cell membranes could, therefore, be involved in the maintenance of tolerance against self.

It has further been documented that these immunoregulative phenomena of antigens could be enhanced by coupling or admixing the same protein antigens to immunogenic or "non-immunogenic" carriers [40]. Among carriers for antigen-specific tolerance induction polyethylene-glycol became particularly popular [41], whereas for antigen-specific immunity coupling to non-related protein carriers like keyhole limpet hemocyanin (KLH), encapsulation in particulate materials [42] or admixture to the protein-absorbing adjuvant $Al(OH)_3$ has been preferred. As vaccine carriers often enhance the antigenic density, the resulting opposed types of immune responses may thus have to do with the different epitope spacing.

Among B-lymphocyte responses, one has also to dissect between the so-called T-lymphocyte-dependent (TD) and T-independent (TI) responses. According to their definition, for immune responses to TD antigens like low-dose-soluble antigen or monovalent haptenated proteins T-cell help has to be provided to induce sufficient immunity [43]. However, T-cell dependence is a relative matter: some antigens, largely TI but still needing residual T-cell help, are called TI-2 antigens. However, in complete T-cell independence, also immune responses comprising high titers of IgM antibodies may be generated by the so-called TI-1 antigens. In this model, polymeric high-molecular-weight antigens (like lipopolysaccharide, LPS) may represent polyclonal B-cell stimulators or – when exposing highly organized, rigid surfaces – be potent-specific crosslinkers of the BCRs. In a classic publication, Dintzis et al. defined in 1976 the *immunon*, that is, minimally 12–20 antigenic determinants spaced in a distance of 10 nm, as the minimal requirement of TI B-cell activation [44]. Later, Bruton's tyrosine kinase (Btk) was found to be associated with these clusters, not only being responsible for B-cell activation in terms of proliferation

and antibody synthesis but also controlling the cytoskeleton and thus having a function in antigen processing and presentation [45]. In further pioneer studies, Dintzis et al. specified that for the optimal spacing of at least approximately 20 haptenic epitopes within an immunon, a minimal threshold size of approximately 100 kDa of the monomeric antigen is required [46]. Therefore, antigens which are too small to display a sufficient number of epitopes to form an immunon can bind B lymphocytes but cannot stimulate them. On the other hand, it has been realized that sometimes large polymeric molecules, although exhibiting a dense epitope display, are not inducing immunity but in contrast tolerance. The explanation was that the distance between epitopes of multivalent antigens can also be too large to allow productive B-cell stimulation [46]. In that case, recognition of several epitopes far apart on the antigen, but coming together on a flexible loop, does not substitute for a rigid, optimal crosslinking. Taken together, crosslinking of the BCR occurs optimally with antigens exhibiting a repetitive (at least 12–20 copies) epitope display in rigid spacing above 5–10 nm. Interestingly, some viruses displaying a crystalline-like surface with perfectly spaced epitopes have been recognized as TI-1 antigens [47, 48]. In both TI cases, the antigenic determinants must be arranged in a properly spaced manner for optimal crosslinking, B-cell activation and IgM immunoglobulin synthesis. The degree of antigen organization is even more important for the magnitude of IgG responses and can be supported by costimulatory B-cell signals like via CD21 [49] and Toll-like receptor-4 (TLR4)–MyD88 complex [50], the latter being also susceptible for stimulation with heat shock protein 60 (HSP60) [51]. Further, the spacing of the virus epitopes is affecting the affinity of the (bivalent) IgG response and its capacity to reduce the infectivity of the virion particle [52].

The B lymphocytes are, therefore, today recognized as pattern recognizers activated not by single epitopes but by the repetitiveness and spatial organization of the antigen [53]. Importantly, the concentration or aggregation state of an antigen, for instance upon chemical modification, can determine its immunogenicity [54]; environmental stress augments expression of pathogenesis-related proteins in plants [55], and in turn, food processing may render immunogenic aggregates of proteins [56]. With increasing concentration of an antigen also the epitope density increases and may significantly improve the recognition and uptake of the antigen by B-cells as well as other professional APCs. This is important, because professional APCs take care for recruitment of specific and bystander T-helper cells and thus enhance the extent of immune responses. Importantly, it is not sufficient that TD antigens are sensed by the specific BCR but simultaneously a second danger signal is received via by TLRs, representing another class of pattern recognition receptors (PRRs) also expressed by the B lymphocytes [57]. In an experimental system using transgenic mice devoid of TLR on their B lymphocytes (but not on DCs), antigen-specific antibody production indeed was deficient and could not be substituted by adoptive transfer of CD4-positive T-cells [58].

Generally, for TD antigens, the given cytokine milieu will determine the consecutive isotype switch, and the immune response can further be promoted by natural [59] or artificial adjuvants and carriers [60, 61].

10.3 Crosslinking – Indispensable for IgE Synthesis and Pathophysiology

We hypothesize that the above reviewed principles for B-cell activation, namely, rigid and dense (but not too dense) epitope display on antigens, will similarly account for IgE production. The rational for this is derived from the fact that in both the sensitization and the effector phase of IgE-mediated responses crosslinking is a critical biological phenomenon. Thereby, the epitopes of an antigen (or allergen if clinically undesired hypersensitivity is meant) must interact with the complementary determining regions (CDRs) of at least two IgE antibodies to induce a biological response in the form of signal transduction, protein synthesis or mediator release, respectively [62, 63].

For the mast cell, being the most typical IgE-binding effector cell, it has been shown that also the antigen amount and contact duration are decisive for the overall signal strength and thus determine whether the cell will degranulate or acquire enhanced survival [64, 65]. In contrast, interaction of two antigenic epitopes with only one homodimeric IgE molecule expressed as membrane IgE (mIgE) by a B-lymphocyte or passively bound to high-affinity FcεRI will not activate but, contrarily, lead to anergy or tolerance by the B-cell or non-reactivity of the effector cell. The same principle obviously accounts for DCs, where polyvalent but not monovalent IgE engagement resulted in internalization of antigens [66].

Therefore, the spacing of epitopes will critically affect antigenicity and allergenicity of an agent with respect to its capacity to induce immunoglobulin synthesis. The single, monoclonal B lymphocyte is uttermost restrictive, because each single immunoglobulin expressed on its membrane will recognize the same epitope. Consequently, as discussed above, recent work suggests that B lymphocytes are pattern recognizers [53]. Primarily, upon antigen contact and TI activation, the B lymphocyte will produce a soluble form of IgM antibodies through alternative splicing and secrete them. However, if simultaneously with repeated antigen contact the CD40 ligation and/or IL-4 and IL-13 stimulation occurs, the specific B lymphocyte has several options to switch toward IgE: (i) direct deletional switching [67, 68] and (ii) sequential switching via gamma 4 [68, 36] or even in an IgM-independent fashion, which was at least demonstrated in mice infested with helminths [37]. The (IgE-producing) εB-lymphocytes undergo somatic hypermutation and affinity maturation in spite of their location outside germinal centers [3]. Thereby, recognition of the original antigen epitopes is improved substantially, rendering outstanding IgE affinities, with equilibrium dissociation constants ($K_D = k_d/k_a$) between 10^{-10} and 10^{-11} M [2]. Obviously, also for the reactivation and expansion of the memory subset of the B lymphocytes at later points of time it is crucial that epitopes are presented in a repetitive manner. Indeed, the antibody response in sensitized mice was successfully re-challenged with a dimeric allergen, but not monomeric allergen [69]. For memory εB lymphocytes, contacts with TLR activators may possibly be important for productive activation too, as previously demonstrated for IgG [50]. Moreover, also the achieved affinity to the epitopes will affect surface binding of

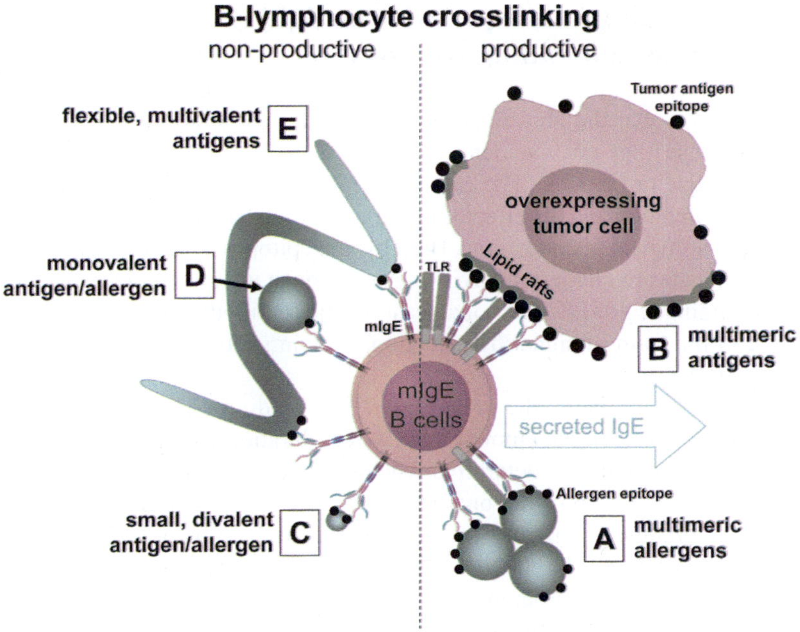

Fig. 10.1 The antigen determines immune reactions through the spacing of its B-cell epitopes. *Right side*: Productive activation (including antibody synthesis) will take place when a multivalent antigen is able to crosslink more than one mIgE by the rigid display of repetitive epitopes. These requirements are fulfilled by multimeric allergens (**A**), and overexpressed tumor antigens, e.g. accumulating in lipid rafts (**B**). Other pattern recognition receptors, as TLR family members, may contribute to the extent of activation. *Left side*: Non-productive activation (cytokine production, prolongued survival, but no IgE synthesis) will take place when mIgE remains monomeric. This may happen upon contact with a too small divalent antigen (**C**), with a single molecular unit of a monovalent antigen (**D**), and upon contact with loosely connected epitopes (**E**)

allergens and level of activation [70, 71]. Contrarily, antigens may also induce tolerance in IgE-producing B lymphocytes, possibly in case of multivalent polymers, improper epitope spacing, high flexibility of antigen, or at too small molecular size of an antigen, being monomeric [72] (Fig. 10.1).

Spacing of allergenic epitopes is also critical for the effector phase of the established immediate-type allergy, when IgE is already bound with high affinity to its receptors on mast cells, eosinophils or basophils. According to the textbook, allergens have to be at least bivalent, but should rather be multivalent to increase their potency to activate FcεRI-bearing effector cells, that is, exposure of more than one IgE epitope (Fig. 10.2). Moreover, the FcεRI signal depends on concentration and affinity of both the antigen and the receptors [73].

Interestingly, activation via FcεRI and TLR-4 both induce a shared core response of gene expression toward Th2 in mast cells [74]. Thereby, also monovalent IgE-allergen interactions can induce signaling and prolong the lifetime of mast cells [64, 74, 75] and induce FcεRI surface expression [76, 77]. The higher the epitope density, the more likely effective crosslinking will occur. Whether or not an allergic

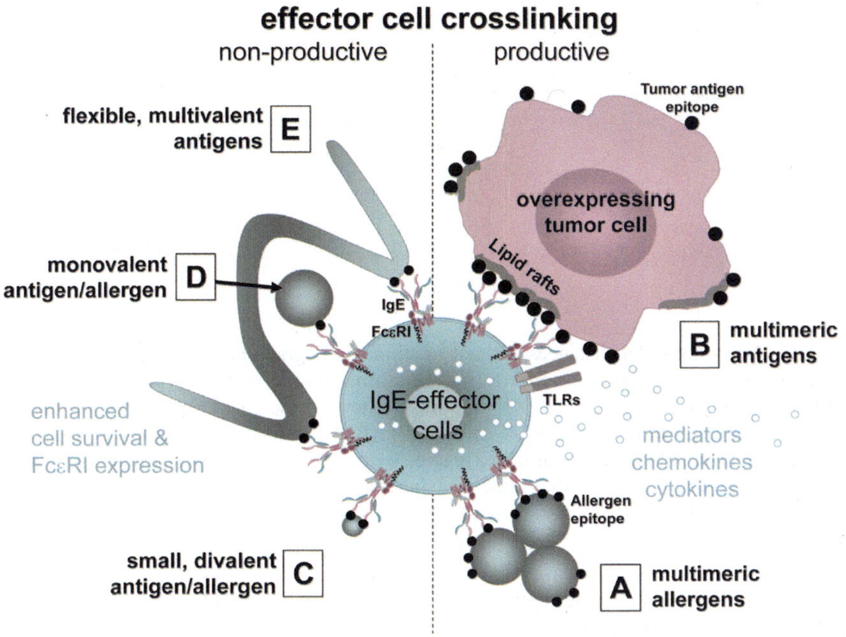

Fig. 10.2 The antigen determines the extent of immediate type inflammation upon crosslinking through the spacing of its B-cell epitopes. A typical effector cell, for instance a mast cell, is illustrated with multiple IgE molecules bound in bent shape to its high affinity receptors FcεRI, constituted of four chains. *Right side*: Productive activation rendering mediator release will take place when a multivalent antigen is able to crosslink more than one FcεRI-bound IgE by the rigid display of repetitive epitopes. These requirements are fulfilled by multimeric allergens (**A**) and overexpressed tumor antigens, e.g. accumulating in lipid rafts. The later may lead to antibody-dependent cellular cytotoxicity (ADCC) or phagocytosis (ADCP) (**B**). Other pattern recognition receptors, as TLR family members (*dark grey bars*), may contribute to the extent of activation. *Left side*: Non-productive activation (cytokine production, prolonged survival) will take place when FcεRI-bound IgE remains monomeric. This may happen upon contact with a too small divalent antigen (**C**), with a single molecular unit of a monovalent antigen (**D**), and upon contact with loosely connected epitopes (**E**)

reaction will be elicited may, however, finally depend on the structural integrity of the allergen and on the distinct spacing of its IgE epitopes (reviewed in [78]).

In early IgE crosslinking studies with rigidly spaced bivalent avidin constructs, molecules with a length of 49.4 Å were poorer triggering agents than those of 92.7 and 135.8 Å; the best cellular degranulation effect was achieved with dimers and polymers from the length of about 80–>240 Å [79] (Fig. 10.3). In contrast, more recent studies indicate a shorter distance of allergen epitopes: performing in vitro studies with double-stranded DNA as a versatile rigid spacer, Paar et al. were able to show that for effective crosslinking of specific IgE on rat basophil leukemia cells, an inter-epitope distance of 44–51 Å was optimal to stimulate degranulation [80].

Further, the interaction of an antibody with its specific epitope depends on the flexibility of the Fab arms, which again depends on the respective immunoglobulin isotype. For the Fab arms of IgE in solution there is limited segmental flexibility, and

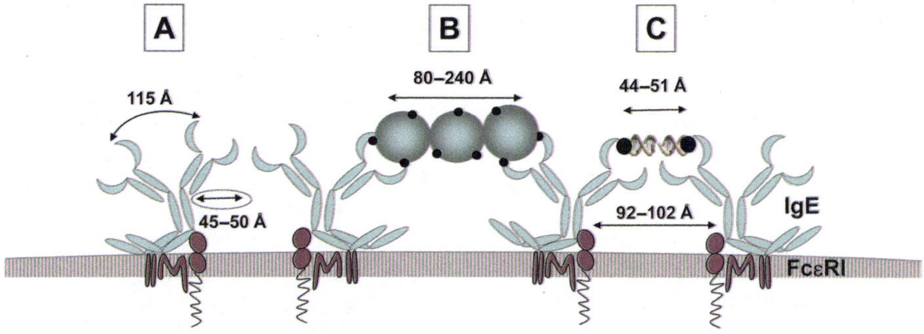

Fig. 10.3 Inter-molecular distances optimal to stimulate degranulation of effector cells via IgE bound to its high affinity receptor, FcεRI. (**A**) The estimated intra-molecular distance between two Fab binding sites is at least 115 Å [88] and thus fits to the calculated upper limit for the radius of FceRI-bound IgE in the range of 45–50 Å [79]. (**B**) Cellular degranulation through antigen-mediated IgE crosslinking was optimally triggered by dimers or polymers from the length of 80 to 240 Å [79], but also (**C**) by smaller proteins using dsDNA as rigid model spacer with a distance of 44–51 Å [80]. The minimal distance between two IgE molecules cross-linked by antigen was estimated in the range of 92–102 Å [79]

Fab arms are not free to undergo extensive "wagging" motions [79] also because of the bent shape of IgE [81], both in solution and on FcεRI [82–84]. This means that the IgE antibody itself cannot adapt the fit to the allergen.

Allergic individuals have a small number of IgE antibodies on the basophil surface (about 40,000 molecules per cell) evenly distributed in non-activated condition [85]. It was speculated by Siraganian et al. that short bivalent haptens are capable of eliciting histamine release because the second FcεRI-bound IgE molecule would move closer through lateral diffusion within the cell membrane [86], today more precisely defined as movements into and within the lipid rafts of detergent-resistant membranes [87]. Resonance energy transfer measurements suggested a minimal distance of 92–102 Å between two cross-linked IgE molecules and an upper limit for the receptor radius of 45–50 Å [79].

On the other hand, the two Fab-binding sites *within one IgE molecule* were calculated to be at least 115 Å apart [88] (Fig. 10.3). It was furthermore shown in this study that flexible bivalent ligands longer than 130 Å form cyclic monomers with IgE in solution, that is intra-molecular bridging, and thereby rather block than induce histamine release. This would mean that, for instance, a small globular allergen dimer like Bet v 1, the major birch pollen allergen, with an estimated diameter of 38 Å could not form intramolecular bridging of Fab sites of the same IgE and is actually also below the optimal distance for cross-link of two separate IgE antibodies.

10.4 AAMPs: Allergen-Associated Molecular Patterns

Motifs recognized by PRRs may be called pathogen-associated molecular patterns (PAMPs) when associated with membranes of infectious agents [89]. We

suggest here that also allergens display repetitive motifs which we accordingly designate allergen-associated molecular patterns (AAMPs). Our suggestion is based on the observation that in many cases allergenic molecules occur as dimers or even multimers, a list growing longer over time (Table 10.1).

The consequence of di- or multimerization is the repetitive display of individual epitopes within the molecular complex. As suggested previously, the repetitive epitope display is important for both the sensitization and the effector phase of type I allergy [69] and may represent the long-sought common characteristic of allergens. Some allergens, especially small proteins, may possess only few or even a single immunodominant B-cell epitope and therefore as a single molecular unit do not fulfill the requirements for crosslinking. Examples are Api m 4 from bee (*Apis mellifera*) venom with only 2.8 kDa (26 amino acid residues) [90] and Amb a 5 from ragweed (*Ambrosia artemisiifolia*) pollen, which shows one very dominant B-cell epitope for human IgG binding [91]; also for the major birch (*Betula verrucosa*) pollen allergen Bet v 1 a single immunodominant murine IgG epitope was identified [92, 26, 93], which was distinct from the epitope of human polyclonal IgE [94]. For such small proteins, multimerization or oligomerization may provide the necessary means for efficient IgE crosslinking. Indeed, for Amb m 4 the formation of tetramers in aqueous solution was confirmed [95, 96] and Bet v 1 also forms dimers and higher oligomers in physiological solution, which is a necessary pre-requisite for its biological allergenic activity [69]. In accordance, Ghosh et al. have recently demonstrated that protein T1, a non-allergenic Bet v 1-homologue, lacks the capacity to dimerize although sharing a high-sequence and structural homology with other members of the Bet v 1 family [97].

When a series of recombinant monoclonal antibodies equipped with a humanized Fcε domain were tested for their efficacy to activate mast cells, the antibody concentration, affinity and clonality affected the degree of effector cell degranulation [98]. As this experiment was based on murine IgG monoclonals originally raised in mice it may, however, be not representative for the human setting. The impact of epitope presentations for the crosslinking of monoclonal IgE antibodies was further tested with synthetic B-epitope peptides of allergen Phl p 1 from timothy grass (*Phleum pratense*) pollen. The polymeric peptide resulted in the highest release of β-hexosaminidase (70% of total release) compared to monomeric peptide (no release) and dimeric peptide (41% of total release) in in vitro experiments [99]. Moreover, although bivalent DNP-antigen was sufficient to bind and crosslink IgE, the best degranulation results were obtained with multivalent DNP-antigen using a rigid DNA display system [80] (Fig. 10.3).

A limited number of epitopes has also been shown for the major allergen from house dust mite (*Dermatophagoides pteronyssinus*), Der p 1, and Amb a 1 from ragweed, where binding of polyclonal IgE from serum of allergic patients was studied with respect to binding affinities and heterogeneity of recognized epitopes [100]. It was observed that in highly sensitized donors only two to three different affinity levels in antibody–antigen binding studies were relevant. The authors conclude from their work that a large proportion of sensitized patients harbor high-affinity IgE antibodies toward the same epitopes and that therefore the final affinity is determined

Table 10.1 Examples of allergens able to form dimers, multimers and higher aggregates (sorted by year of publication)

Allergen (source)[a]	Year of publication	References
Gad c 1 (Baltic codfish)	1967	Aas and Jebsen [140]
Api m 4 (bee venom)	1982	Terwilliger et al. [96]
ABA 1 (Ascaris, nematodes)	1990	McGibbon et al. [142]
A2U (rat urinary allergen)	1992	Bocskei et al. [143]
Mus m 1 (MUP; mouse urinary protein)	1992	Bocskei et al. [143]
Gly m Bd 30 K (soy bean)	1993	Ogawa et al. [144]
Sol i II (fire ant)	1993	Hoffman [145]
Tropomyosin (e.g. fish)	1995	Gimona et al. [146]
Alt a 1 (*Alternaria*, fungi)	1996	De Vouge et al. [147]
Bet v 1 (birch pollen)	1996	Wellhausen et al. [148]
Bos d 2 (BDA20) and Bos d 5 (alpha-lactalbumin), bovine dander	1996	Rautiainen et al. [149]
Ara h 1 (peanut)	1998	Shin et al. [150]
Phl p 1 (grass pollen)	1998	Petersen et al. [151]
Aca s 13 (*Acarus siro*, dust mite)	1999	Eriksson et al. [152]
Equ c 1 (horse dander)	1999	Gregoire et al. [153]
Tropomyosin (seafood)	1999	Reese et al. [102]
ABA-1 (*Ascaris*, nematodes)	2000	Xia et al. [154]
Ara h 1 (peanut)	2000	Maleki et al. [155]
Equ c 1 (horse dander)	2000	Lascombe et al. [156]
Ves v 5 (wasp venom)	2000	Suck et al. [157]
Ole e 1 (olive pollen)	2001	Huecas et al. [141]
Beta-lactoglobulin (bovine milk)	2001	Sakurai et al. [158]
Ara h 2 (peanut)	2002	Sen et al. [159]
Gad m 1 (Atlantic codfish)	2002	Das Dores et al. [160]
Phl p 5b (grass pollen)	2002	Rajashankar et al. [161]
Phl p 7 (grass pollen)	2002	Verdino et al. [162]
Profilin (panallergen)	2002	Wopfner et al. [163]
Phl p 1 (grass pollen)	2003	Ball et al., RCSB Protein Data Bank 1N10 [168]
Cav p 1 (guinea pig dander)	2003	Fahlbusch et al. [164]
Fel d 1 (cat dander)	2003	Gronlund et al. [165]
Bet v 1 (birch pollen)	2005	Schöll et al. [69]
Dac g 5 (grass pollen)	2005	van Oort et al. [166]
Ara h 1 (peanut)	2006	van Boxtel et al. [105]
Der p 1 (house dust mite)	2006	de Halleux et al. [167]
Can f 1 and 2 (dog dander)	2007	Kamata et al. [169]
Bos d 4 (bovine α-lactalbumin), Bos d 5 (β-lactoglobulin) (bovine milk)	2008	Roth-Walter et al. [56]
Bla g 2 (cockroach)	2008	Li et al. [170]
Der p 21 (house dust mite)	2008	Weghofer et al. [171]
Per a 3 (cockroach)	2008	Bellinghausen et al. [103]
Per a 4 (cockroach)	2009	Tan et al. [172]

[a]Codes for allergen molecules are given according to the international allergen nomenclature (http://www.allergen.org/Allergen.aspx).

by the structure of the allergenic epitope rather than by variations of the immune response of the individual. In accordance, our own surface plasmon resonance affinity determinations with purified human polyclonal IgE rendered reactivity profiles like monoclonal antibodies, indicating that the repertoire of allergen-specific IgE antibodies within a single patient may be restricted to a handful high-affinity clones [101].

The IgE crosslinking process – already discussed above – is not only important in the effector phase of type I allergy but also for sensitization with allergens. A much better secondary antibody response is produced when allergens display their epitopes repetitively through multimerization [69] (Fig. 10.1A). Accordingly, dimerization was shown to have a positive effect on the immunogenicity of Dau c 1, a major allergen of carrot (*Daucus carota*) [102]. In these immunization studies of BALB/c mice, the highest IgG titers were reached in serum when the dimer of Dau c 1 was applied compared to monomers or mutated proteins. As professional antigen-presenting cells, like DCs, may be the first to handle allergens, they are in focus in several recent studies. For example, monomeric Per a 3 from American cockroach (*Periplaneta americana*) was demonstrated to be less immunogenic and allergenic than its naturally occurring hexamer structure [103]. When monocyte-derived autologous DCs of sensitized and non-sensitized individuals were pulsed with monomeric Per a 3, the release of mainly Th1 cytokines like IFN-γ was observed; in contrast, hexameric Per a 3 induced higher Th2-cytokine levels only in sensitized patients. Also the leukotriene release from leukocytes of allergic patients was higher with the Per a 3 hexamers. Similarly, without touching the question of multimericity, stimulation of allergic DCs from allergic donors with Bet v 1 and its homologues from food rendered Th2 cytokine production [104].

A number of allergens form even larger oligomers or multimers, like Ara h 1 from peanut (*Arachis hypogea*), which has been thought to be a trimer, but it was revealed that it might even form larger oligomers with a molecular weight of approximately 700 kDa, independent of the salt concentration and therefore of the ionic strength [105]. As mentioned above, the aggregation state of proteins is substantially affected by food processing and other manufacturing processes, as well as environmental pollution.

In addition to the formation of multimeric protein aggregates, the occurrence of repetitive epitopes on the native molecule might enhance the allergenic capacity (Fig. 10.2). An example is Hev b 5 from latex (*Hevea brasiliensis*) [106], where an immunodominant B-cell epitope is repeated three times within the protein sequence and, therefore, makes the allergen multivalent. Also, Bla g 1 from German cockroach (*Blattella germanica*) shows tandem repeats, forming two duplexes within the natural allergen [107], and tropomyosin, for example, from shrimps has repetitive motifs [108]. Molecular motifs as such seem to play an important part in the allergenicity of an antigen [109, 110]. A consensus sequence was recently created from different tropomyosin motifs (tropomyosins from house dust mite, cockroaches, shrimp and other). When it was expressed in *E. coli* and tested for IgE binding with sera of shellfish-allergic patients, binding of IgE to the consensus motif correlated well with binding to the full-length allergen, suggesting that the motif represents the allergenic part of the protein [109, 110].

Refining this approach, Kong et al. used an algorithm combining motifs of known allergens. Using motif length of 35 amino acids and motif number of 500, the algorithm can achieve both a high sensitivity and a high specificity for prediction of allergenicity [111]. In the light of novel proteins continuously introduced by the genetic engineering into our plants and diet, in silico approaches may provide useful means to predict allergenicity and protect sensitized patients.

In summary, the number and spacing of B-cell epitopes and the display of repetitive epitopes determine the induction and outcome of allergic reactions in the sensitized patient and, therefore, may be called AAMPs.

10.5 TAMPs: Tumor-Associated Molecular Patterns

From above it is clear that correct epitope spacing is a marker for foreignness and thus a key event in B-cell activation. Consequently, highly repetitive epitope display like by particulate antigens, but not monovalent-soluble proteins can break B-cell tolerance [112]. This basic principle represents a safety measure against autoimmunity by several means. Soluble antigens which may be secreted or shedded off by cells do rarely elicit a significant immunity. Several tumor types are shedding off their antigens to escape from eventual immune recognition. Among them, soluble forms for the epidermal growth factor receptor (EGFR), human epidermal growth factor receptor-2 (HER-2) and carcinoembryonic antigen (CEA; CEACAM5) have been described and are already used or suggested for diagnostic purposes [113–115]. In experimental conditions, soluble antigens require the addition of adjuvants to form immunogenic aggregates and even then may induce insufficient antibody titers only. Further, some of the body's own molecules which are displaying repetitive motifs are safely locked within the cells and thus are not encountered by B lymphocytes in healthy conditions. Only when exposed through inflammation elicited through physical damage or infections, self-molecules with repetitive epitope display, including proteins (actin, myosin, collagen) or DNA, will become accessible TI antigens and lead to strong IgM autoantibody production, followed by T-cell activation and IgG synthesis. Moreover, inflammatory oxidative stress may modify self-antigens making them even more antigenic, and thereby supporting the breaking of tolerance [116], or supporting upregulation of stress proteins. One example is HSP70, which is overexpressed in colon cancer and promotes antitumor immunity [117].

Thus, repetitive display of self- and modified epitopes is possible in mammalians, and B lymphocytes are indeed infiltrating tumor tissues [118]. Since Taylor and coworkers made the observation that the distribution of membrane immunoglobulins on a B lymphocyte is dynamic [119], one may speculate that low-affinity interactions between autoantigens on tumor cell membranes and the specific BCR may be too weak to allow receptor aggregation and crosslinking. As a result, similarly as with TI-2 antigens, only minimal immunoglobulin production may take place at least in the absence of exogenously added cytokines [120]. However, in settings of antigen overexpression by a tumor cell, the epitope density increases dramatically

and should favor productive B-lymphocyte activation. Indeed, natural antibodies of the IgM, IgG and IgE class toward tumor antigens have been detected, indicating that the epitope display reaches sufficient density to induce B-lymphocyte activation [121].

For instance, the four members of the EGFR family (EGFR/HER-1, HER-2, HER-3, HER-4) lead to signal transduction by various homo- and heterodimerizations and by large-scale clustering within lipid rafts, impacting internalization and signaling processes [122, 123]. There are only a few published attempts to precisely define the intermolecular distances between these tumor antigens, which decrease with the absolute numbers of molecules overexpressed per cell. Moreover, the distances between various EGFR family members depend on the molar ratio to each other and to lipid-raft-specific mono-sialo-ganglioside GM1 [124]. In an early approach, the number of HER-2 molecules was calculated as 10^4–10^6 molecules per cell, depending on the type of tumor [125]. Due to low degree of expression, exact determinations sometimes fail [126]. In addition, the more members of the EGFR family are overexpressed, the more heterodimers could be observed by fluorescence resonance energy transfer (FRET) technology [127], making the composition of antigens on the cell membrane more complex. The authors state that the ratios of EGFR : HER-2 produced "...subtle changes in the average (molecular) distance...." More precisely, the intermolecular distances were recently calculated for EGFR homodimers, which on A431 cells membranes reside in 8 or 5.5 nm distance, as recently revealed by single-molecule imaging combined with fluorescence lifetime imaging [128]. This distance exactly fulfills the minimal requirements for B-cell activation (see above).

A mechanistic problem, however, may be the relatively loose, low-affinity interaction between homo- or heterodimer partners within the lipid rafts resulting in easy dissociation. Nagy et al. have also shown previously that crosslinking of raft lipid GM1 by Cholera toxin subunit B resulted in decrease of HER-2 cluster density as well as of HER-2/HER-3 heteroassociations [124]. Which conditions could, therefore, stabilize the tumor antigen display within the lipid rafts and render higher immunogenicity? As one interesting example, it has been shown that cholesterol, an important constituent of mammalian cell membranes, supports clustering and heterodimerization of EGFR and HER-2 within lipid rafts [129]. Cholesterol contents in tumor versus normal tissues are enhanced [130], and furthermore, the cholesterol content of tumor cell membranes was associated with increased metastatic potential [131]. In contrast, cholesterol depletion impairs microviscosity and thus receptor activation and downstream signaling [132], except EGF receptor [133]. When carcinoma cells were treated with cholesterol or cholesterol esters, their immunogenicity upon transplantation in animal models increased [134, 131]. Although the immunological mechanism was not examined in these pioneer studies, the improved display of tumor-associated antigens in cholesterol-enriched lipid rafts could contribute to the enhanced specific immunogenicity. Recently, IgE antibodies (but no other antibody classes) against a 50-kDa pancreatic cancer antigen were detected in sera of patients suffering from pancreatic cancer. The isolated IgE indeed elicited tumoricidic effects via ADCC [22] (Fig. 10.2). In accordance, it has been shown

that statins through inhibition of cholesterol synthesis impair the attack of CD20-overexpressing lymphoma cells by monoclonal antibody rituximab [135]. Even though the authors suggest a conformational change of CD20 to occur upon cholesterol depletion, the reduced recruition of CD20 into decholesterinated lipid rafts could contribute to the observed effect [136, 137].

Also the glycosylation pattern on tumor cell membrane changes during the disease development, affecting adhesivity and metastatic potential of malignant cells. In principal, the resulting high-molecular glycoproteins could be targets of IgE antibodies. For instance, MUC4 exposes a rigid tandem repeat structure possibly mimicking EGFR-like domains, which could support interaction with HER-2 [138, 139]. Whether natural IgE against heavily glycosylated tumor antigens can be formed in humans and be implicated in the surveillance of cancer has to the best of our knowledge not been investigated to this date.

10.6 Conclusion

Today, mostly parasite antigens and allergens are known as targets of IgE antibodies. However, accumulating evidence indicates that also tumor antigens are recognized by IgE antibodies. Especially against cancer cells, IgE could be beneficial for the following reasons: (i) IgE binds efficiently to FcεRI-bearing tumoricidic effector cells and may exploit them as shuttles into tumor tissues, (ii) IgE recognizes preferentially 3D epitopes and can, therefore, target viable tumor cells and (iii) IgE may exert surveillance functions against tumor stem cells, as due to high-affinity recognition of the antigens it may trace and kill low numbers of malignant cells. An important molecular requirement for IgE synthesis by B lymphocytes is the recognition of epitope patterns. Molecular patterns can be achieved when allergens display the epitopes repetitively such as in aggregated state or when self-antigens are highly overexpressed like on tumor cell membranes. Repetitive epitope display could also largely facilitate the crosslinking of IgE bound by its FcεRs on effector cells and thus support the triggering of immediate inflammation. From the collected evidence we suggest that molecular patterns displayed by allergens or tumor antigens, which we here designated as AAMPs or TAMPs, respectively, are decisive for the synthesis and triggering of IgE antibodies.

Acknowledgments This work was supported by grants of the Austrian Science Fund FWF (P18238-B13, SFB F01808-B13) and by the Ludwig Boltzmann Cluster Oncology, Vienna, Austria. Isabella Pali-Schoell was supported by Herta Firnberg grant T283-B13 of the FWF. Further, we would like to thank Mr. Walter Jarolim, crossip comm, Vienna, Austria, for excellent support in graphic arts.

References

1. Arias MA, Rey Nores JE, Vita N, Stelter F, Borysiewicz LK, Ferrara P, and Labeta MO (2000) Cutting edge: human B cell function is regulated by interaction with soluble CD14: opposite effects on IgG1 and IgE production. J Immunol 164:3480–6

2. Hantusch B, Scholl I, Harwanegg C, Krieger S, Becker WM, Spitzauer S, Boltz-Nitulescu G, and Jensen-Jarolim E (2005) Affinity determinations of purified IgE and IgG antibodies against the major pollen allergens Phl p 5a and Bet v 1a: discrepancy between IgE and IgG binding strength. Immunol Lett 97:81–9
3. Erazo A, Kutchukhidze N, Leung M, Christ AP, Urban JF Jr, Curotto de Lafaille MA, and Lafaille JJ (2007) Unique maturation program of the IgE response in vivo. Immunity 26:191–203
4. Karagiannis SN, Bracher MG, Beavil RL, Beavil AJ, Hunt J, McCloskey N, Thompson RG, East N, Burke F, Sutton BJ, Dombrowicz D, Balkwill FR, and Gould HJ (2008) Role of IgE receptors in IgE antibody-dependent cytotoxicity and phagocytosis of ovarian tumor cells by human monocytic cells. Cancer Immunol Immunother 57:247–63
5. Gould HJ and Sutton BJ (2008) IgE in allergy and asthma today. Nat Rev Immunol 8: 205–17
6. Peavy RD and Metcalfe DD (2008) Understanding the mechanisms of anaphylaxis. Curr Opin Allergy Clin Immunol 8:310–5
7. Tu Y, Salim S, Bourgeois J, Di Leo V, Irvine EJ, Marshall JK, and Perdue MH (2005) CD23-mediated IgE transport across human intestinal epithelium: inhibition by blocking sites of translation or binding. Gastroenterology 129:928–40
8. Hjelm F, Karlsson MC, and Heyman B (2008) A novel B cell-mediated transport of IgE-immune complexes to the follicle of the spleen. J Immunol 180:6604–10
9. Galli SJ, Kalesnikoff J, Grimbaldeston MA, Piliponsky AM, Williams CM, and Tsai M (2005) Mast cells as "tunable" effector and immunoregulatory cells: recent advances. Annu Rev Immunol 23:749–86
10. Galli SJ, Tsai M, and Piliponsky AM (2008) The development of allergic inflammation. Nature 454:445–54
11. Zehnder JL and Galli SJ (1999) Mast-cell heparin demystified. Nature 400:714–5
12. Untersmayr E, Bakos N, Scholl I, Kundi M, Roth-Walter F, Szalai K, Riemer AB, Ankersmit HJ, Scheiner O, Boltz-Nitulescu G, and Jensen-Jarolim E (2005) Anti-ulcer drugs promote IgE formation toward dietary antigens in adult patients. FASEB J 19:656–8
13. Akdis M (2008) T-cell tolerance to inhaled allergens: mechanisms and therapeutic approaches. Expert Opin Biol Ther 8:769–77
14. Francis JN, James LK, Paraskevopoulos G, Wong C, Calderon MA, Durham SR, and Till SJ (2008) Grass pollen immunotherapy: IL-10 induction and suppression of late responses precedes IgG4 inhibitory antibody activity. J Allergy Clin Immunol 121:1120–25 e2
15. Daeron M, Latour S, Malbec O, Espinosa E, Pina P, Pasmans S, and Fridman WH (1995) The same tyrosine-based inhibition motif, in the intracytoplasmic domain of Fc gamma RIIB, regulates negatively BCR-, TCR-, and FcR-dependent cell activation. Immunity 3: 635–46
16. Satoguina JS, Adjobimey T, Arndts K, Hoch J, Oldenburg J, Layland LE, and Hoerauf A (2008) Tr1 and naturally occurring regulatory T cells induce IgG4 in B cells through GITR/GITR-L interaction, IL-10 and TGF-beta. Eur J Immunol 38:3101–13
17. Jarnicki AG, Lysaght J, Todryk S, and Mills KH (2006) Suppression of antitumor immunity by IL-10 and TGF-beta-producing T cells infiltrating the growing tumor: influence of tumor environment on the induction of CD4+ and CD8+ regulatory T cells. J Immunol 177: 896–904
18. Ma HL, Whitters MJ, Jacobson BA, Donaldson DD, Collins M, and Dunussi-Joannopoulos K (2004) Tumor cells secreting IL-13 but not IL-13Ralpha2 fusion protein have reduced tumorigenicity in vivo. Int Immunol 16:1009–17
19. Aspord C, Pedroza-Gonzalez A, Gallegos M, Tindle S, Burton EC, Su D, Marches F, Banchereau J, and Palucka AK (2007) Breast cancer instructs dendritic cells to prime interleukin 13-secreting CD4+ T cells that facilitate tumor development. J Exp Med 204:1037–47
20. Wynn TA (2003) IL-13 effector functions. Annu Rev Immunol 21:425–56

21. Neuchrist C, Kornfehl J, Grasl M, Lassmann H, Kraft D, Ehrenberger K, and Scheiner O (1994) Distribution of immunoglobulins in squamous cell carcinoma of the head and neck. Int Arch Allergy Immunol 104:97–100
22. Fu SL, Pierre J, Smith-Norowitz TA, Hagler M, Bowne W, Pincus MR, Mueller CM, Zenilman ME, and Bluth MH (2008) Immunoglobulin E antibodies from pancreatic cancer patients mediate antibody-dependent cell-mediated cytotoxicity against pancreatic cancer cells. Clin Exp Immunol 153:401–9
23. Jensen-Jarolim E, Achatz G, Turner MC, Karagiannis S, Legrand F, Capron M, Penichet ML, Rodriguez JA, Siccardi AG, Vangelista L, Riemer AB, and Gould H (2008) AllergoOncology: the role of IgE-mediated allergy in cancer. Allergy 63:1255–66
24. Davies DR and Metzger H (1983) Structural basis of antibody function. Annu Rev Immunol 1:87–117
25. Padlan EA, Silverton EW, Sheriff S, Cohen GH, Smith-Gill SJ, and Davies DR (1989) Structure of an antibody-antigen complex: crystal structure of the HyHEL-10 Fab-lysozyme complex. Proc Natl Acad Sci USA 86:5938–42
26. Mirza O, Henriksen A, Ipsen H, Larsen JN, Wissenbach M, Spangfort MD, and Gajhede M (2000) Dominant epitopes and allergic cross-reactivity: complex formation between a Fab fragment of a monoclonal murine IgG antibody and the major allergen from birch pollen Bet v 1. J Immunol 165:331–8
27. Bosshard HR (1996) Epitope mapping by differential chemical modification of antigens. Methods Mol Biol 66:85–95
28. Riemer AB and Jensen-Jarolim E (2007) Mimotope vaccines: epitope mimics induce anti-cancer antibodies. Immunol Lett 113:1–5
29. Szalai K, Jensen-Jarolim E, and Pali-Scholl I (2008) Vaccination strategies based on the mimotope concept. G Ital Dermatol Venereol 143:95–104
30. Knittelfelder R and Jensen-Jarolim E (2009) Mimotope vaccination – from allergy to cancer. Expert Opin Biol Ther 9:1–14
31. Riemer AB, Untersmayr E, Knittelfelder R, Duschl A, Pehamberger H, Zielinski CC, Scheiner O, and Jensen-Jarolim E (2007) Active induction of tumor-specific IgE antibodies by oral mimotope vaccination. Cancer Res 67:3406–11
32. Berglund L, Andrade J, Odeberg J, and Uhlen M (2008) The epitope space of the human proteome. Protein Sci 17:606–13
33. Bell GI (1974) Model for the binding of multivalent antigen to cells. Nature 248:430–1
34. Dintzis HM and Dintzis RZ (1990) Antigens as immunoregulators. Immunol Rev 115:243–50; discussion 251
35. Omori SA, Cato MH, Anzelon-Mills A, Puri KD, Shapiro-Shelef M, Calame K, and Rickert RC (2006) Regulation of class-switch recombination and plasma cell differentiation by phosphatidylinositol 3-kinase signaling. Immunity 25:545–7
36. Monticelli S and Vercelli D (2001) Molecular regulation of class switch recombination to IgE through epsilon germline transcription. Allergy 56:270–8
37. Perona-Wright G, Mohrs K, Taylor J, Zaph C, Artis D, Pearce EJ, and Mohrs M (2008) Cutting edge: Helminth infection induces IgE in the absence of mu- or delta-chain expression. J Immunol 181:6697–701
38. Feldmann M (1972) Induction of immunity and tolerance in vitro by hapten protein conjugates. I. The relationship between the degree of hapten conjugation and the immunogenicity of dinitrophenylated polymerized flagellin. J Exp Med 135:735–53
39. Feldmann M (1972) Induction of immunity and tolerance in vitro by hapten protein conjugates. 3. Hapten inhibition studies of antigen binding to B cells in immunity and tolerance. J Exp Med 136:532–45
40. Katz DH, Hamaoka T, and Benacerraf B (1974) Immunological tolerance in bone marrow-derived lymphocytes. 3. Tolerance induction in primed B cells by hapten conjugates of unrelated immunogenic or "nonimmunogenic" carriers. J Exp Med 139:1464–72

41. Hubbard DA, Lee WY, and Sehon AH (1981) Suppression of the anti-DNP IgE response with tolerogenic conjugates of DNP with polyvinyl alcohol. I. Specific suppression of the anti-DNP IgE response. J Immunol 126:407–13
42. Scholl I, Kopp T, Bohle B, and Jensen-Jarolim E (2006) Biodegradable PLGA particles for improved systemic and mucosal treatment of Type I allergy. Immunol Allergy Clin North Am 26:349–64, ix
43. Feldmann M and Easten A (1971) The relationship between antigenic structure and the requirement for thymus-derived cells in the immune response. J Exp Med 134:103–19
44. Dintzis HM, Dintzis RZ, and Vogelstein B (1976) Molecular determinants of immunogenicity: the immunon model of immune response. Proc Natl Acad Sci USA 73:3671–5
45. Sharma S, Orlowski G, and Song W (2009) Btk regulates B cell receptor-mediated antigen processing and presentation by controlling actin cytoskeleton dynamics in B cells. J Immunol 182:329–39
46. Dintzis RZ, Middleton MH, and Dintzis HM (1983) Studies on the immunogenicity and tolerogenicity of T-independent antigens. J Immunol 131:2196–203
47. Bachmann MF, Hengartner H, and Zinkernagel RM (1995) T helper cell-independent neutralizing B cell response against vesicular stomatitis virus: role of antigen patterns in B cell induction? Eur J Immunol 25:3445–51
48. Fehr T, Skrastina D, Pumpens P, and Zinkernagel RM (1998) T cell-independent type I antibody response against B cell epitopes expressed repetitively on recombinant virus particles. Proc Natl Acad Sci USA 95:9477–81
49. Jegerlehner A, Storni T, Lipowsky G, Schmid M, Pumpens P, and Bachmann MF (2002) Regulation of IgG antibody responses by epitope density and CD21-mediated costimulation. Eur J Immunol 32:3305–14
50. Yang R, Murillo FM, Delannoy MJ, Blosser RL, Yutzy WHt, Uematsu S, Takeda K, Akira S, Viscidi RP, and Roden RB (2005) B lymphocyte activation by human papillomavirus-like particles directly induces Ig class switch recombination via TLR4-MyD88. J Immunol 174:7912–9
51. Cohen-Sfady M, Nussbaum G, Pevsner-Fischer M, Mor F, Carmi P, Zanin-Zhorov A, Lider O, and Cohen IR (2005) Heat shock protein 60 activates B cells via the TLR4-MyD88 pathway. J Immunol 175:3594–602
52. Dimmock NJ and Hardy SA (2004) Valency of antibody binding to virions and its determination by surface plasmon resonance. Rev Med Virol 14:123–35
53. Hinton HJ, Jegerlehner A, and Bachmann MF (2008) Pattern recognition by B cells: the role of antigen repetitiveness versus Toll-like receptors. Curr Top Microbiol Immunol 319: 1–15
54. Gruijthuijsen YK, Grieshuber I, Stocklinger A, Tischler U, Fehrenbach T, Weller MG, Vogel L, Vieths S, Poschl U, and Duschl A (2006) Nitration enhances the allergenic potential of proteins. Int Arch Allergy Immunol 141:265–75
55. Hoffmann-Sommergruber K (2002) Pathogenesis-related (PR)-proteins identified as allergens. Biochem Soc Trans 30:930–35
56. Roth-Walter F, Berin MC, Arnaboldi P, Escalante CR, Dahan S, Rauch J, Jensen-Jarolim E, and Mayer L (2008) Pasteurization of milk proteins promotes allergic sensitization by enhancing uptake through Peyer's patches. Allergy 63:882–90
57. Vos Q, Lees A, Wu ZQ, Snapper CM, and Mond JJ (2000) B-cell activation by T-cell-independent type 2 antigens as an integral part of the humoral immune response to pathogenic microorganisms. Immunol Rev 176:154–70
58. Pasare C and Medzhitov R (2005) Control of B-cell responses by Toll-like receptors. Nature 438:364–68
59. Traidl-Hoffmann C, Mariani V, Hochrein H, Karg K, Wagner H, Ring J, Mueller MJ, Jakob T, and Behrendt H (2005) Pollen-associated phytoprostanes inhibit dendritic cell interleukin-12 production and augment T helper type 2 cell polarization. J Exp Med 201:627–36

60. Brunner R, Wallmann J, Szalai K, Karagiannis P, Altmeppen H, Riemer AB, Jensen-Jarolim E, and Pali-Scholl I (2009) Aluminium per se and in the anti-acid drug sucralfate promotes sensitization via the oral route. Allergy 64:890–7
61. Brunner R, Wallmann J, Szalai K, Karagiannis P, Kopp T, Scheiner O, Jensen-Jarolim E, and Pali-Scholl I (2007) The impact of aluminium in acid-suppressing drugs on the immune response of BALB/c mice. Clin Exp Allergy 37:1566–73
62. Sato M, Adachi T, and Tsubata T (2007) Augmentation of signaling through BCR containing IgE but not that containing IgA due to lack of CD22-mediated signal regulation. J Immunol 178:2901–7
63. Segal DM, Taurog JD, and Metzger H (1977) Dimeric immunoglobulin E serves as a unit signal for mast cell degranulation. Proc Natl Acad Sci USA 74:2993–7
64. Asai K, Kitaura J, Kawakami Y, Yamagata N, Tsai M, Carbone DP, Liu FT, Galli SJ, and Kawakami T (2001) Regulation of mast cell survival by IgE. Immunity 14:791–800
65. Yamasaki S, Ishikawa E, Kohno M, and Saito T (2004) The quantity and duration of FcRgamma signals determine mast cell degranulation and survival. Blood 103:3093–101
66. Maurer D, Fiebiger E, Reininger B, Ebner C, Petzelbauer P, Shi GP, Chapman HA, and Stingl G (1998) Fc epsilon receptor I on dendritic cells delivers IgE-bound multivalent antigens into a cathepsin S-dependent pathway of MHC class II presentation. J Immunol 161:2731–9
67. Shapira SK, Jabara HH, Thienes CP, Ahern DJ, Vercelli D, Gould HJ, and Geha RS (1991) Deletional switch recombination occurs in interleukin-4-induced isotype switching to IgE expression by human B cells. Proc Natl Acad Sci USA 88:7528–32
68. Jabara HH, Loh R, Ramesh N, Vercelli D, and Geha RS (1993) Sequential switching from mu to epsilon via gamma 4 in human B cells stimulated with IL-4 and hydrocortisone. J Immunol 151:4528–33
69. Scholl I, Kalkura N, Shedziankova Y, Bergmann A, Verdino P, Knittelfelder R, Kopp T, Hantusch B, Betzel C, Dierks K, Scheiner O, Boltz-Nitulescu G, Keller W, and Jensen-Jarolim E (2005) Dimerization of the major birch pollen allergen Bet v 1 is important for its in vivo IgE-cross-linking potential in mice. J Immunol 175:6645–50
70. Mongini PK, Blessinger CA, Highet PF, and Inman JK (1992) Membrane IgM-mediated signaling of human B cells. Effect of increased ligand binding site valency on the affinity and concentration requirements for inducing diverse stages of activation. J Immunol 148: 3892–901
71. Kouskoff V, Famiglietti S, Lacaud G, Lang P, Rider JE, Kay BK, Cambier JC, and Nemazee D (1998) Antigens varying in affinity for the B cell receptor induce differential B lymphocyte responses. J Exp Med 188:1453–64
72. Katz DH, Hamaoka T, and Benacerraf B (1973) Induction of immunological tolerance in bone marrow-derived lymphocytes of the IgE antibody class. Proc Natl Acad Sci USA 70:2776–80
73. Rivera J, Cordero JR, Furumoto Y, Luciano-Montalvo C, Gonzalez-Espinosa C, Kovarova M, Odom S, and Parravicini V (2002) Macromolecular protein signaling complexes and mast cell responses: a view of the organization of IgE-dependent mast cell signaling. Mol Immunol 38:1253–8
74. Okumura S, Kashiwakura J, Tomita H, Matsumoto K, Nakajima T, Saito H, and Okayama Y (2003) Identification of specific gene expression profiles in human mast cells mediated by Toll-like receptor 4 and FcepsilonRI. Blood 102:2547–54
75. Kawakami T and Galli SJ (2002) Regulation of mast-cell and basophil function and survival by IgE. Nat Rev Immunol 2:773–86
76. Furuichi K, Rivera J, and Isersky C (1985) The receptor for immunoglobulin E on rat basophilic leukemia cells: effect of ligand binding on receptor expression. Proc Natl Acad Sci USA 82:1522–5
77. Yamaguchi M, Lantz CS, Oettgen HC, Katona IM, Fleming T, Miyajima I, Kinet JP, and Galli SJ (1997) IgE enhances mouse mast cell Fc(epsilon)RI expression in vitro and in vivo: evidence for a novel amplification mechanism in IgE-dependent reactions. J Exp Med 185:663–72

78. Holowka D, Sil D, Torigoe C, and Baird B (2007) Insights into immunoglobulin E receptor signaling from structurally defined ligands. Immunol Rev 217:269–79
79. Kane PM, Holowka D, and Baird B (1988) Cross-linking of IgE-receptor complexes by rigid bivalent antigens greater than 200 A in length triggers cellular degranulation. J Cell Biol 107:969–80
80. Paar JM, Harris NT, Holowka D, and Baird B (2002) Bivalent ligands with rigid double-stranded DNA spacers reveal structural constraints on signaling by Fc epsilon RI. J Immunol 169:856–64
81. Perez-Montfort R and Metzger H (1982) Proteolysis of soluble IgE-receptor complexes: localization of sites on IgE which interact with the Fc receptor. Mol Immunol 19:1113–25
82. Wan T, Beavil RL, Fabiane SM, Beavil AJ, Sohi MK, Keown M, Young RJ, Henry AJ, Owens RJ, Gould HJ, and Sutton BJ (2002) The crystal structure of IgE Fc reveals an asymmetrically bent conformation. Nat Immunol 3:681–6
83. Zheng Y, Shopes B, Holowka D, and Baird B (1991) Conformations of IgE bound to its receptor Fc epsilon RI and in solution. Biochemistry 30:9125–32
84. Zheng Y, Shopes B, Holowka D, and Baird B (1992) Dynamic conformations compared for IgE and IgG1 in solution and bound to receptors. Biochemistry 31:7446–56
85. Becker KE, Ishizaka T, Metzger H, Ishizaka K, and Grimley PM (1973) Surface IgE on human basophils during histamine release. J Exp Med 138:394–409
86. Hook WA, Siraganian RP, and Wahl SM (1975) Complement-induced histamine release from human basophils. I. Generation of activity in human serum. J Immunol 114:1185–90
87. Yamashita T, Yamaguchi T, Murakami K, and Nagasawa S (2001) Detergent-resistant membrane domains are required for mast cell activation but dispensable for tyrosine phosphorylation upon aggregation of the high affinity receptor for IgE. J Biochem 129: 861–8
88. Schweitzer-Stenner R, Licht A, Luscher I, and Pecht I (1987) Oligomerization and ring closure of immunoglobulin E class antibodies by divalent haptens. Biochemistry 26: 3602–12
89. Janeway CA Jr and Medzhitov R (2002) Innate immune recognition. Annu Rev Immunol 20:197–216
90. King TP, Kochoumian L, and Joslyn A (1984) Melittin-specific monoclonal and polyclonal IgE and IgG1 antibodies from mice. J Immunol 133:2668–73
91. Rafnar T, Brummet ME, Bassolino-Klimas D, Metzler WJ, and Marsh DG (1998) Analysis of the three-dimensional antigenic structure of giant ragweed allergen, Amb t 5. Mol Immunol 35:459–67
92. Jensen-Jarolim E, Leitner A, Kalchhauser H, Zurcher A, Ganglberger E, Bohle B, Scheiner O, Boltz-nitulescu G, and Breiteneder H (1998) Peptide mimotopes displayed by phage inhibit antibody binding to bet v 1, the major birch pollen allergen, and induce specific IgG response in mice. FASEB J 12:1635–42
93. Spangfort MD, Mirza O, Ipsen H, Van Neerven RJ, Gajhede M, and Larsen JN (2003) Dominating IgE-binding epitope of Bet v 1, the major allergen of birch pollen, characterized by X-ray crystallography and site-directed mutagenesis. J Immunol 171:3084–90
94. Ganglberger E, Grunberger K, Sponer B, Radauer C, Breiteneder H, Boltz-Nitulescu G, Scheiner O, and Jensen-Jarolim E (2000) Allergen mimotopes for 3-dimensional epitope search and induction of antibodies inhibiting human IgE. Faseb J 14:2177–84
95. Habermann E (1972) Bee and wasp venoms. Science 177:314–22
96. Terwilliger TC, Weissman L, and Eisenberg D (1982) The structure of melittin in the form I crystals and its implication for melittin's lytic and surface activities. Biophys J 37:353–61
97. Ghosh D and Gupta-Bhattacharya S (2008) Structural insight into protein T1, the non-allergenic member of the Bet v 1 allergen family-An in silico analysis. Mol Immunol 45:456–62
98. Christensen LH, Holm J, Lund G, Riise E, and Lund K (2008) Several distinct properties of the IgE repertoire determine effector cell degranulation in response to allergen challenge. J Allergy Clin Immunol 122:298–304

99. Gieras A, Focke-Tejkl M, Ball T, Verdino P, Hartl A, Thalhamer J, and Valenta R (2007) Molecular determinants of allergen-induced effector cell degranulation. J Allergy Clin Immunol 119:384–90
100. Pierson-Mullany LK, Jackola DR, Blumenthal MN, and Rosenberg A (2000) Characterization of polyclonal allergen-specific IgE responses by affinity distributions. Mol Immunol 37:613–20
101. Hantusch B, Schöll I, Harwanegg C, Krieger S, Becker WM, Spitzauer S, Boltz-Nitulescu G, and Jensen-Jarolim E (2005) Affinity determinations of purified IgE and IgG antibodies against the major pollen allergens Phl p 5a and Bet v 1a: discrepancy between IgE and IgG binding strength. Immunol Lett 97:81–9
102. Reese G, Ayuso R, and Lehrer SB (1999) Tropomyosin: an invertebrate pan-allergen. Int Arch Allergy Immunol 119:247–58
103. Bellinghausen I, Haringer B, Lafargue B, Strand D, Konig B, Decker H, and Saloga J (2008) Allergological implication of the quaternary hexameric structure of the cockroach allergen Per a 3. Clin Exp Allergy 38:539–48
104. Smole U, Balazs N, Hoffmann-Sommergruber K, Breiteneder H, and Wagner S (2008) Different polarization of Th responses by dendritic cells (DCs) of birch pollen allergic and non atopic donors pulsed with Bet v 1 and homologous food allergens (XXVII Congress of the European Academy of Allergology and Clinical Immunology, June 7–11, 2008, Barcelona, Spain). Allergy 63:255
105. van Boxtel EL, van Beers MM, Koppelman SJ, van den Broek LA, and Gruppen H (2006) Allergen Ara h 1 occurs in peanuts as a large oligomer rather than as a trimer. J Agric Food Chem 54:7180–6
106. Beezhold DH, Hickey VL, Sutherland MF, and O'Hehir RE (2004) The latex allergen hev B 5 is an antigen with repetitive murine B-cell epitopes. Int Arch Allergy Immunol 134:334–40
107. Pomes A, Vailes LD, Helm RM, and Chapman MD (2002) IgE reactivity of tandem repeats derived from cockroach allergen, Bla g 1. Eur J Biochem 269:3086–92
108. Ayuso R, Lehrer SB, and Reese G (2002) Identification of continuous, allergenic regions of the major shrimp allergen Pen a 1 (tropomyosin). Int Arch Allergy Immunol 127:27–37
109. Marti P, Truffer R, Stadler MB, Keller-Gautschi E, Crameri R, Mari A, Schmid-Grendelmeier P, Miescher SM, Stadler BM, and Vogel M (2007) Allergen motifs and the prediction of allergenicity. Immunol Lett 109:47–55
110. Stadler MB and Stadler BM (2003) Allergenicity prediction by protein sequence. Faseb J 17:1141–43
111. Kong W, Tan TS, Tham L, and Choo KW (2007) Improved prediction of allergenicity by combination of multiple sequence motifs. In Silico Biol 7:77–86
112. Cooke MP, Heath AW, Shokat KM, Zeng Y, Finkelman FD, Linsley PS, Howard M, and Goodnow CC (1994) Immunoglobulin signal transduction guides the specificity of B cell-T cell interactions and is blocked in tolerant self-reactive B cells. J Exp Med 179:425–38
113. Lindblom A and Liljegren A (2000) Regular review: tumour markers in malignancies. Bmj 320:424–27
114. Wu JT (2002) C-erbB2 oncoprotein and its soluble ectodomain: a new potential tumor marker for prognosis early detection and monitoring patients undergoing Herceptin treatment. Clin Chim Acta 322:11–9
115. Voorzanger-Rousselot N and Garnero P (2007) Biochemical markers in oncology. Part I: molecular basis. Part II: clinical uses. Cancer Treat Rev 33:230–83
116. Kurien BT and Scofield RH (2008) Autoimmunity and oxidatively modified autoantigens. Autoimmun Rev 7:567–73
117. Banerjea A, Feakins RM, Nickols CD, Phillips SM, Powar MP, Bustin SA, and Dorudi S (2005) Immunogenic hsp-70 is overexpressed in colorectal cancers with high-degree microsatellite instability. Dis Colon Rectum 48:2322–28
118. Yasuda M, Takenoyama M, Obata Y, Sugaya M, So T, Hanagiri T, Sugio K, and Yasumoto K (2002) Tumor-infiltrating B lymphocytes as a potential source of identifying tumor antigen in human lung cancer. Cancer Res 62:1751–56

119. Taylor RB, Duffus WPH, Raff MC, and de Petris S (1971) Redistribution and pinocytosis of lymphocyte surface immunoglobulin molecules induced by anti immunoglobulin antibody. (New Biology) Nature 233:225–9
120. Pecanha LM, Snapper CM, Finkelman FD, and Mond JJ (1991) Dextran-conjugated anti-Ig antibodies as a model for T cell-independent type 2 antigen-mediated stimulation of Ig secretion in vitro. I. Lymphokine dependence. J Immunol 146:833–9
121. Schwartz-Albiez R, Laban S, Eichmuller S, and Kirschfink M (2008) Cytotoxic natural antibodies against human tumours: an option for anti-cancer immunotherapy? Autoimmun Rev 7:491–5
122. Cheng ZJ, Singh RD, Marks DL, and Pagano RE (2006) Membrane microdomains, caveolae, and caveolar endocytosis of sphingolipids. Mol Membr Biol 23:101–10
123. Brown DA (2006) Lipid rafts, detergent-resistant membranes, and raft targeting signals. Physiology (Bethesda) 21:430–9
124. Nagy P, Vereb G, Sebestyen Z, Horvath G, Lockett SJ, Damjanovich S, Park JW, Jovin TM, and Szollosi J (2002) Lipid rafts and the local density of ErbB proteins influence the biological role of homo- and heteroassociations of ErbB2. J Cell Sci 115:4251–62
125. Rodriguez GC, Boente MP, Berchuck A, Whitaker RS, O'Briant KC, Xu F, and Bast RC Jr (1993) The effect of antibodies and immunotoxins reactive with HER-2/neu on growth of ovarian and breast cancer cell lines. Am J Obstet Gynecol 168:228–32
126. Milenic DE, Garmestani K, Brady ED, Albert PS, Ma D, Abdulla A, and Brechbiel MW (2004) Targeting of HER2 antigen for the treatment of disseminated peritoneal disease. Clin Cancer Res 10:7834–41
127. Ozcelik S, Orr G, Hu D, Chen C-S, Resat H, Harms GS, Opresko LK, Wiley HS, and Colson SD (2004) FRET measurements between small numbers of molecules identifies subtle changes in receptor interactions. Proc SPIE 5323:119
128. Webb SE, Roberts SK, Needham SR, Tynan CJ, Rolfe DJ, Winn MD, Clarke DT, Barraclough R, and Martin-Fernandez ML (2008) Single-molecule imaging and fluorescence lifetime imaging microscopy show different structures for high- and low-affinity epidermal growth factor receptors in A431 cells. Biophys J 94:803–19
129. Orr G, Hu D, Ozcelik S, Opresko LK, Wiley HS, and Colson SD (2005) Cholesterol dictates the freedom of EGF receptors and HER2 in the plane of the membrane. Biophys J 89: 1362–73
130. Dessi S, Batetta B, Pulisci D, Spano O, Anchisi C, Tessitore L, Costelli P, Baccino FM, Aroasio E, and Pani P (1994) Cholesterol content in tumor tissues is inversely associated with high-density lipoprotein cholesterol in serum in patients with gastrointestinal cancer. Cancer 73:253–8
131. Skornick Y, Kurman CC, and Sindelar WF (1984) Active immunization of hamsters against pancreatic carcinoma with lipid-treated cells or their shed antigens. Cancer Res 44: 946–8
132. Wang XQ and Paller AS (2006) Lipid rafts: membrane triage centers. J Invest Dermatol 126:951–3
133. Chen X and Resh MD (2002) Cholesterol depletion from the plasma membrane triggers ligand-independent activation of the epidermal growth factor receptor. J Biol Chem 277:49631–7
134. Shinitzky M, Skornick Y, and Haran-Ghera N (1979) Effective tumor immunization induced by cells of elevated membrane-lipid microviscosity. Proc Natl Acad Sci USA 76:5313–6
135. Winiarska M, Bil J, Wilczek E, Wilczynski GM, Lekka M, Engelberts PJ, Mackus WJ, Gorska E, Bojarski L, Stoklosa T, Nowis D, Kurzaj Z, Makowski M, Glodkowska E, Issat T, Mrowka P, Lasek W, Dabrowska-Iwanicka A, Basak GW, Wasik M, Warzocha K, Sinski M, Gaciong Z, Jakobisiak M, Parren PW, and Golab J (2008) Statins impair antitumor effects of rituximab by inducing conformational changes of CD20. PLoS Med 5:e64
136. Janas E, Priest R, Wilde JI, White JH, and Malhotra R (2005) Rituxan (anti-CD20 antibody)-induced translocation of CD20 into lipid rafts is crucial for calcium influx and apoptosis. Clin Exp Immunol 139:439–46

137. Janas E, Priest R, and Malhotra R (2005) Functional role of lipid rafts in CD20 activity? Biochem Soc Symp:165–75
138. Chaturvedi P, Singh AP, and Batra SK (2008) Structure, evolution, and biology of the MUC4 mucin. Faseb J 22:966–81
139. Chaturvedi P, Singh AP, Chakraborty S, Chauhan SC, Bafna S, Meza JL, Singh PK, Hollingsworth MA, Mehta PP, and Batra SK (2008) MUC4 mucin interacts with and stabilizes the HER2 oncoprotein in human pancreatic cancer cells. Cancer Res 68:2065–70
140. Aas K, and Jebsen JW (1967) Studies of hypersensitivity to fish. Partial purification and crystallization of a major allergenic component of cod. Int Arch Allergy Appl Immunol 32:1–20
141. Huecas S, Villalba M, and Rodriguez R (2001) Ole e 9, a major olive pollen allergen is a 1,3-beta-glucanase. Isolation, characterization, amino acid sequence, and tissue specificity. J Biol Chem 276:27959–66
142. McGibbon AM, Christie JF, Kennedy MW, and Lee TD (1990) Identification of the major Ascaris allergen and its purification to homogeneity by high-performance liquid chromatography. Mol Biochem Parasitol 39:163–71
143. Bocskei Z, Groom CR, Flower DR, Wright CE, Phillips SE, Cavaggioni A, Findlay JB, and North AC (1992) Pheromone binding to two rodent urinary proteins revealed by X-ray crystallography. Nature 360:186–8
144. Ogawa T, Tsuji H, Bando N, Kitamura K, Zhu YL, Hirano H, and Nishikawa K (1993) Identification of the soybean allergenic protein, Gly m Bd 30 K, with the soybean seed 34-kDa oil-body-associated protein. Biosci Biotechnol Biochem 57:1030–3
145. Hoffman DR (1993) Allergens in Hymenoptera venom XXIV: the amino acid sequences of imported fire ant venom allergens Sol i II, Sol i III, and Sol i IV. J Allergy Clin Immunol 91:71–8
146. Gimona M, Watakabe A, and Helfman DM (1995) Specificity of dimer formation in tropomyosins: influence of alternatively spliced exons on homodimer and heterodimer assembly. Proc Natl Acad Sci USA 92:9776–80
147. De Vouge MW, Thaker AJ, Curran IH, Zhang L, Muradia G, Rode H, and Vijay HM (1996) Isolation and expression of a cDNA clone encoding an Alternaria alternata Alt a 1 subunit. Int Arch Allergy Immunol 111:385–95
148. Wellhausen A, Schoning B, Petersen A, and Vieths S (1996) IgE binding to a new cross-reactive structure: a 35 kDa protein in birch pollen, exotic fruit and other plant foods. Z Ernahrungswiss 35:348–55
149. Rautiainen J, Pentikainen J, Rytkonen M, Linnala-Kankkunen A, Pelkonen J, Virtanen T, and Mantyjarvi R (1996) Molecular analysis of allergenic proteins in bovine dander. Allergy 51:378–82
150. Shin DS, Compadre CM, Maleki SJ, Kopper RA, Sampson H, Huang SK, Burks AW, and Bannon GA (1998) Biochemical and structural analysis of the IgE binding sites on Ara h1, an abundant and highly allergenic peanut protein. J Biol Chem 273:13753–9
151. Petersen A, Schramm G, Schlaak M, and Becker WM (1998) Post-translational modifications influence IgE reactivity to the major allergen Phl p 1 of timothy grass pollen. Clin Exp Allergy 28:315–21
152. Eriksson TL, Whitley P, Johansson E, van Hage-Hamsten M, and Gafvelin G (1999) Identification and characterisation of two allergens from the dust mite Acarus siro, homologous with fatty acid-binding proteins. Int Arch Allergy Immunol 119:275–81
153. Gregoire C, Tavares GA, Lorenzo HK, Dandeu JP, David B, and Alzari PM (1999) Crystallization and preliminary crystallographic analysis of the major horse allergen Equ c 1. Acta Crystallogr D Biol Crystallogr 55(Pt 4):880–2
154. Xia Y, Spence HJ, Moore J, Heaney N, McDermott L, Cooper A, Watson DG, Mei B, Komuniecki R, and Kennedy MW (2000) The ABA-1 allergen of Ascaris lumbricoides: sequence polymorphism, stage and tissue-specific expression, lipid binding function, and protein biophysical properties. Parasitology 120(Pt 2):211–24

155. Maleki SJ, Kopper RA, Shin DS, Park CW, Compadre CM, Sampson H, Burks AW, and Bannon GA (2000) Structure of the major peanut allergen Ara h 1 may protect IgE-binding epitopes from degradation. J Immunol 164:5844–9
156. Lascombe MB, Gregoire C, Poncet P, Tavares GA, Rosinski-Chupin I, Rabillon J, Goubran-Botros H, Mazie JC, David B, and Alzari PM (2000) Crystal structure of the allergen Equ c 1. A dimeric lipocalin with restricted IgE-reactive epitopes. J Biol Chem 275: 21572–7
157. Suck R, Weber B, Kahlert H, Hagen S, Cromwell O, and Fiebig H (2000) Purification and immunobiochemical characterization of folding variants of the recombinant major wasp allergen Ves v 5 (antigen 5). Int Arch Allergy Immunol 121:284–91
158. Sakurai K, Oobatake M, and Goto Y (2001) Salt-dependent monomer-dimer equilibrium of bovine beta-lactoglobulin at pH 3. Protein Sci 10:2325–35
159. Sen M, Kopper R, Pons L, Abraham EC, Burks AW, and Bannon GA (2002) Protein structure plays a critical role in peanut allergen stability and may determine immunodominant IgE-binding epitopes. J Immunol 169:882–7
160. Das Dores S, Chopin C, Villaume C, Fleurence J, and Gueant JL (2002) A new oligomeric parvalbumin allergen of Atlantic cod (Gad mI) encoded by a gene distinct from that of Gad cI. Allergy 57(Suppl 72):79–83
161. Rajashankar K, Bufe A, Weber W, Eschenburg S, Lindner B, and Betzel C (2002) Structure of the functional domain of the major grass-pollen allergen Phlp 5b. Acta Crystallogr D Biol Crystallogr 58:1175–81
162. Verdino P, Westritschnig K, Valenta R, and Keller W (2002) The cross-reactive calcium-binding pollen allergen, Phl p 7, reveals a novel dimer assembly. Embo J 21:5007–16
163. Wopfner N, Willeroidee M, Hebenstreit D, van Ree R, Aalbers M, Briza P, Thalhamer J, Ebner C, Richter K, and Ferreira F (2002) Molecular and immunological characterization of profilin from mugwort pollen. Biol Chem 383:1779–89
164. Fahlbusch B, Rudeschko O, Schlott B, Henzgen M, Schlenvoigt G, Schubert H, and Kinne RW (2003) Further characterization of IgE-binding antigens from guinea pig hair as new members of the lipocalin family. Allergy 58:629–34
165. Gronlund H, Bergman T, Sandstrom K, Alvelius G, Reininger R, Verdino P, Hauswirth A, Liderot K, Valent P, Spitzauer S, Keller W, Valenta R, and van Hage-Hamsten M (2003) Formation of disulfide bonds and homodimers of the major cat allergen Fel d 1 equivalent to the natural allergen by expression in Escherichia coli. J Biol Chem 278: 40144–51
166. van Oort E, Dieker MC, de Heer PG, Peltre G, Aalberse RC, and van Ree R (2005) The major grass pollen group 5 allergen from Dactylis glomerata and its C-terminal split product both behave as dimers: implications for allergen standardization. Int Arch Allergy Immunol 136:113–22
167. de Halleux S, Stura E, VanderElst L, Carlier V, Jacquemin M, and Saint-Remy JM (2006) Three-dimensional structure and IgE-binding properties of mature fully active Der p 1, a clinically relevant major allergen. J Allergy Clin Immunol 117:571–6
168. Ball T, Leistler B, Valenta R, and Almo SC (2003) X-ray crystal structure of Phl p 1, a major timothy grass pollen allergen. RCSB Protein Data Bank 1N10
169. Kamata Y, Miyanomae A, Nakayama E, Miyanomae T, Tajima T, Nishimura K, Tada T, and Hoshi H (2007) Characterization of dog allergens Can f 1 and Can f 2. 2. A comparison of Can f 1 with Can f 2 regarding their biochemical and immunological properties. Int Arch Allergy Immunol 142:301–8
170. Li M, Gustchina A, Alexandratos J, Wlodawer A, Wunschmann S, Kepley CL, Chapman MD, and Pomes A (2008) Crystal structure of a dimerized cockroach allergen Bla g 2 complexed with a monoclonal antibody. J Biol Chem 283:22806–14
171. Weghofer M, Dall'Antonia Y, Grote M, Stocklinger A, Kneidinger M, Balic N, Krauth MT, Fernandez-Caldas E, Thomas WR, van Hage M, Vieths S, Spitzauer S, Horak F, Svergun DI, Konarev PV, Valent P, Thalhamer J, Keller W, Valenta R, and Vrtala S (2008)

Characterization of Der p 21, a new important allergen derived from the gut of house dust mites. Allergy 63:758–67

172. Tan YW, Chan SL, Ong TC, Yit le Y, Tiong YS, Chew FT, Sivaraman J, and Mok YK (2009) Structures of Two Major Allergens, Bla g 4 and Per a 4, from Cockroaches and Their IgE Binding Epitopes. J Biol Chem 284:3148–57

Chapter 11
The Role of Th2-Mediated Anti-Tumor Immunity in Tumor Surveillance and Clearance

Ljubov Simson, Julia I. Ellyard, and Christopher R. Parish

Abstract The concept that the immune system has the potential to recognize tumor cells and either eliminate them (tumor immune surveillance) or select for immune-resistant variants (immunoediting) has gained a resurgence of interest by the scientific community in the last decade. To date, much of the research on the immune response to cancer has focused on the response of cytotoxic $CD8^+$ T lymphocytes to tumor-specific antigens and the production of Th1 cytokines by $CD4^+$ and $CD8^+$ T cells. In contrast, Th2-mediated immunity has traditionally been viewed as enhancing tumor growth, both by promoting angiogenesis and by inhibiting cell-mediated immunity and subsequent tumor cell killing. Although components of Th2-mediated immunity have been shown to promote tumor growth, there is also an expanding body of evidence demonstrating the anti-tumor activity of $CD4^+$ Th2 cells, particularly in collaboration with tumor-infiltrating granulocytes, such as eosinophils. In this chapter we examine all the key components of type 2 immunity and their effects on tumor growth. Based on this collective data, there exists great potential for the development of Th2-mediated immunotherapies that harness the anti-tumor activity of eosinophils, alternatively activated macrophages and the antigen–IgE–receptor axis.

11.1 Introduction

The fundamental requirement for the co-operation between the innate and the adaptive immune systems for effective tumor identification and tumor eradication is widely accepted. Importantly, the role of the immune system in the surveillance of transformed cells has seen a resurgence of interest in the last 10 years, with a substantial body of data in mice and humans supporting a role for the immune system in host protection from tumor development and in shaping tumor immunogenicity [1]. Tumor immune surveillance and immune editing are processes whereby the

---

L. Simson (✉)
Centre for Biomedical, Molecular and Chemical Research, University of Canberra, ACT, Australia
e-mail: luby.simson@canberra.edu.au

M.L. Penichet, E. Jensen-Jarolim (eds.), *Cancer and IgE*,
DOI 10.1007/978-1-60761-451-7_11,

immune system has the inherent capacity to recognize, modify and induce the elimination of transformed cells within the body. Additionally, host immune status has been identified as critical in controlling the spread and growth of metastatic tumors [1]. By increasing our understanding of the anti-tumor immune responses, cancer immunotherapy aims to harness those specific immune responses most effective at producing tumor elimination.

Until recently, most tumor eradication studies have focused on the role of the adaptive dendritic cell (DC)-driven $CD8^+$ cytotoxic T-lymphocyte (CTLs) response to tumor-associated antigens (TAAs) following recognition of tumor antigens presented by MHC class I molecules on transformed cells. Many types of vaccines incorporating peptide antigens, proteins, DNA and whole tumor cells, as well as adoptive transfer of tumor-reactive CTLs, have been evaluated, although generally these approaches have had limited clinical success [2, 3]. The lack of success encountered by these strategies highlight the many problems associated with generating CTL-mediated anti-tumor immunity, including the fact that "successful" tumors have often been "immunoselected" or "immunoedited" to evade recognition by CTLs [4]. The fact remains that the ability of the host to generate an effective innate immune response against the tumor is crucial for the subsequent development of an adaptive immunity and an effective CTL response, with the adaptive immune response also recruiting innate effector cells, including natural killer (NK) cells, neutrophils, mast cells, macrophages and eosinophils, into tumors [5]. These observations have stimulated the search for more effective approaches to cancer immunotherapy.

11.2 $CD4^+$ T cells – The Th1 and Th2 Paradigm in Tumor Biology

In the last decade there has been renewed interest in anti-tumor immune responses mediated by $CD4^+$ T cells. Studies have highlighted the role of $CD4^+$ T cells in both the activation of innate effector cells in the primary response and the subsequent co-operation with innate cells in tumor cell killing [6]. Unlike CTLs, $CD4^+$ T cells can respond to MHC class I negative tumors, recognizing TAAs presented on MHC class II molecules by bystander antigen-presenting cells (APCs), a process found to be less susceptible to immunoediting and subsequent immunoselection [6, 7]. Studies using either a $CD4^+$ T-cell activating cancer vaccine [8] or in vitro-generated tumor antigen-specific $CD4^+$ T cells [9, 10] have shown that $CD4^+$ T cells can clear established tumors from mice, with both Th1 and Th2 cytokines being implicated in the tumor eradication process. Importantly, recent studies by Mautner et al. of a patient with renal cell carcinoma highlighted the potential of harnessing $CD4^+$ T cells against MHC class II-restricted tumor antigens in an immunotherapy strategy [11].

Studies from our own laboratory have demonstrated a critical role for antigen-specific $CD4^+$ T cells exhibiting a cytokine profile characteristic of Th2 cells, in

the clearance of established B16 melanoma metastasis [12]. However, in contrast to previous studies [9], $CD4^+$ Th1 cells had a limited effect at inducing tumor clearance [12]. The advantage of $CD4^+$ Th2 cells is that they have the potential to directly enhance antibody-mediated tumor immunity as well as innate anti-tumor immune responses by directly recruiting tumoricidal myeloid cells, including mast cells, macrophages and eosinophils, into the tumor site, a process dependent on the production of Th2-associated cytokines, such as interleukin (IL)-4 [13–16]. Since the establishment of the classification of $CD4^+$ T cells as Th1 or Th2 based on their cytokine expression [17], there has been a strongly held conviction that maintaining a Th1/Th2 immune balance favoring Th1-mediated cellular immunity is linked to a positive clinical prognosis in cancer patients [18, 19]. However, more recent studies in humans and in animal models clearly illustrate that Th2-mediated cellular and chemical mediators have tumor immune surveillance and tumor clearance potential [20–23]. This chapter aims to focus on the mechanisms of Th2-mediated anti-tumor immunity.

11.3 Key Cellular and Chemical Mediators Involved in Th2-Mediated Tumor Immunity

Clinical and laboratory-based evidence is mounting to highlight the potential of Th2-mediated immune responses in initiating and effecting anti-tumor activity, particularly through Th2-mediated cytokines/chemokines, activated eosinophils, alternatively activated macrophages (aaMacs), Tc2 cells, B cells and mast cells loaded with anti-tumor IgE (Table 11.1, Fig. 11.1). In addition, Th2-mediated immunity has the potential to be harnessed as a cancer immunotherapy strategy. The key cellular and chemical mediators involved in Th2-mediated tumor immunity will be discussed below.

11.3.1 Th2 Cytokines

As a key regulator of humoral and adaptive immunity, the role of IL-4 in tumor biology has been studied most extensively. IL-4 is a pleiotropic cytokine produced by activated $CD4^+$ Th2 cells, mast cells, basophils and eosinophils. Murine studies, using IL-4-secreting tumors [13], directly injecting IL-4 into tumors [15] or injecting IL-4 around the tumor draining lymph node [13], have demonstrated a role for this pleiotropic cytokine in tumor clearance. In these studies, tumor clearance was found to directly correlate with the infiltration of eosinophils and macrophages into the tumor site [13–15]. In addition, neutralization of IL-4 with an anti-IL-4 monoclonal antibody resulted in the loss of the eosinophil and macrophage infiltrates and a concurrent loss of anti-tumor immunity, results which were found to be less evident following the neutralization of IL-5 using an anti-IL-5 monoclonal antibody [15]. Although B cells, NK cells and mast cells do not appear to be required for IL-4-mediated tumor clearance [15], $CD8^+$ T cells have been reported to be

Table 11.1 The key factors involved in Th2-mediated immunity and their effect on tumor growth

Factor	Tumor growth	Key observations	References
IL-4	Inhibit	IL-4 induces tumor clearance via infiltrating granulocytes and is anti-angiogenic.	13–15, 25, 27, 28,29
	Enhance	Inhibition of tumor apoptosis.	26
IL-13	Inhibit	IL-13 induces granulocyte-mediated tumor clearance.	36,37,43
		IL-13Rα2 cytotoxin constructs induce tumor clearance.	41,42
	Enhance	NKT cell-derived IL-13 inhibits CTL activation via macrophage secretion of TGF-β.	38
		IL-13 as an autocrine factor in Hodgkin's lymphoma.	40
IL-24/mda-7	Inhibit	IL-24 promotes tumor growth suppression, apoptosis and radiosensitization.	53–55
		Ad.IL-24 therapy successful in several cancers.	54,56–58
IL-25/IL-17E	Inhibit	IL-25 promotes expansion of Th2-mediated tumor immune responses.	61
		Tumor clearance mediated by Virulizin linked to IL-25-induced eosinophilia and macrophage influx.	62–64
Eosinophils	Inhibit	Role in IL-4-mediated tumor clearance in mice and can directly kill tumor cells in vitro.	8,9,12,13,15,16,24
		Eosinophil-mediated tumor clearance.	67,72,74
		Eosinophils implicated in tumor immune surveillance.	23
		High eosinophil counts in tumors are associated with a good prognosis.	66–70
	Enhance	Eosinophils may promote tumor angiogenesis.	78
		High eosinophil counts in tumors associated with poor prognosis.	75–77
aaMacs	Inhibit	aaMac-derived arginase-1-mediated arginine depletion inhibits tumor growth.	89–95
	Enhance	Arginase-1 can inhibit CTL function and anti-tumor activity.	96
B-cells	Inhibit	B cell deficient mice have a decreased tumor growth.	99–101
		Antigen-IgE-FcεR1 axis can induce ADCC and tumor clearance.	114–116
	Enhance	B cells inhibit CTL-mediated tumor clearance through IgG-mediated formation of IC.	102,105,106
Mast cells	Inhibit	Mast-cell deficiency linked to increased tumor growth and inhibition of tumor apoptosis.	122,123
	Enhance	Mast cell infiltration associated with poor prognosis.	119,120
Tc2 cells	Inhibit	IL-4-secreting Tc2 cells can induce tumor clearance.	127,128,130
	Enhance	Tc2 cells secreting high levels of IL-10 can inhibit tumor clearance.	131

IL, interleukin; NK, natural killer; CTL, cytotoxic T lymphocyte; TGF-β, tumor necrosis factor β; Tc2, type-2 $CD8^+$ T cell; ADCC, antibody-dependent cellular cytotoxicity; IC, immune complex

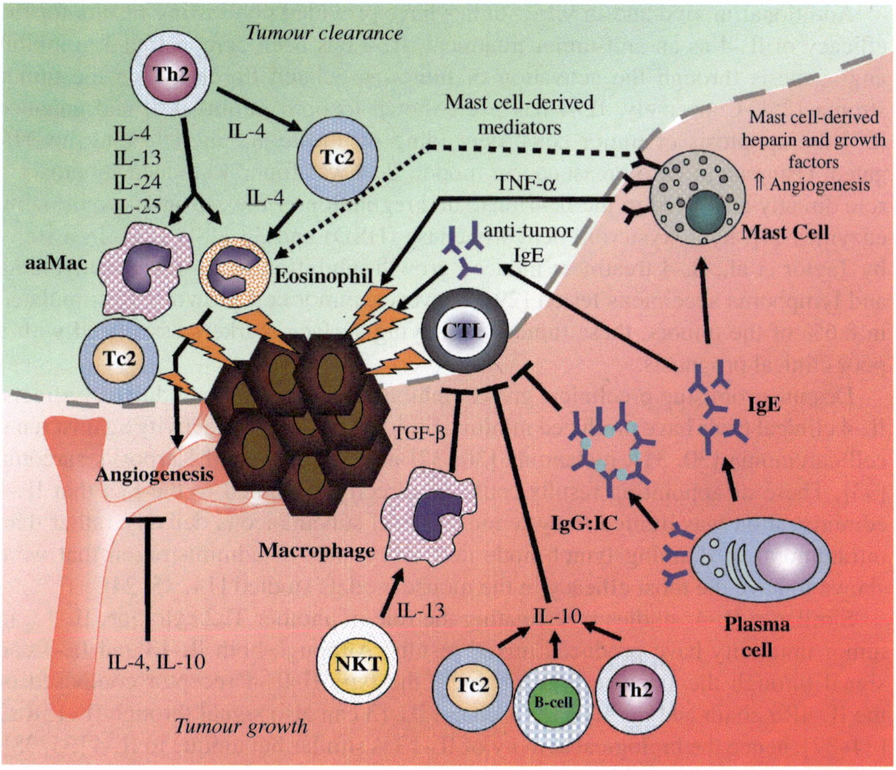

Fig. 11.1 The "yin and yang" of Th2-mediated inflammation within tumors. The model shows how different components of Th2-mediated immunity can either enhance tumor clearance (*light/green zone*) or promote tumor growth (*darker/red zone*). Secretion of IL-4, IL-13, IL-24 or IL-25 by $CD4^+$ Th2 cells can induce an influx of eosinophils and alternatively activated macrophages (aaMacs) into the tumor and promote anti-tumor cytotoxic activity. Similarly, IL-4-secreting $CD8^+$ Tc2 cells may induce the direct killing of tumor cells, although less effectively than $CD8^+$ CTL cells, in addition to collaborating with eosinophils and macrophages to induce tumor clearance. Mast-cell mediators, such as TNF-α, have also been shown to have a direct anti-tumor effect. Conversely, NKT cell-derived IL-13 can induce TGF-β secretion by $CD11b^+$ macrophages, inhibiting CTL-mediated anti-tumor activity by interfering with antigen processing and presentation, similar to immunosuppressive IL-10, produced by Th2, Tc2 and B cells. Plasma cells can promote tumor growth by the secretion of anti-tumor antibodies that form immune complexes (ICs), in particular, IgG-mediated ICs that interfere with CTL-mediated tumor cell lysis, and together with tissue-remodeling leukocytes, such as eosinophils and macrophages, promote tumor angiogenesis. Anti-tumor IgE, however, can be harnessed for both passive and active tumor immunotherapy, resulting in subsequent tumor clearance. Also, IgE-mediated activation of mast cells can result in mast cell degranulation, the activation of eosinophils by mast-cell-derived mediators and resultant enhanced tumor clearance. On the other hand, mast-cell-derived heparin and growth factors, as well as eosinophils, have been linked with enhanced angiogenesis. Based on figure published in *Tissue Antigens* by Ellyard, Simson and Parish [20]

either essential [24] or not required [15]. $CD8^+$ T-cell efficacy in IL-4-mediated tumor clearance has more recently been related to direct or indirect interactions with eosinophils, rather than CTL activity, a process which will be more thoroughly discussed later in this chapter.

Additional in vivo and in vitro studies have provided contrasting results for the efficacy of IL-4 as an anti-tumor treatment. IL-4 has been demonstrated to inhibit angiogenesis through the activation of tumor-associated fibroblasts in the tumor stroma [25]. Conversely, IL-4 has been shown to both inhibit [26] and enhance [27] the apoptosis of tumor cells, depending on the tumor model being investigated. Using an in vitro breast cancer model, IL-4 was found to induce apoptosis, a role directly attributed to the IL-4-mediated regulation of the estrogen synthesizing enzymes 17β-hydroxysteroid dehydrogenase (HSD) and 3β-HSD [28]. In a study by Taylor et al., IL-4 treatment induced growth inhibition in 52–60% of myeloma and lymphoma specimens tested [29]. However, tumor cell growth was stimulated in 8.6% of the tumors, these tumors displaying surface markers associated with a poor clinical prognosis.

Despite promising preclinical growth inhibitory and immunomodulatory effects, IL-4 clinical trials have produced minimal biologic and clinical activity against renal cell carcinoma [30, 31], melanoma [30, 32] and AIDS-related Karposi's sarcoma [33]. These disappointing results could be directly attributed to the fact that IL-4 administration was limited to systemic or distal subcutaneous delivery rather than intratumoral or draining lymph node delivery, routes of administration that were shown to have the most efficacy in the mouse models studied [14, 15, 24].

Similar to IL-4, studies investigating the role of another Th2 cytokine, IL-13, in tumor immunity have produced mixed results. Although both IL-13 and IL-4 can signal through the same receptor, namely the type II IL-4 receptor composed of the IL-4Rα chain and the IL-13Rα1 chain, IL-13 can also signal through IL-13Rα2 [34–37]; hence the biological activity of IL-13 is similar but unique to IL-4 [35, 38]. Overexpression of IL-13 by tumor cells has been shown to induce tumor clearance, with Gr-1^+ and MAC-3^+ expression identifying the tumor-infiltrating leukocytes as neutrophils and macrophages [36, 37]. However, the expression of Gr-1^+ on eosinophils, coupled with the known role of eosinophils in IL-13-mediated inflammation [39], suggests that eosinophils may also be effector cells in IL-13-mediated tumor clearance, as observed for IL-4. In contrast, transfection of a soluble IL-13Rα2 decoy receptor into the tumor cells or administration of the receptor as a soluble fusion protein had no effect on the growth of B16F1 melanoma and Meth A fibrosarcoma tumors [38]. Furthermore, studies by Terabe et al. have indicated that IL-13 plays a role in $CD4^+$ NKT cell-mediated suppression of tumor immune surveillance [38]. IL-13 has also been identified as an autocrine growth factor for Reed–Sternberg cells in Hodgkin's lymphoma [40].

Interestingly, IL-13Rα2 but not IL-13Rα1 is overexpressed in a variety of human cancer cells derived from glioblastoma, squamous cell carcinoma of head and neck, breast cancer, colon cancer, renal cell carcinoma, pancreatic cancer and AIDS-associated Kaposi's sarcoma [41, 42]. However, the stable transfection of the IL-13Rα2 in human breast and pancreatic cancer cell lines identified a significant inhibition in the tumorigenicity of the IL-13Rα2-expressing tumors in immunodeficient mice, with IL-13 produced by infiltrating neutrophils combined with tumor cell-derived IL-8 producing an anti-tumor effect [43]. The use of targeted therapy employing an IL-13Rα2 cytotoxin construct has shown promising preclinical tumor

cytotoxicity in vitro and in vivo [41, 42], but clinical trials using an IL-13Rα2 cytotoxin have shown no significant effect on tumor growth [44]. It remains clear that although IL-13Rα2 expression is elevated in some cancers, the role of IL-13 in tumor growth varies greatly between tumor types.

Previous reports suggesting that Th2-type cytokines inhibit anti-tumor immunity in vivo [45–47] and in vitro [48] had attributed this effect to IL-10-mediated immune suppression. However, it has now become clear that IL-10 has the potential to regulate both Th1-type and Th2-type cytokine responses [49]. On the other hand, the melanoma differentiation association gene (mda)-7, or IL-24, has been identified as a unique tumor suppressor in the IL-10 family of cytokines and is classified as a Th2 cytokine, being produced by monocytes and Th2 cells [50]. The two heterodimeric IL-24 receptors, IL-22R1/IL-20R2 and IL-20R1/IL20R2 [51], are expressed in human lymphoid organs such as spleen and thymus, as well as by peripheral blood leukocytes and normal melanocytes [52]. In vitro, IL-24 has been shown to selectively induce growth suppression, apoptosis and radiosensitization of a diverse range of human cancer cells, without causing similar effects in normal cells [53]. Intratumoral and peritumoral treatment of prostate cancer tumors in athymic nude mice using a replication-incompetent adenovirus expressing IL-24 (Ad.IL-24) was found to completely eradicate primary tumors as well as tumors created at a distal site to treatment [54]. Similarly, Ad.IL24 transduction of human breast cancer cells resulted in G(2)/M phase cell cycle arrest and apoptotic cell death, which correlated with the secretion of the IL-24 protein. Tumor cell killing by IL-24 was also dependent on binding to the IL-20R1/IL-20R2 heterodimeric receptor complex expressed by tumor cells [55].

Importantly, the efficacy of Ad.IL-24 as a gene therapy for cancer has been validated in terminal prostate cancer patients [54]. These studies also identified the ability of Ad.IL-24 to induce a "potent bystander apoptosis-inducing effect" in adjacent tumor cells not initially receiving this gene product, whereas normal cells are unaffected [56]. Based on its profound cancer tropism, Ad.IL-24 has been evaluated in a phase I clinical trial in patients with melanomas and other solid cancers. These studies document that mda-7/IL-24 is well tolerated and demonstrates evidence of significant clinical activity [57]. Recent in vitro studies have observed that certain cancers, including pancreatic and colorectal cancer cells, are resistant to monotherapy with Ad.IL-24; however, combinatorial treatment with chemo- or radiotherapy, small-molecule inhibitors and anti-tumor monoclonal antibodies have improved the efficacy of treatment and improved success in resistant tumors [54, 58].

Unlike other members of the IL-17 family of cytokines, IL-25/IL-17E is found to be secreted by activated Th2 cells, rather than the recently discovered Th17 lineage of helper T cells [59]. Furthermore, Th2 memory cells express high levels of IL-25R [59, 60], which following IL-25 binding promotes cell expansion and Th2 cytokine production by Th2 central memory cells activated by a variety of stimuli, such as thymic stromal lymphopoietin (TSLP)-activated DCs, homeostatic cytokines or T-cell receptor triggering [61]. IL-25 regulates hematopoietic and immune functions, stimulating the development of eosinophils and B lymphocytes [61]. The fact that IL-25 overexpression results in high levels of circulating eosinophils, IL-4, IL-5,

eotaxin and IgE suggests that IL-25 may be a pro-inflammatory cytokine favoring Th2-type immune responses [60]. Recent clinical studies by Liu et al. have shown that Virulizin®, a novel biological response modifier extracted from bovine bile, has produced significant anti-tumor efficacy in a variety of human tumor xenograft models including melanoma, pancreatic cancer, breast cancer, ovarian cancer and prostate cancer [62]. Interestingly, tumor clearance is directly linked to IL-25-induced eosinophilia and macrophage infiltration into the tumor environment [63, 64].

11.3.2 Eosinophils and Eosinophil-Derived Mediators

The eosinophil remains as one of the most enigmatic cells in the immune system, a pleiotropic multifunctional leukocyte involved directly and indirectly in the modulation of innate and adaptive immunity. However, the true immunological role(s) of the eosinophil is yet to be fully elucidated. In the clinic, the development of blood eosinophilia and the localization of high eosinophils numbers within the tumor stroma and necrotic core of solid tumors, or tumor-associated tissue eosinophilia (TATE), have been observed since the 1950s [65]. The previously held belief that eosinophils act as ineffectual bystanders in the tumor environment has come under great scrutiny, with several clinical studies showing a direct correlation between eosinophil infiltration and a favorable patient prognosis, suggesting a true effector cell role for the eosinophil in tumor clearance. Thus, high infiltrating eosinophil levels have been associated with a positive prognosis in pulmonary adenocarcinoma, nasopharyngeal and esophageal squamous cell carcinoma, head, neck, gastric and prostate cancer [66–70]. As an extension of earlier studies, Takanami et al. found a significant difference in the rate of patient survival between patients whose tumors had high levels of eosinophils, as identified by the eosinophil-specific antibody EG2, and those patients with low numbers of eosinophils, suggesting the importance of a large eosinophil infiltrate into the tumor for the mediation of a positive clinical outcome [70].

Our own previous studies in mouse models have demonstrated that tumor-specific $CD4^+$ T cells, exhibiting a cytokine secretion profile characteristic of Th2 cells, are capable of clearing established lung and visceral metastases of the B16-F1 CTL-resistant melanoma [12]. Clearance of B16 metastases by the Th2 cells was found to be completely dependent on the eosinophil chemokine, eotaxin, with degranulating eosinophils within the tumors being associated with tumor regression [12]. Tumor clearance was also partially dependent on the transcription activator signal transducer and activator of transcription 6 (STAT6) that is important in IL-4 and IL-13 signaling through the type II IL-4R [12], suggesting that these Th2 cytokines play a supportive role in eosinophil-mediated tumor eradication. Additional in vivo studies have since confirmed that eosinophils can exhibit potent anti-tumor activity when recruited into established tumors [8, 9, 12–15, 24].

For the first time, we recently established an important role for eosinophils in tumor immune surveillance [23]. The key findings were that genetically modified

mice that have enhanced levels of circulating eosinophils were extremely resistant to tumor induction by the carcinogen, methylcholanthrene (MCA), with most tumors that arose having remarkably slow growth rates leading to a dormant tumor state [23]. In contrast, eosinophil-deficient IL-5/CCL11$^{-/-}$ and ΔdblGATA strains were highly susceptible to tumor induction at high and low concentrations of MCA in the total absence of eosinophils. Further studies are currently aimed at clarifying whether eosinophil-mediated tumor immune surveillance primarily involves either adaptive or innate immune responses or whether both are needed to establish effective tumor control.

Once recruited into the tumor environment, eosinophils have the ability to harness both direct and indirect mechanisms to induce tumor clearance. Direct tumor killing can be mediated via the release of granule-associated cytotoxic proteins, including major basic protein (MBP), eosinophil peroxidase (EPO), eosinophil cationic protein (ECP) and eosinophil-derived neurotoxin (EDN), which are capable of inducing tissue damage and dysfunction [71] and have been linked to tumor cell apoptosis [72]. In addition, tumor-specific antibodies may earmark tumor cells for killing by eosinophils via mechanisms similar to those demonstrated in studies of immunity to helminthic parasites [73]. In vivo experiments using either an eotaxin-expressing melanoma (Simson and Parish – unpublished observation) or an eotaxin-expressing hepatocellular carcinoma [74] have revealed that although eosinophils are successfully recruited into the tumors, there is little effect on tumor growth unless the tumors are grown in IL-5 transgenic recipients, confirming the potential importance of IL-5 in tumor eradication.

However, modeling eosinophil-mediated tumor cytotoxicity in-vitro has highlighted the complex nature of this process. Studies by Furbert-Harris et al. were able to demonstrate that eosinophils harvested from allergic individuals, and the conditioned media of cell-lines established from these cells, were able to inhibit prostate tumor growth in vitro [67]. We have also reported that in vitro mouse eosinophils can directly induce the killing of MCA-induced fibrosarcoma cells [23], a process significantly enhanced when eosinophils were used from Th2-induced inflammatory exudates [23].

Conversely, high levels of infiltrating eosinophils have also been associated with a negative clinical prognosis in some cancer patients [75–77]. It has been proposed that eosinophils have the potential to promote tumor growth by inducing angiogenesis. Several factors that are known to promote angiogenesis, including vascular endothelial growth factor (VEGF), fibroblast growth factor-2 (FGF-2), tumor necrosis factor (TNF)-α, granulocyte–macrophage colony-stimulating factor (GM-CSF) and IL-8, are synthesized by eosinophils and stored in their granules [78]. In one study, human peripheral blood eosinophils were able to induce rat aortic endothelial cell proliferation and angiogenesis in the chick embryo chorioallantoic membrane, a process partially mediated through VEGF [78]. However, a study by Tataroglu et al. evaluating non-small-cell lung carcinoma biopsies found no correlation between eosinophil, macrophage or mast-cell content and tumor angiogenesis, as confirmed by vascular density and microvessel quantification [15, 79].

Interestingly, although clinical prognostic score studies in classical Hodgkin lymphoma focus on the evaluation of eosinophil and mast-cell tumor infiltration, a recent retrospective analysis revealed eosinophil predominance to have no prognostic value that could be used in clinical practice although a tendency for a correlation between mast-cell infiltration with overall survival was identified [80]. Thus, to date, no direct role for eosinophils in tumor angiogenesis has been identified.

A synopsis of these studies suggests that the tumor microenvironment in which eosinophils are recruited plays a role in determining the physiological outcomes. Hence, a specific combination of activation signals is required to achieve effective eosinophil-mediated tumor clearance, enabling a degree of regulation when considering the high toxicity of eosinophil-derived mediators. Furthermore, our recent in vivo studies suggest that Th2-recruited myeloid cells, other than eosinophils, may be involved in providing both the appropriate activation environment and are also directly involved in tumor eradication (Ellyard, Simson, Parish – in submission). In many studies highlighting the anti-tumor role of eosinophils, a concurrent influx of macrophages, has been observed [8, 12, 13, 16, 24] and will be discussed in the following section. Hence, the relationship between eosinophils and other immune cells known to be involved in tumor clearance and immune surveillance is of considerable interest. In addition, the signals required for the recruitment of eosinophils into the tumor microenvironment and the subsequent mechanisms employed by eosinophils to induce tumor cell death warrant further investigation.

11.3.3 Alternatively Activated Macrophages

As previously highlighted, the Th2-mediated infiltration of eosinophils into the tumor stroma is often associated with a corresponding influx of macrophages into the tumor microenvironment [13, 15, 24], suggesting that macrophages may also play a role in Th2-mediated tumor clearance. However, tumor-associated macrophages (TAMs) have often been associated with increased tumor growth, tumor angiogenesis and a suppression of anti-tumor $CD8^+$ T-cell responses, equating with a poor clinical prognosis [80]. Conversely, macrophages have been demonstrated to elicit the direct killing of tumor cells in vitro and in vivo [8, 81, 82]. Thus the role of macrophages remains controversial and, as with many other immune cells including the eosinophil, may differ depending on the tumour microenvironment.

Macrophages are one of the most heterogeneous cells of the body, with differentiation from monocyte precursors being determined by tissue-related and immune-related stimuli [83]. Macrophage-mediated cytotoxicity is traditionally associated with IFN-γ-activated type-1 macrophages and mediated through nitric oxide [84], TNF-α [85, 86], cytolytic proteases [85] and the generation of reactive oxygen species such as hydrogen peroxide and superoxide following activation of antibody-dependent cellular cytotoxicity (ADCC) [86, 87]. Alternatively activated macrophages (aaMacs) are elicited through a Th2-mediated IL-4/IL-13 environment [83], resulting in the upregulated expression of the mannose receptor and

MHC class II, enhanced endocytosis and antigen presentation, and production of the chemokines CCL22 and CCL17. The IL-4/IL13-induced production of the intracellular enzyme, arginase-1, and the reduced production and release of nitric oxide through arginase-1 suppression of nitric oxide synthase (NOS)-2 [83] are characteristic features of aaMacs.

Recent studies by Anthony et al. revealed that aaMacs effectively mediate the IL-4-induced clearance of the gastrointestinal parasite *Heligmosomoides polygyrus* in mice, a process dependent on the production of arginase-1 [88]. Recent studies in our laboratory have illustrated, for the first time, the ability of Th2-activated aaMacs to induce tumor eradication in vitro (Ellyard, Simson, Parish – unpublished results). In this study it was found that macrophages in a type-2 inflammatory infiltrate, when exposed to either IL-4 or IL-13, became cytotoxic for B16-F1 melanoma cells via a mechanism dependent on arginase-1-mediated depletion of L-arginine in the tumor cell microenvironment (Ellyard, Simson, Parish – unpublished results). The sensitivity of many tumour cells to arginase-1-mediated L-arginine depletion in vitro is well documented [89–94]. In fact, pegylated arginase deaminase, an enzyme known to induce the depletion of L-arginine, is now being developed as a potential anticancer agent and has entered phase II and phase III clinical trials [95].

The debate continues regarding the role of macrophages in tumor progression in vivo, with some studies suggesting that the tumor microenvironment suppresses TAM-mediated cytotoxicity. In fact TAM-derived arginase-1 has been linked to the inhibition of CTL-mediated immune surveillance, L-arginine depletion resulting in the inhibition of CD3 expression and subsequent T-cell activation and proliferation [96]. In addition, many clinical studies have correlated a high number of TAMs within the tumor microenvironment with a poor patient prognosis [80, 97]. It should be noted that in most clinical studies the TAM phenotype, namely identifying infiltrating macrophages as IFN-γ-activated type-1 macrophages or aaMacs, has not been evaluated. Based on our own studies, a considerable number of aaMacs need to be present for effective L-arginine depletion and resultant tumor cytotoxicity. In fact, when L-arginine depletion was incomplete, the aaMacs actually enhanced tumor cell proliferation (Ellyard, Simson, Parish – unpublished results). Furthermore, whether macrophages, through the production of arginase-1, also play a role in Th2-mediated tumour clearance in vivo remains to be fully elucidated.

11.3.4 B Cells, IgG and IgE

An important function of $CD4^+$ T cells with a Th2-cytokine phenotype is to provide "help" for antigen-specific B cells and facilitate IgG1 and IgE antibody responses. Clinical and experimental data indicate that chronic inflammation, often antibody-induced, results in the recruitment and activation of innate immune cells within the tumor environment, which can promote cancer development [98]. In fact, increased humoral immunity has been reported to be a factor in several chronic inflammatory diseases, such as ulcerative colitis, asbestosis, HCV-related cirrhosis and chronic obstructive airway disease, and several autoimmune diseases [98]. Mouse studies

support this view, B-cell deficient mice displaying a higher resistance to colon carcinoma, B16 melanoma and EL4 thymoma [99, 100], in addition to an enhanced T-cell response to melanoma vaccines and an increased resistance to subsequent tumor challenge [101]. However, as has already been discussed in this chapter, most innate cells and their released mediators are also able to effectively induce tumor clearance in the appropriate tumor microenvironment.

The mechanism of B-cell-mediated inhibition of anti-tumor immunity is likely to be multifactorial. B-cell-mediated anti-tumor antibodies, in particular those of the IgG class, have been shown to enhance tumor growth by inhibiting CTL-mediated tumor killing and by forming immune complexes (ICs) within tumors [102]. ICs have been associated with increased tumor burden and poor prognosis in several cancers [103, 104], a process unrelated to specific antigens. Interestingly, receptors for the Fc portion of IgG, namely FcγRs, have been identified as inducers of IC-mediated inflammation and subsequent downregulation of anti-tumor immune responses [105]. In addition, IgG has been shown to complex with latent transforming growth factor (TGF)-β, resulting in the inhibition of CTL-mediated anti-tumor responses [106].

The role of IgE-mediated allergy (atopy) in cancer etiology is covered extensively in other chapters of this monograph. Numerous epidemiological studies have evaluated the association between allergy, in particular atopic disorders, and an enhanced capacity for tumor immune surveillance [107–110]. In summary, case–control studies, measuring allergen-specific IgE in patients with cancer, have reported conflicting results [111–113]. However, recent studies have effectively harnessed the antigen–IgE–FcRI axis in tumor targeting strategies based on the strong affinity of IgE for FcRI even in the absence of antigen [114]. Passive immunotherapy with a chimeric IgE antibody against an ovarian tumor-specific antigen resulted in IgE-mediated tumor clearance by infiltrating macrophages, tumor elimination being mediated via FcεRI ADCC and CD23 antibody-dependent cellular phagocytosis (ADCP) [114]. In addition, eosinophils were identified as potent effector cells in this model. Interestingly, a direct comparison between the efficacy of IgG- and IgE-mediated tumor clearance revealed that IgE chimeric antibodies were able to more effectively inhibit tumor growth [114, 115]. Related studies have focused on using IgE-loaded tumor cells as tumor vaccines, with the tumor clearance induced by these vaccines being via both innate effector mechanisms and eosinophil-dependent induction of tumor-specific T-cell immunity [116].

11.3.5 Mast Cells and Mast-Cell Mediators

The role of mast cells in tumor biology is extensively covered in Chapter 6 of this book; consequently, this section will only briefly highlight the potential interaction of these myeloid cells and their mediators with other Th2-mediated effector cells in tumor immunity.

Mast cells are regarded as playing an important role in adaptive and innate host defense against parasites and bacteria [117], in addition to being recognized as the

key effector cell in IgE-mediated allergic responses [118]. The potential of mast cells to actively promote tumor angiogenesis, a process mediated by mast-cell-derived heparin [119], VEGF, FGF-2 IL-8, TNF-α and matrix metalloproteinase (MMP)-9, is well documented [120]. Consistent with these activities, the majority of epidemiological evidence suggests that the presence of higher mast-cell numbers within tumors is associated with a poor prognosis [121]. Conversely, recent studies clarifying the prognostic value of tumor-localized mast cells in classical Hodgkin lymphoma confirmed a correlation between higher mast-cell infiltration and overall improvement in patient survival [122]. However, the role of mast cells in systemic tumor immunity remains poorly understood. To examine the role of mast cells in intestinal tumorigenesis, mast-cell-deficient Sash mice were crossed with the Min mouse, a genetic model of intestinal neoplasia [123]. The resulting mast-cell-deficient Min–Sash mice developed 50% more adenomas than littermate controls, and the tumors were 33% larger in these mice. Mast-cell deficiency did not affect tumor cell proliferation, but tumor cell apoptosis was significantly reduced in mast-cell-deficient mice. Interestingly, although tumor-infiltrating neutrophil, macrophage and T-cell populations remained similar between the Min and the Min–Sash mice, eosinophil infiltration was greatly reduced in the tumors of Min–Sash mice [123].

11.3.6 Tc2 Cells

Similar to $CD4^+$ T cells, $CD8^+$ T cells can be classified into two distinct types of effector cells based on their cytokine secretion profile following antigen encounter [124, 125]. Type 1 $CD8^+$ T cells (Tc1) secrete IFN-γ, IL-2 and TNF-α and type 2 $CD8^+$ T cells (Tc2) predominately produce IL-4, IL-5 and IL-10 [124]. The role of Tc1 $CD8^+$ CTLs in tumor clearance is largely IFN-γ-mediated, while cytotoxicity is primarily mediated through the Fas/Fas ligand or perforin/granzyme signaling pathways [126]. Although the anti-tumor activity of Tc1 cells is outside the scope of this chapter, of interest are several recent studies aimed at clarifying the role of Tc2 cells in anti-tumor immunity. Transfer of OVA-specific Tc2 effector cells into an OVA-transfected B16-melanoma model was found to induce perforin-dependent tumor regression and enhanced survival of mice [127]. Interestingly, the use of gene-deficient mice confirmed that anti-tumor activity was dependent on effector cell-derived IL-4 and IL-5. In addition, Tc1-mediated IFN-γ release was also upregulated in surviving Tc2-treated hosts [127]. In a related study, although Tc2 cells were found to induce tumor clearance in an EG7 thymoma model, Tc2 cells were reported to be 5- to 25-fold less effective in inducing an equivalent anti-tumor effect to Tc1 cells [128].

Studies by Dobrzanki et al. suggested that Tc2 cells may facilitate tumor rejection through their interaction with other leukocytes such as macrophages, NK cells and eosinophils [127], although only eosinophils were found to infiltrate tumors at significant levels [127, 129]. However, as previously reported in this chapter, a role for $CD8^+$ T cells in Th2-mediated or IL-4-mediated tumor clearance is well

established, with eosinophils and macrophages deemed to be effector cells in this process [9, 10, 14, 24]. Furthermore, in a supporting study, adoptive transfer of IL-4 producing $CD8^+$ T cells cleared established lung metastasis via a process dependent on $CD8^+$ T-cell-derived IL-4 and host NK cells and partially dependent on granulocytes [130].

Conversely, several studies have found that Tc2 cells lack the capacity to induce effective anti-tumor immunity. TCR-transgenic $CD8^+$ T cells were activated in vitro to generate cytotoxic Th1 and Tc2 cells, which were adoptively transferred into syngeneic hosts, and their ability to protect against tumor challenge was compared. Tc1 cells were able to significantly delay tumor growth, whereas Tc2 cells from IFN-γ-deficient donors had no effect. In a separate study, tumor-specific Tc2 cells were found to be significantly less effective than Tc1 cells in mediating perforin-dependent lysis of tumor cells in vitro, had a significantly lower capacity for in vivo survival after adoptive T-cell transfer, and were significantly less effective at eradicating established tumors in animals [131]. One consistent factor in studies highlighting the reduced anti-tumor activity of Tc2 cells is the production of high levels of IL-10 in the tumor microenvironment, an observation not reported in models where effective Tc2-mediated tumor clearance occurred. The immunosuppressive effects of IL-10 in anti-tumor immunity are well documented and may counteract the anti-tumor potential of Tc2 cells.

11.4 Conclusion

Historically Th2-mediated immunity has been associated with the inhibition of anti-tumor immunity, both by promoting tumor angiogenesis and by suppressing cell-mediated immunity and effective tumor clearance. However, a more thorough analysis of the scientific literature and our own observations highlight the potential role for Th2-mediated immune effector cells and their mediators in tumor immune surveillance and tumor clearance (summarized in Table 11.1 and Fig. 11.1). Of particular interest are eosinophils and aaMacs which, through their innate responsiveness or recruitment and activation by the adaptive immune system, have the potential to act as potent anti-tumor effector cells. Most importantly, the tumor microenvironment and its milieu of cells and mediators play a primary role in determining the efficacy of global anti-tumor immunity and must be fully evaluated in the design and implementation of Th2-mediated tumor immunotherapies.

Acknowledgments This work was supported by a National Health and Medical Research Council of Australia (NHMRC) Program grant. L.S. is a recipient of a NHMRC Peter Doherty Postdoctoral Fellowship and ACT Health and Medical Research Grant.

References

1. Dunn, G.P., L.J. Old, and R.D. Schreiber. 2004. The three Es of cancer immunoediting. *Annu Rev Immunol* 22:329–360.
2. Tey, S.K., C.M. Bollard, and H.E. Heslop. 2006. Adoptive T-cell transfer in cancer immunotherapy. *Immunol Cell Biol* 84:281–289.

3. Rammensee, H.G. 2006. Some considerations on the use of peptides and mRNA for therapeutic vaccination against cancer. *Immunol Cell Biol* 84:290–294.
4. Urosevic, M., and R. Dummer. 2008. Human leukocyte antigen-G and cancer immunoediting. *Cancer Res* 68:627–630.
5. Brigati, C., D.M. Noonan, A. Albini, and R. Benelli. 2002. Tumors and inflammatory infiltrates: friends or foes? *Clin Exp Metastasis* 19:247–258.
6. Parish, C.R. 2003. Cancer immunotherapy: the past, the present and the future. *Immunol Cell Biol* 81:106–113.
7. Sant, A.J., F.A. Chaves, S.A. Jenks, K.A. Richards, P. Menges, J.M. Weaver, and C.A. Lazarski. 2005. The relationship between immunodominance, DM editing, and the kinetic stability of MHC class II: peptide complexes. *Immunol Rev* 207:261–278.
8. Hung, K., R. Hayashi, A. Lafond-Walker, C. Lowenstein, D. Pardoll, and H. Levitsky. 1998. The central role of CD4(+) T cells in the antitumor immune response. *J Exp Med* 188: 2357–2368.
9. Nishimura, T., K. Iwakabe, M. Sekimoto, Y. Ohmi, T. Yahata, M. Nakui, T. Sato, S. Habu, H. Tashiro, M. Sato, and A. Ohta. 1999. Distinct role of antigen-specific T helper type 1 (Th1) and Th2 cells in tumor eradication in vivo. *J Exp Med* 190:617–627.
10. Ossendorp, F., E. Mengede, M. Camps, R. Filius, and C.J. Melief. 1998. Specific T helper cell requirement for optimal induction of cytotoxic T lymphocytes against major histocompatibility complex class II negative tumors. *J Exp Med* 187:693–702.
11. Mautner, J., E.M. Jaffee, and D.M. Pardoll. 2005. Tumor-specific CD4+ T cells from a patient with renal cell carcinoma recognize diverse shared antigens. *Int J Cancer* 115:752–759.
12. Mattes, J., M. Hulett, W. Xie, S. Hogan, M.E. Rothenberg, P. Foster, and C. Parish. 2003. Immunotherapy of cytotoxic T cell-resistant tumors by T helper 2 cells: an eotaxin and STAT6-dependent process. *J Exp Med* 197:387–393.
13. Modesti, A., L. Masuelli, A. Modica, G. D'Orazi, S. Scarpa, M.C. Bosco, and G. Forni. 1993. Ultrastructural evidence of the mechanisms responsible for interleukin-4-activated rejection of a spontaneous murine adenocarcinoma. *Int J Cancer* 53:988–993.
14. Musiani, P., A. Allione, A. Modica, P.L. Lollini, M. Giovarelli, F. Cavallo, F. Belardelli, G. Forni, and A. Modesti. 1996. Role of neutrophils and lymphocytes in inhibition of a mouse mammary adenocarcinoma engineered to release IL-2, IL-4, IL-7, IL-10, IFN-alpha, IFN-gamma, and TNF-alpha. *Lab Invest* 74:146–157.
15. Tepper, R.I., R.L. Coffman, and P. Leder. 1992. An eosinophil-dependent mechanism for the antitumor effect of interleukin-4. *Science* 257:548–551.
16. Tepper, R.I., P.K. Pattengale, and P. Leder. 1989. Murine interleukin-4 displays potent anti-tumor activity in vivo. *Cell* 57:503–512.
17. Mosmann, T.R., H. Cherwinski, M.W. Bond, M.A. Giedlin, and R.L. Coffman. 2005. Two types of murine helper T cell clone. I. Definition according to profiles of lymphokine activities and secreted proteins. 1986. *J Immunol* 175:5–14.
18. Becker, Y. 2006. Molecular immunological approaches to biotherapy of human cancers – a review, hypothesis and implications. *Anticancer Res* 26:1113–1134.
19. Shurin, M.R., L. Lu, P. Kalinski, A.M. Stewart-Akers, and M.T. Lotze. 1999. Th1/Th2 balance in cancer, transplantation and pregnancy. *Springer Semin Immunopathol* 21: 339–359.
20. Ellyard, J.I., L. Simson, and C.R. Parish. 2007. Th2-mediated anti-tumour immunity: friend or foe? *Tissue Antigens* 70:1–11.
21. Ito, N., Y. Suzuki, Y. Taniguchi, K. Ishiguro, H. Nakamura, and S. Ohgi. 2005. Prognostic significance of T helper 1 and 2 and T cytotoxic 1 and 2 cells in patients with non-small cell lung cancer. *Anticancer Res* 25:2027–2031.
22. Kidd, P. 2003. Th1/Th2 balance: the hypothesis, its limitations, and implications for health and disease. *Altern Med Rev* 8:223–246.
23. Simson, L., J.I. Ellyard, L.A. Dent, K.I. Matthaei, M.E. Rothenberg, P.S. Foster, M.J. Smyth, and C.R. Parish. 2007. Regulation of carcinogenesis by IL-5 and CCL11: a potential role for eosinophils in tumor immune surveillance. *J Immunol* 178:4222–4229.

24. Pericle, F., M. Giovarelli, M.P. Colombo, G. Ferrari, P. Musiani, A. Modesti, F. Cavallo, F. Di Pierro, F. Novelli, and G. Forni. 1994. An efficient Th2-type memory follows CD8+ lymphocyte-driven and eosinophil-mediated rejection of a spontaneous mouse mammary adenocarcinoma engineered to release IL-4. *J Immunol* 153:5659–5673.
25. Schuler, T., S. Kornig, and T. Blankenstein. 2003. Tumor rejection by modulation of tumor stromal fibroblasts. *J Exp Med* 198:1487–1493.
26. Conticello, C., F. Pedini, A. Zeuner, M. Patti, M. Zerilli, G. Stassi, A. Messina, C. Peschle, and R. De Maria. 2004. IL-4 protects tumor cells from anti-CD95 and chemotherapeutic agents via up-regulation of antiapoptotic proteins. *J Immunol* 172:5467–5477.
27. Falkensammer, C., K. Johrer, H. Gander, R. Ramoner, T. Putz, A. Rahm, R. Greil, G. Bartsch, and M. Thurnher. 2006. IL-4 inhibits the TNF-alpha induced proliferation of renal cell carcinoma (RCC) and cooperates with TNF-alpha to induce apoptotic and cytokine responses by RCC: implications for antitumor immune responses. *Cancer Immunol Immunother* 55:1228–1237.
28. Nagai, S., and M. Toi. 2000. Interleukin-4 and breast cancer. *Breast Cancer* 7:181–186.
29. Taylor, C.W., T.M. Grogan, and S.E. Salmon. 1990. Effects of interleukin-4 on the in vitro growth of human lymphoid and plasma cell neoplasms. *Blood* 75:1114–1118.
30. Margolin, K., F.R. Aronson, M. Sznol, M.B. Atkins, R. Gucalp, R.I. Fisher, M. Sunderland, J.H. Doroshow, M.L. Ernest, J.W. Mier, J.P. Dutcher, E.R. Gaynor and G.R. Weiss. 1994. Phase II studies of recombinant human interleukin-4 in advanced renal cancer and malignant melanoma. *J Immunother Emphasis Tumor Immunol* 15:147–153.
31. Stadler, W.M., M.E. Rybak, and N.J. Vogelzang. 1995. A phase II study of subcutaneous recombinant human interleukin-4 in metastatic renal cell carcinoma. *Cancer* 76: 1629–1633.
32. Whitehead, R.P., J.M. Unger, J.W. Goodwin, M.J. Walker, J.A. Thompson, L.E. Flaherty, and V.K. Sondak. 1998. Phase II trial of recombinant human interleukin-4 in patients with disseminated malignant melanoma: a Southwest Oncology Group study. *J Immunother* 21:440–446.
33. Tulpule, A., B. Joshi, N. DeGuzman, B.M. Espina, R. Mocharnuk, O. Prakash, D. Templeton, A.M. Levine, and P.S. Gill. 1997. Interleukin-4 in the treatment of AIDS-related Kaposi's sarcoma. *Ann Oncol* 8:79–83.
34. Caput, D., P. Laurent, M. Kaghad, J.M. Lelias, S. Lefort, N. Vita, and P. Ferrara. 1996. Cloning and characterization of a specific interleukin (IL)-13 binding protein structurally related to the IL-5 receptor alpha chain. *J Biol Chem* 271:16921–16926.
35. Zhang, J.G., D.J. Hilton, T.A. Willson, C. McFarlane, B.A. Roberts, R.L. Moritz, R.J. Simpson, W.S. Alexander, D. Metcalf, and N.A. Nicola. 1997. Identification, purification, and characterization of a soluble interleukin (IL)-13-binding protein. Evidence that it is distinct from the cloned Il-13 receptor and Il-4 receptor alpha-chains. *J Biol Chem* 272:9474–9480.
36. Lebel-Binay, S., B. Laguerre, F. Quintin-Colonna, H. Conjeaud, M. Magazin, B. Miloux, F. Pecceu, D. Caput, P. Ferrara, and D. Fradelizi. 1995. Experimental gene therapy of cancer using tumor cells engineered to secrete interleukin-13. *Eur J Immunol* 25:2340–2348.
37. Ma, H.L., M.J. Whitters, B.A. Jacobson, D.D. Donaldson, M. Collins, and K. Dunussi-Joannopoulos. 2004. Tumor cells secreting IL-13 but not IL-13Ralpha2 fusion protein have reduced tumorigenicity in vivo. *Int Immunol* 16:1009–1017.
38. Terabe, M., J.M. Park, and J.A. Berzofsky. 2004. Role of IL-13 in regulation of anti-tumor immunity and tumor growth. *Cancer Immunol Immunother* 53:79–85.
39. Singer, M., J. Lefort, and B.B. Vargaftig. 2002. Granulocyte depletion and dexamethasone differentially modulate airways hyperreactivity, inflammation, mucus accumulation, and secretion induced by rmIL-13 or antigen. *Am J Respir Cell Mol Biol* 26:74–84.
40. Skinnider, B.F., U. Kapp, and T.W. Mak. 2002. The role of interleukin 13 in classical Hodgkin lymphoma. *Leuk Lymphoma* 43:1203–1210.
41. Kawakami, K. 2005. Cancer gene therapy utilizing interleukin-13 receptor alpha2 chain. *Curr Gene Ther* 5:213–223.

42. Kioi, M., S.R. Husain, D. Croteau, S. Kunwar, and R.K. Puri. 2006. Convection-enhanced delivery of interleukin-13 receptor-directed cytotoxin for malignant glioma therapy. *Technol Cancer Res Treat* 5:239–250.
43. Kawakami, K., M. Kawakami, P.J. Snoy, S.R. Husain, and R.K. Puri. 2001. In vivo overexpression of IL-13 receptor alpha2 chain inhibits tumorigenicity of human breast and pancreatic tumors in immunodeficient mice. *J Exp Med* 194: 1743–1754.
44. Jarboe, J.S., K.R. Johnson, Y. Choi, R.R. Lonser, and J.K. Park. 2007. Expression of interleukin-13 receptor alpha2 in glioblastoma multiforme: implications for targeted therapies. *Cancer Res* 67:7983–7986.
45. Dummer, W., B.C. Bastian, N. Ernst, C. Schanzle, A. Schwaaf, and E.B. Brocker. 1996. Interleukin-10 production in malignant melanoma: preferential detection of IL-10-secreting tumor cells in metastatic lesions. *Int J Cancer* 66:607–610.
46. Salazar-Onfray, F., M.N. Lopez, and A. Mendoza-Naranjo. 2007. Paradoxical effects of cytokines in tumor immune surveillance and tumor immune escape. *Cytokine Growth Factor Rev* 18:171–182.
47. Sharma, S., M. Stolina, Y. Lin, B. Gardner, P.W. Miller, M. Kronenberg, and S.M. Dubinett. 1999. T cell-derived IL-10 promotes lung cancer growth by suppressing both T cell and APC function. *J Immunol* 163:5020–5028.
48. Matsuda, M., F. Salazar, M. Petersson, G. Masucci, J. Hansson, P. Pisa, Q.J. Zhang, M.G. Masucci, and R. Kiessling. 1994. Interleukin 10 pretreatment protects target cells from tumor- and allo-specific cytotoxic T cells and downregulates HLA class I expression. *J Exp Med* 180:2371–2376.
49. Commins, S., J.W. Steinke, and L. Borish. 2008. The extended IL-10 superfamily: IL-10, IL-19, IL-20, IL-22, IL-24, IL-26, IL-28, and IL-29. *J Allergy Clin Immunol* 121:1108–1111.
50. Kreis, S., D. Philippidou, C. Margue, and I. Behrmann. 2008. IL-24: a classic cytokine and/or a potential cure for cancer? *J Cell Mol Med* 12:2505–2510.
51. Wang, M., Z. Tan, R. Zhang, S.V. Kotenko, and P. Liang. 2002. Interleukin 24 (MDA-7/MOB-5) signals through two heterodimeric receptors, IL-22R1/IL-20R2 and IL-20R1/IL-20R2. *J Biol Chem* 277:7341–7347.
52. Sauane, M., R.V. Gopalkrishnan, D. Sarkar, Z.Z. Su, I.V. Lebedeva, P. Dent, S. Pestka, and P.B. Fisher. 2003. MDA-7/IL-24: novel cancer growth suppressing and apoptosis inducing cytokine. *Cytokine Growth Factor Rev* 14:35–51.
53. Su, Z., L. Emdad, M. Sauane, I.V. Lebedeva, D. Sarkar, P. Gupta, C.D. James, A. Randolph, K. Valerie, M.R. Walter, P. Dent, and P.B. Fisher. 2005. Unique aspects of mda-7/IL-24 antitumor bystander activity: establishing a role for secretion of MDA-7/IL-24 protein by normal cells. *Oncogene* 24:7552–7566.
54. Sarkar, D., I.V. Lebedeva, Z.Z. Su, E.S. Park, L. Chatman, N. Vozhilla, P. Dent, D.T. Curiel, and P.B. Fisher. 2007. Eradication of therapy-resistant human prostate tumors using a cancer terminator virus. *Cancer Res* 67:5434–5442.
55. Zheng, M., D. Bocangel, B. Doneske, A. Mhashilkar, R. Ramesh, K.K. Hunt, S. Ekmekcioglu, R.B. Sutton, N. Poindexter, E.A. Grimm, and S. Chada. 2007. Human interleukin 24 (MDA-7/IL-24) protein kills breast cancer cells via the IL-20 receptor and is antagonized by IL-10. *Cancer Immunol Immunother* 56:205–215.
56. Sauane, M., Z.Z. Su, P. Gupta, I.V. Lebedeva, P. Dent, D. Sarkar, and P.B. Fisher. 2008. Autocrine regulation of mda-7/IL-24 mediates cancer-specific apoptosis. *Proc Natl Acad Sci USA* 105:9763–9768.
57. Lebedeva, I.V., D. Sarkar, Z.Z. Su, R.V. Gopalkrishnan, M. Athar, A. Randolph, K. Valerie, P. Dent, and P.B. Fisher. 2006. Molecular target-based therapy of pancreatic cancer. *Cancer Res* 66:2403–2413.
58. Pataer, A., W. Hu, L. Xiaolin, S. Chada, J.A. Roth, K.K. Hunt, and S.G. Swisher. 2008. Adenoviral endoplasmic reticulum-targeted mda-7/interleukin-24 vector enhances human cancer cell killing. *Mol Cancer Ther* 7:2528–2535.

59. Lee, J., W.H. Ho, M. Maruoka, R.T. Corpuz, D.T. Baldwin, J.S. Foster, A.D. Goddard, D.G. Yansura, R.L. Vandlen, W.I. Wood, and A.L. Gurney. 2001. IL-17E, a novel proinflammatory ligand for the IL-17 receptor homolog IL-17Rh1. *J Biol Chem* 276:1660–1664.
60. Fort, M.M., J. Cheung, D. Yen, J. Li, S.M. Zurawski, S. Lo, S. Menon, T. Clifford, B. Hunte, R. Lesley, T. Muchamuel, S.D. Hurst, G. Zurawski, M.W. Leach, D.M. Gorman, and D.M. Rennick. 2001. IL-25 induces IL-4, IL-5, and IL-13 and Th2-associated pathologies in vivo. *Immunity* 15:985–995.
61. Wang, Y.H., P. Angkasekwinai, N. Lu, K.S. Voo, K. Arima, S. Hanabuchi, A. Hippe, C.J. Corrigan, C. Dong, B. Homey, Z. Yao, S. Ying, D.P. Huston, and Y.J. Liu. 2007. IL-25 augments type 2 immune responses by enhancing the expansion and functions of TSLP-DC-activated Th2 memory cells. *J Exp Med* 204:1837–1847.
62. Liu, C., E.S. Ferdinandi, G. Ely, and S.S. Joshi. 2000. Virulizin-2gamma, a novel immunotherapeutic agent, in treatment of human pancreatic cancer xenografts. *Int J Oncol* 16:1015–1020.
63. Benatar, T., M.Y. Cao, Y. Lee, H. Li, N. Feng, X. Gu, V. Lee, H. Jin, M. Wang, S. Der, J. Lightfoot, J.A. Wright, and A.H. Young. 2008. Virulizin((R)) induces production of IL-17E to enhance antitumor activity by recruitment of eosinophils into tumors. *Cancer Immunol Immunother* 57:1757–1769.
64. Du, C., N. Feng, H. Jin, V. Lee, M. Wang, J.A. Wright, and A.H. Young. 2003. Macrophages play a critical role in the anti-tumor activity of Virulizin. *Int J Oncol* 23:1341–1346.
65. Schmidt, K.E. 1952. [High grade blood eosinophilia associated with malignant tumors]. *Arztl Wochensch* 7:1184–1185.
66. Fujii, M., T. Yamashita, R. Ishiguro, M. Tashiro, and K. Kameyama. 2002. Significance of epidermal growth factor receptor and tumor associated tissue eosinophilia in the prognosis of patients with nasopharyngeal carcinoma. *Auris Nasus Larynx* 29:175–181.
67. Furbert-Harris, P., D. Parish-Gause, I. Laniyan, K.A. Hunter, J. Okomo-Awich, T.R. Vaughn, K.C. Forrest, C. Howland, A. Abdelnaby, and O.A. Oredipe. 2003. Inhibition of prostate cancer cell growth by activated eosinophils. *Prostate* 57:165–175.
68. Ishibashi, S., Y. Ohashi, T. Suzuki, S. Miyazaki, T. Moriya, S. Satomi, and H. Sasano. 2006. Tumor-associated tissue eosinophilia in human esophageal squamous cell carcinoma. *Anticancer Res* 26:1419–1424.
69. Iwasaki, K., M. Torisu, and T. Fujimura. 1986. Malignant tumor and eosinophils. I. Prognostic significance in gastric cancer. *Cancer* 58:1321–1327.
70. Takanami, I., K. Takeuchi, and M. Gika. 2002. Immunohistochemical detection of eosinophilic infiltration in pulmonary adenocarcinoma. *Anticancer Res* 22: 2391–2396.
71. Gleich, G.J., and C.R. Adolphson. 1986. The eosinophilic leukocyte: structure and function. *Adv Immunol* 39:177–253.
72. Newton, D.L., and S.M. Rybak. 1998. Unique recombinant human ribonuclease and inhibition of Kaposi's sarcoma cell growth. *J Natl Cancer Inst* 90:1787–1791.
73. Nutten, S., J.P. Papin, G. Woerly, D.W. Dunne, J. MacGregor, F. Trottein, and M. Capron. 1999. Selectin and Lewis(x) are required as co-receptors in antibody-dependent cell-mediated cytotoxicity of human eosinophils to Schistosoma mansoni schistosomula. *Eur J Immunol* 29:799–808.
74. Kataoka, S., Y. Konishi, Y. Nishio, K. Fujikawa-Adachi, and A. Tominaga. 2004. Antitumor activity of eosinophils activated by IL-5 and eotaxin against hepatocellular carcinoma. *DNA Cell Biol* 23:549–560.
75. Moezzi, J., N. Gopalswamy, R.J. Haas, Jr., R.J. Markert, S. Suryaprasad, and M.S. Bhutani. 2000. Stromal eosinophilia in colonic epithelial neoplasms. *Am J Gastroenterol* 95: 520–523.
76. van Driel, W.J., P.C. Hogendoorn, F.W. Jansen, A.H. Zwinderman, J.B. Trimbos, and G.J. Fleuren. 1996. Tumor-associated eosinophilic infiltrate of cervical cancer is indicative for a less effective immune response. *Hum Pathol* 27:904–911.

77. von Wasielewski, R., S. Seth, J. Franklin, R. Fischer, K. Hubner, M.L. Hansmann, V. Diehl, and A. Georgii. 2000. Tissue eosinophilia correlates strongly with poor prognosis in nodular sclerosing Hodgkin's disease, allowing for known prognostic factors. *Blood* 95: 1207–1213.
78. Puxeddu, I., D. Ribatti, E. Crivellato, and F. Levi-Schaffer. 2005. Mast cells and eosinophils: a novel link between inflammation and angiogenesis in allergic diseases. *J Allergy Clin Immunol* 116:531–536.
79. Tataroglu, C., A. Kargi, S. Ozkal, N. Esrefoglu, and A. Akkoclu. 2004. Association of macrophages, mast cells and eosinophil leukocytes with angiogenesis and tumor stage in non-small cell lung carcinomas (NSCLC). *Lung Cancer* 43:47–54.
80. Lewis, C.E., and J.W. Pollard. 2006. Distinct role of macrophages in different tumor microenvironments. *Cancer Res* 66:605–612.
81. Corthay, A., D.K. Skovseth, K.U. Lundin, E. Rosjo, H. Omholt, P.O. Hofgaard, G. Haraldsen, and B. Bogen. 2005. Primary antitumor immune response mediated by CD4+ T cells. *Immunity* 22:371–383.
82. Yim, C.Y., N.R. Bastian, J.C. Smith, J.B. Hibbs, Jr., and W.E. Samlowski. 1993. Macrophage nitric oxide synthesis delays progression of ultraviolet light-induced murine skin cancers. *Cancer Res* 53:5507–5511.
83. Gordon, S. 2003. Alternative activation of macrophages. *Nat Rev Immunol* 3:23–35.
84. Stuehr, D.J., and C.F. Nathan. 1989. Nitric oxide. A macrophage product responsible for cytostasis and respiratory inhibition in tumor target cells. *J Exp Med* 169:1543–1555.
85. Bingle, L., N.J. Brown, and C.E. Lewis. 2002. The role of tumour-associated macrophages in tumour progression: implications for new anticancer therapies. *J Pathol* 196:254–265.
86. Klimp, A.H., E.G. de Vries, G.L. Scherphof, and T. Daemen. 2002. A potential role of macrophage activation in the treatment of cancer. *Crit Rev Oncol Hematol* 44:143–161.
87. Johnson, W.J., Z. Steplewski, T.J. Matthews, T.A. Hamilton, H. Koprowski, and D.O. Adams. 1986. Cytolytic interactions between murine macrophages, tumor cells, and monoclonal antibodies: characterization of lytic conditions and requirements for effector activation. *J Immunol* 136:4704–4713.
88. Anthony, R.M., J.F. Urban, Jr., F. Alem, H.A. Hamed, C.T. Rozo, J.L. Boucher, N. Van Rooijen, and W.C. Gause. 2006. Memory T(H)2 cells induce alternatively activated macrophages to mediate protection against nematode parasites. *Nat Med* 12:955–960.
89. Currie, G.A., L. Gyure, and L. Cifuentes. 1979. Microenvironmental arginine depletion by macrophages in vivo. *Br J Cancer* 39:613–620.
90. Higuchi, M., N. Higashi, H. Taki, and T. Osawa. 1990. Cytolytic mechanisms of activated macrophages. Tumor necrosis factor and L-arginine-dependent mechanisms act synergistically as the major cytolytic mechanisms of activated macrophages. *J Immunol* 144:1425–1431.
91. Holcenberg, J.S. 1981. Enzyme therapy of cancer, future studies. *Cancer Treat Rep* 65(Suppl 4):61–65.
92. Park, I.S., S.W. Kang, Y.J. Shin, K.Y. Chae, M.O. Park, M.Y. Kim, D.N. Wheatley, and B.H. Min. 2003. Arginine deiminase: a potential inhibitor of angiogenesis and tumour growth. *Br J Cancer* 89:907–914.
93. Singh, R., S. Pervin, A. Karimi, S. Cederbaum, and G. Chaudhuri. 2000. Arginase activity in human breast cancer cell lines: N(omega)-hydroxy-L-arginine selectively inhibits cell proliferation and induces apoptosis in MDA-MB-468 cells. *Cancer Res* 60:3305–3312.
94. Yeatman, T.J., G.L. Risley, and M.E. Brunson. 1991. Depletion of dietary arginine inhibits growth of metastatic tumor. *Arch Surg* 126:1376–1381; discussion 1381–1372.
95. Feun, L., and N. Savaraj. 2006. Pegylated arginine deiminase: a novel anticancer enzyme agent. *Expert Opin Investig Drugs* 15:815–822.
96. Rodriguez, P.C., D.G. Quiceno, J. Zabaleta, B. Ortiz, A.H. Zea, M.B. Piazuelo, A. Delgado, P. Correa, J. Brayer, E.M. Sotomayor, S. Antonia, J.B. Ochoa, and A.C. Ochoa. 2004. Arginase I production in the tumor microenvironment by mature myeloid cells inhibits T-cell receptor expression and antigen-specific T-cell responses. *Cancer Res* 64:5839–5849.

97. Pollard, J.W. 2004. Tumour-educated macrophages promote tumour progression and metastasis. *Nat Rev Cancer* 4:71–78.
98. Tan, T.T., and L.M. Coussens. 2007. Humoral immunity, inflammation and cancer. *Curr Opin Immunol* 19:209–216.
99. Barbera-Guillem, E., M.B. Nelson, B. Barr, J.K. Nyhus, K.F. May, Jr., L. Feng, and J.W. Sampsel. 2000. B lymphocyte pathology in human colorectal cancer. Experimental and clinical therapeutic effects of partial B cell depletion. *Cancer Immunol Immunother* 48:541–549.
100. Shah, S., A.A. Divekar, S.P. Hilchey, H.M. Cho, C.L. Newman, S.U. Shin, H. Nechustan, P.M. Challita-Eid, B.M. Segal, K.H. Yi, and J.D. Rosenblatt. 2005. Increased rejection of primary tumors in mice lacking B cells: inhibition of anti-tumor CTL and TH1 cytokine responses by B cells. *Int J Cancer* 117:574–586.
101. Perricone, M.A., K.A. Smith, K.A. Claussen, M.S. Plog, D.M. Hempel, B.L. Roberts, J.A. St George, and J.M. Kaplan. 2004. Enhanced efficacy of melanoma vaccines in the absence of B lymphocytes. *J Immunother* 27:273–281.
102. Barbera-Guillem, E., K.F. May, Jr., J.K. Nyhus, and M.B. Nelson. 1999. Promotion of tumor invasion by cooperation of granulocytes and macrophages activated by anti-tumor antibodies. *Neoplasia* 1:453–460.
103. Aziz, M., T.K. Das, and A. Rattan. 1997. Role of circulating immune complexes in prognostic evaluation and management of genitourinary cancer patients. *Indian J Cancer* 34:111–120.
104. Das, T.K., M. Aziz, A. Rattan, and R. Sherwani. 1995. Prognostic significance of circulating immune complexes in malignant tumours of head and neck. *J Indian Med Assoc* 93:3–7.
105. Schmidt, R.E., and J.E. Gessner. 2005. Fc receptors and their interaction with complement in autoimmunity. *Immunol Lett* 100:56–67.
106. Rowley, D.A., and R.M. Stach. 1998. B lymphocytes secreting IgG linked to latent transforming growth factor-beta prevent primary cytolytic T lymphocyte responses. *Int Immunol* 10:355–363.
107. Dai, Q., W. Zheng, B.T. Ji, X.O. Shu, F. Jin, J.L. Zhu, and Y.T. Gao. 1995. Prior immunity-related medical conditions and pancreatic-cancer risk in Shanghai. *Int J Cancer* 63:337–340.
108. Eriksson, N.E., A. Holmen, B. Hogstedt, Z. Mikoczy, and L. Hagmar. 1995. A prospective study of cancer incidence in a cohort examined for allergy. *Allergy* 50:718–722.
109. McWhorter, W.P. 1988. Allergy and risk of cancer. A prospective study using NHANESI followup data. *Cancer* 62:451–455.
110. Volkers, N. 1999. Wheezing, sneezing, and cancer risk - still an open door. *J Natl Cancer Inst* 91:1916–1918.
111. Melbye, M., K.E. Smedby, T. Lehtinen, K. Rostgaard, B. Glimelius, L. Munksgaard, C. Schollkopf, C. Sundstrom, E.T. Chang, P. Koskela, H.O. Adami, and H. Hjalgrim. 2007. Atopy and risk of non-Hodgkin lymphoma. *J Natl Cancer Inst* 99:158–166.
112. Wang, H., D. Rothenbacher, M. Low, C. Stegmaier, H. Brenner, and T.L. Diepgen. 2006. Atopic diseases, immunoglobulin E and risk of cancer of the prostate, breast, lung and colorectum. *Int J Cancer* 119:695–701.
113. Wiemels, J.L., J.K. Wiencke, J. Patoka, M. Moghadassi, T. Chew, A. McMillan, R. Miike, G. Barger, and M. Wrensch. 2004. Reduced immunoglobulin E and allergy among adults with glioma compared with controls. *Cancer Res* 64:8468–8473.
114. Karagiannis, S.N., M.G. Bracher, R.L. Beavil, A.J. Beavil, J. Hunt, N. McCloskey, R.G. Thompson, N. East, F. Burke, B.J. Sutton, D. Dombrowicz, F.R. Balkwill, and H.J. Gould. 2008. Role of IgE receptors in IgE antibody-dependent cytotoxicity and phagocytosis of ovarian tumor cells by human monocytic cells. *Cancer Immunol Immunother* 57:247–263.
115. Gould, H.J., G.A. Mackay, S.N. Karagiannis, C.M. O'Toole, P.J. Marsh, B.E. Daniel, L.R. Coney, V.R. Zurawski, Jr., M. Joseph, M. Capron, M. Gilbert, G.F. Murphy, and R. Korngold. 1999. Comparison of IgE and IgG antibody-dependent cytotoxicity in vitro and in a SCID mouse xenograft model of ovarian carcinoma. *Eur J Immunol* 29:3527–3537.

116. Reali, E., J.W. Greiner, A. Corti, H.J. Gould, F. Bottazzoli, G. Paganelli, J. Schlom, and A.G. Siccardi. 2001. IgEs targeted on tumor cells: therapeutic activity and potential in the design of tumor vaccines. *Cancer Res* 61:5517–5522.
117. Erb, K.J., J.W. Holloway, and G. Le Gros. 1996. Mast cells in the front line. Innate immunity. *Curr Biol* 6:941–942.
118. Parish, W.E. 1967. Release of histamine and slow reacting substance with mast cell changes after challenge of human lung sensitized passively with reagin in vitro. *Nature* 215:738–739.
119. Roche, W.R. 1985. Mast cells and tumour angiogenesis: the tumor-mediated release of an endothelial growth factor from mast cells. *Int J Cancer* 36:721–728.
120. Ribatti, D., E. Crivellato, A.M. Roccaro, R. Ria, and A. Vacca. 2004. Mast cell contribution to angiogenesis related to tumour progression. *Clin Exp Allergy* 34:1660–1664.
121. Beer, T.W., L.B. Ng, and K. Murray. 2008. Mast cells have prognostic value in Merkel cell carcinoma. *Am J Dermatopathol* 30:27–30.
122. Keresztes, K., Z. Szollosi, Z. Simon, I. Tarkanyi, Z. Nemes, and A. Illes. 2007. Retrospective analysis of the prognostic role of tissue eosinophil and mast cells in Hodgkin's lymphoma. *Pathol Oncol Res* 13:237–242.
123. Sinnamon, M.J., K.J. Carter, L.P. Sims, B. Lafleur, B. Fingleton, and L.M. Matrisian. 2008. A protective role of mast cells in intestinal tumorigenesis. *Carcinogenesis* 29:880–886.
124. Sad, S., R. Marcotte, and T.R. Mosmann. 1995. Cytokine-induced differentiation of precursor mouse CD8+ T cells into cytotoxic CD8+ T cells secreting Th1 or Th2 cytokines. *Immunity* 2:271–279.
125. Noble, A., P.A. Macary, and D.M. Kemeny. 1995. IFN-gamma and IL-4 regulate the growth and differentiation of CD8+ T cells into subpopulations with distinct cytokine profiles. *J Immunol* 155:2928–2937.
126. Lowin, B., M. Hahne, C. Mattmann, and J. Tschopp. 1994. Cytolytic T-cell cytotoxicity is mediated through perforin and Fas lytic pathways. *Nature* 370:650–652.
127. Dobrzanski, M.J., J.B. Reome, and R.W. Dutton. 2001. Role of effector cell-derived IL-4, IL-5, and perforin in early and late stages of type 2 CD8 effector cell-mediated tumor rejection. *J Immunol* 167:424–434.
128. Helmich, B.K., and R.W. Dutton. 2001. The role of adoptively transferred CD8 T cells and host cells in the control of the growth of the EG7 thymoma: factors that determine the relative effectiveness and homing properties of Tc1 and Tc2 effectors. *J Immunol* 166:6500–6508.
129. Dobrzanski, M.J., J.B. Reome, and R.W. Dutton. 1999. Therapeutic effects of tumor-reactive type 1 and type 2 CD8+ T cell subpopulations in established pulmonary metastases. *J Immunol* 162:6671–6680.
130. Rodolfo, M., C. Zilocchi, P. Accornero, B. Cappetti, I. Arioli, and M.P. Colombo. 1999. IL-4-transduced tumor cell vaccine induces immunoregulatory type 2 CD8 T lymphocytes that cure lung metastases upon adoptive transfer. *J Immunol* 163:1923–1928.
131. Ye, Z., C. Tang, S. Xu, B. Zhang, X. Zhang, T. Moyana, J. Yang, and J. Xiang. 2007. Type 1 CD8+ T cells are superior to type 2 CD8+ T cells in tumor immunotherapy due to their efficient cytotoxicity, prolonged survival and type 1 immune modulation. *Cell Mol Immunol* 4:277–285.

Subject Index

M.L. Penichet, E. Jensen-Jarolim (eds.), *Cancer and IgE*,
DOI 10.1007/978-1-60761-451-7, © Springer Science+Business Media, LLC 2010

9781607614500

Made in the USA
Monee, IL
05 November 2026

67914355R00056